DATE DUE

JE 25 '97	OC 12 '04		
SE 24 '97			
DE 19 '97			
MR 5 '98			
OC 15 '98			
MY 27 '99			
JY 14 '99			
OC 5 '99			
NO 2 '00			
DE 7 '01			
AP 15 '02			
AP 22 '02			
MY 13 '02			
JE 10 '02			
MY 15 '03			
JE 5 '03			

DEMCO 38-296

UNDERSTANDING AIDS

UNDERSTANDING AIDS

A Guide for Mental Health Professionals

SETH C. KALICHMAN

American Psychological Association
Washington, DC

American Psychological Association
750 First Street, NE
Washington, DC 20002

Copies may be ordered from
APA Order Department
P.O. Box 2710
Hyattsville, MD 20784

In the UK and Europe, copies may be ordered from
American Psychological Association
3 Henrietta Street
Covent Garden, London
WC2E 8LU England

Typeset in Minion by University Graphics, Inc., York, PA

Printer: Braun-Brumfield, Inc., Ann Arbor, MI
Cover Designer: Supon Design Group, Washington, DC
Cover Illustrator: Elizabeth Wolf, Washington, DC
Technical/Production Editor: Olin J. Nettles

Library of Congress Cataloging-in-Publication Data
Kalichman, Seth C.
    Understanding AIDS : a guide for mental health professionals /
    Seth C. Kalichman.
        p.   cm.
    Includes bibliographical references and index.
    ISBN 1-55798-284-8
    1. AIDS (Disease) 2. AIDS (Disease)—Psychological aspects.
    3. AIDS (Disease)—Social aspects. 4. AIDS (Disease)—Patients—
    Counseling of. 5. Mental health personnel. I. Title.
    RC607.A26K356   1995
    616.97′92′0019—dc20   94-46870
                                                               CIP

British Cataloguing-in-Publication Data
A CIP record is available from the British Library

Printed in the United States of America

This book is dedicated to
Hannah Fay,
in the hope that she will
know of AIDS
only as we now know
of polio.

Contents

Foreword

HIV is here to stay. Great strides have been made in preventing new infections, and the day will come when an effective vaccine will be added to the arsenal of preventive strategies. But the recent disheartening news about the pace of vaccine development and ongoing difficulties in securing sufficient resources for HIV prevention mean that people with HIV will need care from professionals qualified to meet their numerous and complicated needs.

The easiest work in HIV is behind us, and the really difficult work lies ahead. A headline appeared recently in the *San Francisco Examiner* that read, "AIDS Loses Urgency in Nation's List of Worries." Two days later, another headline ran: "AIDS is Leading Cause of Death For Ages 25–44." Together, these headlines sum up the enormous challenges in front of us. The AIDS epidemic marches on. It continues to devastate the vulnerable populations of the United States and of the world.

The HIV epidemic has taken many people from us. But the HIV epidemic is also an inspiring story of care and commitment. Dr. Kalichman's volume, *Understanding AIDS: A Guide for Mental Health Professionals*, speaks to this care and commitment. It outlines many of the problems so evident in AIDS, but it also presents hope, in that it demonstrates what can be done. It points to the fact that people with HIV experience devastation in most of their organ systems, as well as in their psychological and social welfare. It demonstrates that treatments and interventions are available to maintain health as long as possible. It demonstrates that quality of life can be maintained, even when health declines. It demonstrates that individuals with HIV and AIDS can be helped in very specific ways and that they can have good lives even in the presence of their disabilities.

This book is remarkable in its comprehensiveness. No one can work with people with HIV and AIDS without having an understanding of the biological, psychological, and social factors at work. This book reminds mental health professionals that they need to understand the basic patho-physiology of the disease. It reminds them that they need to be well conversant with developments in treatments so that they can help their patients make wise health care choices. It reminds them that they need to understand the myriad causes of cognitive, emotional, and behavioral difficulties people with HIV may experience, so that they can provide the best care possible for individuals with this complicated disease.

This book is important in bridging the often artificial gap between primary prevention and care. It reminds the provider that good care and good prevention go hand in hand, and that attention to issues of prevention is necessary in any comprehensive care plan. It also reminds the provider that a wide variety of strategies are available and can be used, depending on the needs of the patient.

The HIV epidemic has changed our world. It has devastated many of us and many of our communities. But there have been positive benefits as well. There now exists a vast network of community-based organizations devoted to HIV prevention in various vulnerable communities. We are now talking about things that were not talked about so openly before the epidemic: topics like homosexuality, oral and anal sex, adolescent and teen sexuality, the relative merits of teenage sex education, the importance and stability of same-sex partnerships, the wonderful caregiving so evident in traumatized communities, and the lives of injection drug users. No one can pretend any more that these topics are not important.

Committed and caring mental health professionals are essential in the fight to prevent the further spread of HIV and in the struggle to help individuals with the disease maintain quality of life. As Prior Walter, the main character with AIDS in Tony Kushner's *Angels in America* says, "This disease will be the end of us, but not nearly all, and the dead will be commemorated and will struggle on with the living. We are not going away. We won't die secret deaths any longer. The world only spins forward. We will be citizens. The time has come." This text, and the mental health professionals who use it, are key to helping the world spin forward, to helping the time come when all citizens experience the best that can be offered.

THOMAS J. COATES, PhD
Director, Center for AIDS Prevention Studies
University of California, San Francisco

Acknowledgments

*U*nderstanding AIDS would not have been possible without the help of many people to whom I am deeply indebted. I received helpful comments and encouragement early in the development of this project from Tom Coates, PhD, who reviewed the original proposal. Joe Ricker, PhD, a neuropsychologist, and Laura Radke, MD, an infectious disease physician, reviewed chapters for technical accuracy in their areas of expertise. Ann O'Leary, PhD, John C. Markowitz, MD, and Margaret Nettles, PhD, provided detailed and extensive reviews of sections in their respective areas of expertise. The insightful comments of these highly valued researchers made substantial contributions to the refinement and completeness of the text. I am fortunate to have written this book at the Center for AIDS Intervention Research (CAIR), supported by National Institute of Mental Health (NIMH) Center grant P30 MH52776. My colleagues Kathy Sikkema, PhD, and Tony Somlai, EdD, provided countless suggestions and resources; Allan Hauth assured that I had available to me all of the current research, including the more than 700 references cited; Tami Payne assisted me in preparing the manuscript and verifying the accuracy of the reference list; and Jeff Kelly, PhD, David Ostrow, MD, David Rompa, and Michael Morgan provided helpful suggestions and pointed me to many valuable resources. Michael Lange is thanked for providing me with consultation on the history of epidemics, and Laura, Jen, Cheryl Gregg, and Deb of the Knickerbocker are appreciated for providing me with the space to write. I also wish to thank Judith Rabkin, PhD, for her many thoughtful comments. I am always indebted to Moira, my parents, and the rest of my family for their endless patience and support. I am also indebted to the men and women who participated in the "Health Needs Assessment" interviews, which helped clarify issues and assure external validity of the presentation of research findings. I also wish to thank Olin J.

Nettles of APA Books for his excellent work as production editor. Finally, Ted Baroody and Julia Frank-McNeil of APA Books are once again thanked for their continued support and encouragement that made this book a reality.

Introduction

The uncertainties of human immunodeficiency virus (HIV) infection and its relentless progression to acquired immunodeficiency syndrome (AIDS) place enormous burdens on those affected. Like all life-threatening illnesses, HIV infection drains intrapersonal, interpersonal, and material resources (Haney, 1984; G. M. Reed, Taylor, & Kemeny, 1993) and cannot be thought of as a single, stressful life event, but rather as an unremitting force with an uncertain course. At the time of this writing, more than one million people in the United States are thought to be infected with HIV, over 400,000 have been diagnosed with AIDS, and 243,000 people have died of AIDS-related conditions.

Mental health professionals serving clients with HIV infection confront a myriad of challenges directly related to HIV disease processes, medical interventions targeting HIV infection and its associated illnesses, and the social problems within which HIV infection is often embedded. Although counselors and therapists are not expected to be expert in the medical aspects of AIDS, it is critical that professionals who provide services to HIV-infected persons have a basic understanding of the syndrome and its manifestations. Because medical aspects of HIV infection directly affect the psychological experiences of HIV-infected persons, available psychotherapeutic interventions must be sensitive to the biomedical underpinnings of HIV disease. For these reasons, the biological and medical aspects of HIV infection and AIDS are the focus of Part One of this book. HIV and its actions against the immune system are discussed first, emphasizing viral and transmission characteristics of HIV that are most relevant to symptomatology and psychological responses. In chapter 2, medical aspects of HIV infection and AIDS are discussed, highlighting the psychosocial implications of HIV testing, the natural history of HIV infection and AIDS, and medical treatments. Chapter 3 discusses the psychosocial stressors that both accompany and potentially complicate the course of HIV infection.

Part Two reviews the psychological, neuropsychological, and social aspects of HIV infection. Although much is shared with other life-threatening diseases, several psychosocial characteristics are unique to HIV infection and AIDS. Unlike most other life-threatening diseases, HIV infection primarily strikes young and middle-aged adults and involves extreme social isolation, disruptions to social and sexual relationships, prejudices, and discrimination that leads to lost employment, housing evictions, and disengagement from family and friends. Chapter 4 reviews the literature concerning the psychological sequelae of HIV infection across phases of disease, focusing on negative emotions and maladaptive behaviors. Chapter 5 reviews studies of the central nervous system involvement in HIV infection and its implications for cognitive functioning, neuropsychological impairment, and everyday living. Chapter 6 discusses the adverse social consequences of HIV infection, focusing on social stigmatization and isolation.

Part Three reviews the coping processes exhibited by persons with HIV infection and the means by which mental health professionals may facilitate their adjustment. Specifically, these three chapters focus on HIV-related coping, social support, and psychotherapy. Chapter 7 overviews the coping processes identified among people with HIV infection. The roles of meaning, control, and self-esteem, known to be important in coping with cancer, are discussed with reference to HIV and AIDS. Specific coping strategies are discussed, as are the influences of optimism and spirituality in coping. Chapter 8 discusses social support and HIV infection, focusing on both the structural and functional aspects of support over the course of HIV infection. Social support interventions are also reviewed. Finally, chapter 9 focuses on HIV-related counseling and psychotherapy, including discussions of clinical assessment, HIV-related psychotherapy, themes in psychotherapy that arise with HIV-positive clients, and psychopharmacological treatments. A section on issues of particular relevance to treating women with HIV, as well as an illustrative case example, are included. Confidentiality in therapy and sexual risk reduction counseling are also discussed.

Understanding AIDS was written to provide a broad overview of HIV infection and AIDS based on the empirical literature for psychologists, psychiatrists, counselors, psychotherapists, social workers, and other mental health professionals. The book is not solely intended for practitioners who wish to specialize in caring for persons affected by HIV. Rather, my hope is that all clinicians will have adequate knowledge and sensitivity to HIV–AIDS and its related issues. Because the research literature is rapidly expanding, and because some empirical studies may have missed their mark in explaining aspects of HIV-related experiences, 63 men and women of diverse ethnic and HIV-risk backgrounds were interviewed as part of the research for this book. Their experiences help place the empirical literature in proper perspective.

PART ONE

Virology, Epidemiology, and Clinical Manifestations

Thus, the disease, which apparently had forced on us the solidarity of a beleaguered town, disrupted at the same time long-established communities and sent men out to live, as individuals, in relative isolation. This, too, added to the general feeling of unrest.

(Albert Camus, *The Plague, 1948, p. 160*)

1

The HIV–AIDS Pandemic

The devastation of worldwide epidemics, including syphilis, smallpox, leprosy, influenza, tuberculosis, and polio, are well recorded throughout history. As an example, the epidemic that became known as the Black Death, a combination of bubonic, spectemic, and pneumonic plague, swept across 14th-century Europe, between 1347 and 1352, killing an estimated one third of Europe's population (Kishlansky, Geary, & O'Brien, 1991; Ziegler, 1969). Although today the word *plague* refers to a specific class of infectious disease, plagues are considered historically as widespread contagious diseases associated with significant rates of death (C. L. Thomas, 1977). Thus, *plague* is the appropriate rubric under which to discuss massive and widespread loss of life that is due to any infectious disease. Through the destruction of masses, epidemics alter the structure of societies. Beyond the scope of any previous global epidemic, HIV infection, the cause of AIDS, has reached the proportions of a pandemic, having infected millions and promising to infect millions more.

Understanding how HIV rapidly spread to its current status of a global health threat is just beginning. There is substantial evidence that HIV infection has occurred in Africa for at least the past 30 years (Gallo, 1988). Antibodies specific to HIV were identified in stored blood specimens collected from regions of central Africa dating back to the 1950s (Gallo, 1987). However, HIV infection went unnoticed because it was overshadowed by numerous other fatal illnesses that afflict developing countries. AIDS also remained hidden because its clinical manifestations are expressed as other more readily recognizable infectious diseases (R. M. Anderson & May, 1992).

The exact origin of HIV and its introduction to humans is unknown, but there is much speculation and theorizing about where and how HIV infection first developed. One proposed explanation for HIV is that it was well established in all areas of the world but has only recently been recognized. However, this theory has not been well substantiated. A second proposition holds that HIV evolved through the mutation of an older and nonpathogenic virus. Virologists, however, have dismissed this as a plausible explanation for HIV on the basis of specific characteristics of the virus and its relationship to other viruses (Gallo, 1988). A third and widely discussed possible origin of HIV is zoonosis, the recent entry of a non-human virus into human populations. This is a plausible explanation for the emergence of HIV because similar viruses exist in old-world apes that live in areas that surround African regions where HIV is endemic. Still, zoonosis has not been universally accepted as the source of HIV. The most widely held view of HIV is that it represents a virus that developed in humans in Central Africa and only recently spread because of social changes, most importantly global travel and transcontinental commerce. Epidemiological data provide the strongest support for this last theory (Gallo, 1988; Mann, Tarantola, & Netter, 1992).

The first identified cases of AIDS occurred in the spring of 1981, when the Centers for Disease Control and Prevention (CDC) reported that five young, previously healthy, homosexually active men in Los Angeles exhibited a rare type of upper respiratory infection, *Pneumocystis carinii* pneumonia (CDC, 1981b; Fauci et al., 1984; Gallo, 1987). One month later, the CDC reported another 10 cases of this illness and 26 cases of Kaposi's sarcoma, a rare cancer of connective and vascular tissues. All of these unusual cases occurred in New York City, San Francisco, and Los Angeles among previously healthy young homosexual men (CDC, 1981a). By the end of 1981, the number of AIDS cases grew to 257, and to over 2,000 cases by the end of 1983, setting into motion the rapid accumulation of over 100,000 AIDS cases in the first decade of the epidemic (Elford, Bor, & Summers, 1991; Fauci et al., 1984) and reaching 360,000 cases by the end of 1993. A new case of AIDS is reported in the United States every 15 minutes, more than 5,000 people in the world become infected with HIV each day, and a person in the world dies of AIDS complications every 30 minutes (Teguis & Ahmed, 1992).

Evidence that AIDS is caused by a new human virus emerged between late 1983 and early 1984. Considered the most rapid progression of scientific advances in response to a new disease in the history of biology and medicine, the accelerated rate of investigation into the cause of AIDS is represented in volumes of research. The 24 published papers on HIV–AIDS in 1982 is in contrast with 8,300 articles published in 1990 (Elford et al., 1991). The proliferation of HIV–AIDS research is also shown by the emergence of several scientific and professional journals dedicated solely to publishing AIDS-related articles (e.g., *AIDS, Journal of Acquired Immune Deficiency Syndromes, AIDS Education and Prevention, International Journal of STD and AIDS, AIDS Patient Care,* and *AIDS Care)*, as well as the annual International Conference on AIDS, which included over 5,000 presentations in 1993. Articles concerning various aspects of HIV and AIDS regularly appear in scientific and professional journals across disciplines. Between 1981 and 1990, there were more than 32,700 HIV-related scientific articles published (Elford et al., 1991).

DISCOVERY OF THE HUMAN IMMUNODEFICIENCY VIRUS

Human immunodeficiency virus belongs to a group of viruses called retroviruses, specifically to a subgroup of *cytopathic lentiviruses* (Z. F. Rosenberg & Fauci, 1991). Lentiviruses integrate their genetic material with a cell's genetic material through the complicated process of *reverse transcription* (see Appendix A for a glossary of terms). There are several known retroviruses in the animal kingdom, including the visna virus found in sheep, feline immunodeficiency virus in cats, and avian sarcoma virus in chickens (Fauci, 1988; Gallo, 1988). Retroviruses are often communicable, as is the case with feline leukemia virus, which causes immune deficiency and malignancies (Gallo, 1986). Whereas animal retroviruses have been known since the early part of the century and pose no threat to humans, human retroviruses have only recently been identified (Gallo, 1988).

The first human retrovirus was discovered by Robert Gallo and his associates at the National Cancer Institute. Amid great controversy as to whether or not it was even possible for retroviruses to exist in humans, Gallo's lab identified the human T-cell lymphotropic virus type-I (HTLV-I) in the late 1970s. The clinical importance of HTLV-I is that it causes a type of leukemia involving T-helper lymphocyte cells, which play an integral role in the human immune system (Gallo, 1986, 1991). HTLV-I does not cause AIDS, but results in a depletion of T- helper cells that are the same target of the virus that does cause AIDS (CDC, 1992t). HTLV-I also causes progressive myelopathy, a disease of the spinal cord, and lymphomas in some infected persons (McCutchan, 1990). Subsequently, Gallo's lab discovered a second human leukemia-causing retrovirus, HTLV-II (Gallo, 1991), establishing the likelihood that other undiscovered human retroviruses exist. The discovery of two leukemia-causing human retroviruses held answers to many questions raised nearly a decade later by AIDS.

On the basis of epidemiologic evidence and disease symptoms, it was believed that AIDS resulted from a viral infection (Levy, Kaminsky, Morrow, et al., 1985). Because the disease shares several characteristics with HTLV-I and HTLV-II, including the fact that it results in a loss of T-helper lymphocyte cells and that it is spread through blood, perinatal exchange, and sexual contact, AIDS appeared to be caused by a human retrovirus (Gallo, 1991). Between 1983 and 1984, the virus that causes AIDS was discovered by three laboratories and given three different names: *lymphadenopathy associated virus* (LAV), discovered by Luc Montagnier of the Pasteur Institute of France; *human T-cell lymphotropic virus type-III* (HTLV-III), identified by Gallo at the National Cancer Institute; and *AIDS-associated retrovirus* (ARV), discovered by Jay Levy of the Cancer Research Institute of the University of California at San Francisco. All three virus isolates were essentially the same in terms of structure, apparent mechanisms of transmission, and disease manifestations. It is now believed that these early discoveries were actually variants of the same virus; they were therefore renamed in 1986, by a subcommittee on the taxonomy of viruses, the *human immunodeficiency virus type-1* (HIV-1; Fauci, 1986; Gallo, 1987; Levy, 1992).[1]

---

[1]A great deal of controversy has surrounded which lab first discovered the virus that causes AIDS. Patent rights to the antibody test and the royalties for the test complicated matters further. Although still unsettled for some, the consensus is now that researchers at the Pasteur Institute in France should be credited with the initial identification and isolation of what is now referred to as HIV-1.

Subsequently, a second AIDS-causing virus common in West Africa, HIV-2, was discovered in 1986 (CDC, 1992o). The differences between HIV-1 and HIV-2 are mostly on the molecular level, with few differences in clinical symptomatology. It is thought that HIV-2 is evolutionarily related to HIV-1, because the two viruses share several molecular and pathogenic characteristics (Gallo & Montagnier, 1988). However, HIV-2 has not spread across populations to cause disease at nearly the magnitude of HIV-1, and remains relatively contained to West Africa (Gallo, 1988). As of 1992, there were only 32 cases of HIV-2 infection reported in the United States, and most were among West African immigrants (CDC, 1992o). Concern about potential increases in North American HIV-2 cases has lead to mandated screening for HIV-2 antibodies in addition to HIV-1 antibodies in the national blood supply (S. A. Myers, Prose, & Bartlett, 1993). Although HIV-2 may become a greater health threat in the future, HIV-1 accounts for the vast majority of AIDS cases in the world (Glasner & Kaslow, 1990).

There is a great deal of diversity found among laboratory isolates of HIV-1, both when samples are taken from different infected persons as well as when isolates come from a single patient (Levy, Kaminsky, et al., 1985). The variation within infected persons makes HIV particularly difficult for the immune system to manage because alterations in its biochemistry evade targeted immune responses (A. G. Fisher et al., 1988). Similar but distinct HIV-1 substrains cause deterioration of the immune system because each variant of the virus kills T-helper cells (R. M. Anderson & May, 1992). The profusion of biochemically different strains of HIV-1 poses great obstacles to developing effective treatment as well as a preventive vaccine (Fauci, 1986; Gallo, 1987).

In summary, there are two known groups of human retroviruses, the leukemia-causing retroviruses, HTLV-I and HTLV- II, and the viruses that cause AIDS, HIV-1 and HIV-2. Both are transmitted through close intimate contacts where blood, semen, or vaginal fluids are exchanged; both share T-helper cells as a common pathogenic target; they both become dormant and integrated into the genetic material of infected cells; and they are both related to viruses found in old-world primates. These commonalities suggest that HTLVs and HIVs have a convergent evolution (Gallo, 1988). However, the clinical manifestations of HTLV and HIV are distinctly different, with the HTLVs causing leukemia, characterized by un-

11

restrained growth and proliferation of white blood cells (Thomas, 1977), and the HIVs causing profound deterioration of the immune system because of loss and dysfunction of T-helper lymphocytes. The global AIDS epidemic is the result of HIV-1 infection. How HIV-1 destroys central components of the immune system is the key to understanding AIDS.[2]

VIRAL CYCLE OF HIV

Viruses typically consist of a core of genetic material, almost always deoxyribonucleic acid (DNA), and a surrounding protein coat. However, retroviruses have at their genetic core a strand of ribonucleic acid (RNA). Following infection of a target cell, the RNA is converted into DNA through a process of reverse transcription that relies on the enzyme *reverse transcriptase*. The new viral DNA then either proliferates in the infected cell or integrates itself directly with the cell DNA. The ability of retroviral RNA to transcribe itself into a DNA copy and integrate with host cell DNA is the hallmark of a retrovirus. The virus can then lay dormant for long periods of time, safely hidden within host cells; the process also allows the virus to assemble, package, and replicate itself as a free virus, using the host cell's resources (Fauci, 1986).

The viral cycle of HIV has eight principal steps, shown in Figure 1.1: (a) Upon entry into the bloodstream of an infected person, HIV becomes attached to the membrane of a target cell. HIV is highly selective in its binding properties, only targeting cells that express a surface molecule designated cluster determinant 4 (CD_4), that usually acts as a receptor cite for infectious agents (antigens; Fauci, 1988). T-helper lymphocytes are one type of cell that expresses the surface molecule CD_4, which has an extremely high affinity for an HIV envelope surface protein, *gp*120. In fact, the binding between HIV *gp*120 and CD_4 is stronger than between CD_4 and most non-HIV infectious agents (Hamburg, Koenig, & Fauci, 1990; Rosenberg & Fauci, 1991). (b) After binding with the cell membrane, the virus enters the host cell by means of the same CD_4 surface molecule involved in viral attachment. (c) Once in the cell, the viral core genetic material, RNA, is reverse transcribed into a DNA copy. Reverse transcription of RNA to DNA is dependent on the enzyme reverse transcriptase, a

---

[2]From this point forward, HIV will refer to HIV-1 infection unless otherwise noted.

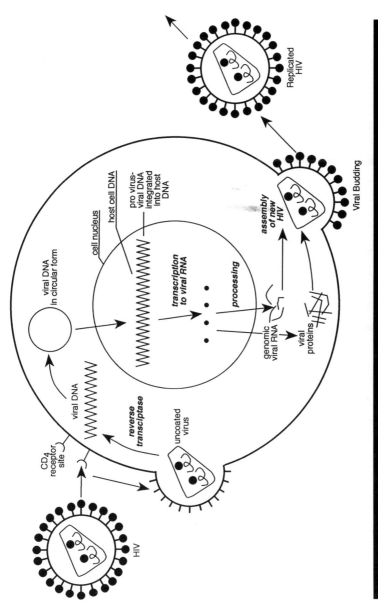

Figure 1.1

The viral replication cycle of HIV. Retroviruses containing RNA bind to CD_4 surface receptors and enter the T-helper cell. HIV RNA is reverse transcribed to DNA, which then integrates itself with the host cell's DNA, taking over all functional aspects of the cell.

process that is distinctive to retroviruses, not found in DNA viruses (Fauci et al., 1984; McCutchan, 1990). (d) The retroviral DNA usually becomes integrated with the genetic material of the host cell. (e) The integrated viral DNA, or proviral DNA, works in the cell to transcribe viral messenger-RNA, which serves to produce more retrovirus (Fauci, 1988). (f) Viral messenger-RNA produces structural proteins for the production of HIV RNA and envelope proteins. (g) The new viral RNA is encapsulated as the core of newly produced proteins in the assembly of new HIV. (h) Replicated virus particles eventually bud and release from the host cell, infecting a multitude of new host cells (McCutchan, 1990). Thus, the natural flow of genetic information, from DNA to RNA, is reversed in the case of retroviruses, flowing from RNA to DNA (Gallo, 1986), making retroviruses extremely difficult to understand and treat.

Shortly after infection with HIV, there is a brief period of intense viral replication, where HIV multiplies and disseminates rapidly. This period is characterized by mass quantities of virus, or *viremia*, and is followed by a decline in virus replication (Tindall, Imrie, Donovan, Penny, & Cooper, 1992). When not replicating, HIV hides within cells in a latent phase. HIV can exist in latent form in T-helper lymphocytes, as well as other infected cells, for long periods of time. Latent HIV infection occurs while the viral genetic material (provirus) is integrated with the host cell DNA, constituting a silent infection, undetectable by the body's immune system (Bednarik & Folks, 1992; Fauci, 1986; Weber & Weiss, 1988). Viral latency should not, however, be confused with clinically asymptomatic periods. Although during viral latency there is often an absence of clinical symptoms (Laurence, 1992), viral replication is occurring in host cells during asymptomatic periods (Maddox, 1993). Thus, HIV can be latent during periods of symptomatic illness and can actively replicate during asymptomatic periods.

Activation of dormant HIV in T-helper lymphocytes can occur under a number of conditions. The slow and persistent progression of immunologic destruction and clinical symptomatology characteristic of HIV infection results from its complex genetic regulation as well as the interaction between HIV, its host cell, and networks of modulating infectious cofactors (Laurence, 1992). Several other infectious agents likely facilitate HIV activation, including herpes simplex virus type-2, HTLV-I, HTLV-II, Epstein–Barr virus, and hepatitis B virus (Hamburg et al., 1990; Hirsch,

Schooley, Ho, & Kaplan, 1984; Laurence, 1992; Pantaleo, Graziosi, & Fauci, 1993). Thus, stimulation of the immune system and activation of HIV are intricately connected (Rosenberg & Fauci, 1991). When activated, proviral DNA in host cells transcribe messenger-RNA, which in turn initiates protein synthesis and the assembling of new HIV (Fauci, 1988; Gallo, 1987).

HIV AND THE IMMUNE SYSTEM

T-helper lymphocytes are destroyed when HIV irrupts, or buds, from host cells (Gallo, 1988; Weber & Weiss, 1988). However, there are a number of mechanisms in addition to viral budding that destroy lymphocytes. For example, when HIV irrupts from an infected cell, the virus sheds fragments of envelope protein *gp*120, which adhere to the CD_4 surface molecules of neighboring T-helper cells. HIV *gp*120 binding with the membrane of uninfected T-helper cells can cause several adverse effects. First, *gp*120 adheres uninfected T-helper cells together, forming a giant multinucleated clump of functionally incapacitated cells called *syncytia* (Fauci, 1988; Gallo & Montagnier, 1988; Weber & Weiss, 1988). Syncytia have been found in the lymphatic systems and brains of HIV-infected patients (Hamburg et al., 1990). Another effect of *gp*120 bound to the surface of T-helper cells is that it triggers an immune response against the cell itself (Pantaleo et al., 1993). When *gp*120 is detected as a foreign particle by the immune system, it is destroyed along with the uninfected lymphocytes (Fauci, 1988; Gallo, 1988). In addition to total cell destruction, HIV can interfere with the fundamental T-helper cell functions. For example, unintegrated DNA within infected cells can have significant effects on T-helper lymphocytes (Hamburg et al., 1990). Several other means by which HIV destroys T-helper cells have been well established (Pantaleo et al., 1993).

Quantitative loss of T-helper lymphocytes was the earliest and most widely cited immunologic abnormality resulting from HIV infection, and it is the depletion of T-helper cells that results in the profound immune suppression of AIDS (Fauci, 1988). T-helper lymphocytes rapidly decline by a factor of one third in the first 12 to 18 months after the occurrence of HIV infection, with a subsequently slower rate of cell loss, approximately 80 T-helper cells per unit measure per year, over the course of several years (McCutchan, 1990). A second accelerated period of T-helper cell decline usually occurs prior to the onset of clinical conditions of AIDS. The close association among persistent effects of HIV infection, loss of T-helper cells, and immunosuppression provides the strongest evidence that HIV is the cause of AIDS (Fahey et al., 1984). Studies consistently show that the progression of HIV infection can be monitored through T-helper lymphocyte counts in conjunction with other markers of immune system functioning (e.g., Hutchinson et al., 1991). For example, independent of declines in the numbers of other immune cells, T-helper cell counts below 200/mm^3 are a reliable marker for development of full-blown AIDS (Fahey et al., 1984; Hamburg et al., 1990; Schoub, 1994) and have, therefore, been included as a diagnostic criterion in revised case definitions of AIDS (e.g., CDC, 1992h).

In addition to absolute numbers of T-helper cells, the ratio between T-helper and T-suppressor (CD$_8$) cells is a key indicator of immune system functioning (Schechter et al., 1990). Healthy people have more T-helper lymphocytes at any given time than T-suppressor cells, with 60% of peripheral lymphocytes being T-helper cells and 30% T-suppressor cells (Fauci et al., 1984). However, with HIV infection, the ratio is often inverted. Although other infections result in increases in the number of T-suppressor cells relative to T-helper cells, HIV causes the inversion because of the loss of T-helper cells as opposed to an increase in T-suppressor cells (Fahey et al., 1984). This immune system abnormality suppresses immunity and results in a substantial increased susceptibility to infectious diseases.

Aside from direct damage to T-helper cells, immune dysfunction occurs as a result of indirect effects of HIV infection on immune functioning. As a part of the cell-mediated branch of the immune system that deals with infection-causing microorganisms, T-helper lymphocytes coordinate immune responses to viruses (McCutchan, 1990). T-helper cells become impaired when HIV envelope proteins adhere to their cell membrane (Rosenberg & Fauci, 1991), disrupting the normal cell signaling and feedback systems (Antoni, Schneiderman, et al., 1990). Progressive T-helper cell dysfunction therefore accounts for immunological disturbances caused by HIV infection, which ultimately interfere with multiple branches of immunologic functioning (Antoni, Schneiderman, et al., 1990; Fauci, 1988; McCutchan, 1990). The widespread and diffuse effects of HIV were at first surprising because it selectively infects a single type of immune cell, the T-helper lymphocyte. However, the effects of HIV infection are pronounced because the loss of T-helper cells and accompanying cell disturbances result in functional deficiencies across several branches of the immune system (Fauci, 1986, 1988).

Although the primary target of HIV is the T-helper lymphocyte, several other immune system cells are indirectly affected by HIV infection (see Table 1.1). For example, although there is not a significant loss of T-suppressor cells and natural killer cells, these immune cells are functionally impaired because of the mediating role played by T-helper cells in coordinating immune system responses (Fauci, 1988). Also of particular importance are the monocyte macrophages, which also express the CD_4 surface molecule to which HIV selectively binds. Monocyte macrophage cells are phagocytic; they engulf and destroy infectious agents. Thus, HIV may enter macrophages after binding with the CD_4 surface molecule, or HIV may be engulfed by the cells through phagocytosis. HIV-infected macrophages are unable to attack and destroy other microorganisms (Hamburg et al., 1990). While inside of macrophages, HIV is also protected from immunologic responses (Rosenberg & Fauci, 1991). It is widely held that macrophages harbor, transport, and disseminate HIV throughout the body, particularly to the lungs and brain (Fauci, 1986, 1988; Gallo, 1988; Hamburg et al., 1990; Rosenberg & Fauci, 1991).

Table 1.1

Summary of HIV Mechanisms That Cause Immune Impairment

Impairment	Description
HIV budding	HIV reproduced in cells erupt and infect a multitude of new target cells
Syncytia	HIV envelope proteins adhere to the receptor area of one cell, which then adheres to another until a cluster of immune cells are bound together
gp120 binding	HIV envelope proteins bound to a cell membrane can cause impaired cell functioning
Autoimmune responses	Virus components bound to cell membranes can trigger an immune response that eventually attacks the infected immune cells

Although the scientific community has mostly accepted HIV as the cause of AIDS, there have been alternative etiological theories. For example, molecular biologist Peter Duesberg, of the University of California at Berkeley, has suggested that AIDS is the end result of a synergism of health-related problems of which HIV infection plays only a minor role. Appearing mostly in the popular press (e.g., Guccione, 1993), Duesberg's views and those of others have stimulated a wide-scale debate on the cause of AIDS. Alternative perspectives discount HIV as being a sufficient cause of disease and place greater weight on combinations of other infectious agents and life-style factors that may impede immune functioning, such as substance abuse and malnutrition (Root-Bernstein 1990, 1992, 1993). Theories of AIDS that de-emphasize the role of HIV are becoming increasingly popular among lay persons and activist groups but have, thus far, lacked scientific verification.

In summary, although many unanswered questions remain, much has been learned about HIV infection. The link between HIV, on the one hand, and immunologic impairment and AIDS, on the other, is well established. As the immune system is suppressed and deteriorates, the body becomes susceptible to infectious diseases that are normally controlled by immune responsiveness. HIV affects immunity through several pathways, including the direct loss of T-helper lymphocyte cells, indirect effects on T-helper cell functions, and impairment of other immune system cells whose functions are mediated by T-helper cells. Similar to other retroviruses, such as HTLV-I and HTLV-II, HIV is contracted through only a few very specific behavioral practices.

ROUTES OF HIV TRANSMISSION

Early epidemiological studies demonstrated that AIDS was the result of a communicable disease. Because the first U.S. AIDS cases almost exclusively involved homosexually active men, the causal agent, not yet known to be a virus, was quickly thought to be contracted through sexual practices. At that time, any possible means of contracting the disease through intimate as well as casual contact were not quickly dismissed, and there was much speculation about how a person might get AIDS. Hysteria was commonplace and understandable given that the cause of a new and devastating illness was unknown. Careful epidemiological study over the past decade, however, has provided several conclusive findings. To date, HIV and HIV-infected cells have only been isolated in substantial quantities from human blood, vaginal secretions, semen, and breast milk, with significantly lower quantities in other body fluids such as saliva and urine (Glasner & Kaslow, 1990; Levy, 1992). Thus, there are four primary modes of HIV transmission: person-to-person through fluid-exchanging sexual behaviors; use of HIV-contaminated injection equipment; mother to infant during pregnancy, labor and delivery, or breast feeding; and through transfusion with infected blood or blood products (Glasner & Kaslow, 1990).

Figure 1.2 presents the percentages of U.S. adult AIDS cases attributed to the most frequent HIV transmission categories. Figure 1.3 presents the percentages of worldwide adult AIDS cases attributed to modes of HIV transmission. As shown, the U.S. epidemic has been characterized by homosexual activity among men, whereas heterosexual contact accounts for the majority of AIDS cases worldwide. Many HIV infections result from multiple exposure risks. Table 1.2 summarizes the most common routes of HIV transmission, each of which is described below.

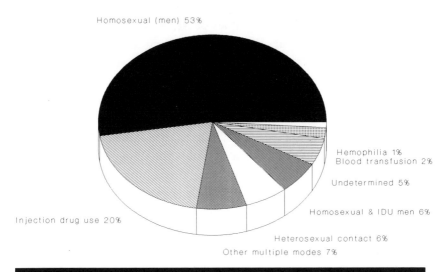

Homosexual (men) 53%

Hemophilia 1%
Blood transfusion 2%

Undetermined 5%

Homosexual & IDU men 6%

Injection drug use 20%

Heterosexual contact 6%

Other multiple modes 7%

Figure 1.2

Proportion of U.S. AIDS cases attributable to various HIV transmission routes ($N = 355,936$; December, 1993).

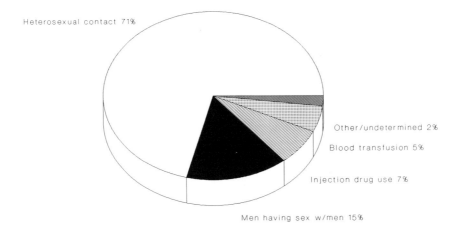

Heterosexual contact 71%

Other/undetermined 2%

Blood transfusion 5%

Injection drug use 7%

Men having sex w/men 15%

Figure 1.3

Proportion of world AIDS cases attributable to various HIV transmission routes (Mann et al., 1992).

Anal Intercourse

Anal intercourse was the first identified route of HIV transmission in North America. Among homosexually active men, anal intercourse is the primary reason for the large number of AIDS cases in this population. Longitudinal cohort studies of gay men residing in U.S. HIV epidemic centers showed close associations between the practice of anal intercourse and HIV infection. For example, Kingsley et al. (1987) followed 2,507 homosexually active men enrolled in the Multicenter AIDS Cohort Study and found that receptive anal intercourse was the primary sexual behavior related to HIV infection. Receptive anal intercourse is the only homosexual practice that is definitively associated with contracting HIV. The risk of becoming infected with HIV accelerates in direct proportion to the number of receptive anal intercourse partners men report (Kingsley et al., 1987). Men who engaged in receptive anal intercourse with one partner over the Kingsley et al. study period were three times more likely to be HIV antibody positive than were men who did not practice receptive anal intercourse, and men with five or more such partners demonstrated an 18-fold increase in risk. Kingsley et al. further showed that men who reduced their practice of receptive anal intercourse substantially reduced their risk for HIV infection.

Prospective studies of gay men have also shown increased risks of infection when there is rectal tissue damage during anal intercourse (O'Brien, Shaffer, & Jaffe, 1992). Chmiel et al. (1987) found that rectal trauma resulting from anal sex provides highly efficient access for HIV to enter the bloodstream. Ninety percent of men in the large Chmiel et al. sample who experienced rectal injuries or bleeding caused by anal sex acts were HIV infected. In another longitudinal study, Keet, van Lent, Sandfort, Coutinho, and van Griensven (1992) followed 102 men who contracted HIV infection and found that the majority attributed becoming infected to having engaged in anal intercourse. Thus, there is conclusive evidence that anal sexual intercourse affords highly efficient transmission of HIV, and the risk seems highest for receptive partners with rectal trauma. It should be noted, however, that proceptive, or insertive, anal in-

Table 1.2

Routes of HIV Transmission

Risk behavior	Transmission mechanism
Anal intercourse	Infected semen or blood enters the anal/rectal mucosa or penis through absorption or micro-openings
Vaginal intercourse	Infected vaginal fluids, semen, or blood enter the vaginal or penile mucosa or through micro-openings
Oral–genital contact	Infected semen or vaginal fluids enter bloodstream through micro-openings in oral cavity, or infected cells enter vagina or penis through micro-openings
Perinatal transmission	Transplacental transfer of virus during gestation, transfer of virus or maternal blood during labor/delivery, breast feeding
Injection drug use	Use of needles and other injection equipment previously used by an infected person; virus or infected cells directly enter blood stream
Blood transfusion—receiving blood products	Principal risk in U.S. occurred prior to 1984 blood screening programs; blood or blood parts from an infected person enter bloodstream

tercourse also carries substantial risk for HIV infection and should not be dismissed as a low-risk sexual activity.

Risk associated with anal intercourse results from the high degree of vascularization of anal–rectal tissue and its relatively thin mucosal lining. The practice of anal intercourse is not found exclusively among homosexually active men. Gayle and D'Angelo (1991) reported that 25% of female adolescents engage in anal intercourse and that anal intercourse is often practiced among adolescents as a method of avoiding pregnancy and "maintaining virginity." Padian et al. (1987) found that anal intercourse was frequently engaged in by women infected with HIV, and this was most commonly the case when their partner was bisexual. Finally, in a national sample of men, of which only 2% reported homosexual activity, Billy, Tanfer, Grady, and Klepinger (1993) found that 20% of respondents reported engaging in anal intercourse, further supporting the common practice of anal intercourse among heterosexual couples.

Vaginal Intercourse

Penile–vaginal intercourse accounts for the greatest number of cases of HIV infection in the world (Mann et al., 1992). Heterosexual transmission of HIV, primarily through vaginal intercourse, has been widely documented in North America (Fauci et al., 1984; Padian, 1988, 1990), and transmission between men and women is bidirectional (J. B. Glaser, Strange, & Rosati, 1989). During the course of one prospective study, approximately 10% to 20% of 307 women married to HIV infected men contracted HIV infection (Padian, Shiboski, & Jewell, 1991). Although HIV transmission from women to men occurs during vaginal intercourse, the rates of transmission are not as high as those for men to women (Padian et al., 1991; Potts, Anderson, & Baily, 1991). One study that followed 730 couples with one HIV-positive partner found that the risk of male-to-female infection is 2.3 times greater then female-to-male transmission (Nicolosi et al., 1994). Exact rates of male-to-female and female-to-male HIV transmission are not known, but two reasons for higher male-to-female efficiency may be the greater mucosal surface area of the female genital tract (Glasner & Kaslow, 1990) and the large number of potentially infected cells in seminal fluids (Levy, 1992). Although there may be differential rates of infection for receptive and proceptive partners, as in anal intercourse, there are no exact probabilities for calculating risk for HIV infection from vaginal intercourse.

It is well documented that HIV infection can occur after a single heterosexual exposure (Mays, 1988). In a classic example of how rapidly HIV can be spread among heterosexuals, Clumeck et al. (1989) discussed one African man living in Belgium who infected 11 of 18 of his female sexual partners. A portion of these women, in turn, reported subsequent sexual contact with other men who may have also become infected. Thus, like penile–anal intercourse, vaginal intercourse carries high risk for HIV infection.

Oral–Genital Contact

Among sexual behaviors that involve the exchange of semen or vaginal fluids, the most controversial in terms of risk for HIV is oral–genital contact. Unlike anal and vaginal intercourse, oral–genital contact has not been definitively linked to HIV transmission (Chmiel et al., 1987; Kingsley et al., 1987; Padian et al., 1987). However, there are cases of HIV-infected men who report oral–genital contact and deny engaging in anal or vaginal intercourse as well as any other known risks for HIV transmission. Rozenbaum, Gharakhanian, Cardon, Duval, and Coulaud (1988) studied five men who denied engaging in anal or vaginal intercourse and who tested positive for HIV antibodies subsequent to a negative antibody test three months earlier. Similarly, a prospective study in Amsterdam reported four men who allegedly contracted HIV solely through oral–genital sex (Keet et al., 1992).

Lower rates of HIV infection via oral–genital contact may be accounted for by several factors, including minimal exposure to the bloodstream through the oral cavity. Additional factors may therefore increase the risk of oral–genital transmission of HIV, such as lacerations, trauma, or open sores in the mouth, including those caused by gingivitis, herpes infections, cracked lips, and canker sores. However, it should be noted that there is no evidence that such potential ports of entry are necessary for oral HIV transmission to occur. Another factor contributing to apparent low rates of oral–genital transmission is that oral sex does not necessarily occur in isolation from other forms of sexual contact. Thus, although oral–genital contact appears to carry lower risks for HIV transmission than do anal and vaginal intercourse, it is not possible to say that oral sex with semen or vaginal fluid exchange constitutes a low-risk sexual behavior.

Condom Use and Other Protection Against HIV Transmission

Once HIV was established as the cause of AIDS and it was determined that HIV was transmitted through sexual contact, tests were conducted to evaluate the effectiveness of condoms as barriers against HIV transmission. Laboratory tests conclusively showed that latex condoms are impermeable to HIV and other retroviruses (Conant, Hardy, Sernatinger, Spicer, & Levy, 1986). The effectiveness of latex condoms as a primary means of preventing HIV transmission has resulted in the widespread dissemination of condoms and mass media promotion of condom use. To further increase the use of barrier methods of protection, and to offset power differentials in condom-use decision making in heterosexual relationships, the United States government approved a vaginal insertive condom-like lubricated polyurethane sheath (Gollub & Stein, 1993; Potts et al., 1991). There is also considerable evidence that some spermicidal applications, in particular nonoxynol-9, have virucidal effects and may add to the protective value of condoms. Laboratory studies have shown that some spermicides have virus-deactivating properties by disrupting the viral envelope (M. J. Rosenberg, Holmes, and the World Health Organization Working Group on Virucides, 1993). Spermicides therefore offer an additional level of protection against HIV infection when used in proper combination with latex condoms, but provide no protection when used alone (CDC, 1993g; Howe, Minkoff, & Duerr, 1994).

Population-based surveys consistently show that frequency of condom use tends to be quite low even among persons with identifiable high-risk behavior histories. In a nationally representative study, Tanfer, Grady, Klepinger, and Billy (1993) found that nearly two thirds of sexually active men did not use condoms at all in the previous month. One study of inner-city women living in Chicago found that women with high-risk behavior histories were no more likely to use condoms than women at lower behavioral risk, and overall rates of condom use averaged below 50% of vaginal intercourse occasions (Kalichman, Hunter, & Kelly, 1992). Among homosexually active men, Kelly et al. (1992) reported that men who engaged in unprotected anal intercourse were not intending to use condoms in the future. Condom use is also infrequent among injection drug users, with 46% of men who inject drugs reporting never using condoms with their steady sexual partners and 52% never using them with casual partners (CDC, 1992a, 1992b). Individuals with multiple sexual partners are more likely to use condoms than those who have a long-term sexual partner, even among injection drug users who are at risk of infection from sharing needles (Upchurch et al., 1992). Likewise, prostitutes are less likely to use condoms with their steady partner than with their clients (CDC, 1987a). Thus, even among persons at high risk for HIV infection, condom use is infrequent.

It should be noted that when latex condoms are used they reduce risk but do not eliminate risk for HIV infection. Failure of condoms to protect against HIV, as well as other sexually transmitted infections and pregnancy, has been widely documented. Condom failure frequently occurs during vaginal intercourse (Grady, Klepinger, Billy, & Tanfer, 1993; Richters, Donovan, & Gerofi, 1993) and anal intercourse (Golombok, Sketchley, & Rust, 1989). A national survey found that over a 6-month period, 13% of men using condoms experienced breaks or tears, and 14% had condoms slip off during intercourse (Grady et al., 1993). As many as 79% of heterosexual couples who consistently use condoms experience breaks (Hatcher et al., 1988). One study showed that even with consistent use of condoms, HIV infection occurred among 17% of heterosexual couples with one HIV-infected partner, compared with 82% for those who inconsistently used condoms (Hatcher et al., 1988). Condom failure is also common among homosexual men, with 31% reporting condom breaks at least once during anal intercourse (Golombok et al., 1989). Similarly, a study of over 500 male prostitutes in San Francisco found that 58% experienced condom breaks and 47% had condoms slip off, usually during anal intercourse (Waldorf & Lauderback, 1993). With respect to the female condom, there is an overall estimated 26% failure rate for pregnancy, and the failure rate is 11% when used consistently and correctly (CDC, 1993g). Further research is needed to know the effects of the female condom on disease prevention.

Small, undetectable tears in latex condoms permit HIV transmission because HIV is considerably smaller than other sexually transmitted viruses, including herpes simplex virus and cytomegalovirus (Feldblum &

Fortney, 1988). Thus, it is not only essential that condoms be used, but that they be used properly, including using a new condom for each occurrence of sexual intercourse, keeping the condom on for the entire sexual act from start to finish, leaving an adequate reservoir at the tip to collect semen, ensuring that there is no air between the condom and penis, and using adequate and proper lubrication to reduce strain on the latex (CDC, 1993g).

A common factor in condom failure is the use of improper lubricants. Because oil-containing products, even if water-soluble, quickly deteriorate and degrade latex, only oil-free, water-based lubricants should be used to lubricate latex condoms (Voeller, Coulson, Bernstein, & Nakamura, 1989). Unfortunately, the mistaken use of oil-containing lubricants is common, with 60% of homosexually active men reporting use of oil-containing products during anal intercourse (D. J. Martin, 1992). It is common for people to mistake water-soluble products, which may contain oils, with the necessary water-based lubricants. Thus, although condom-use promotion is essential to prevent the spread of HIV, condoms are not foolproof and require instruction for proper use.

Perinatal Transmission

Pregnant women infected with HIV can transmit the virus to their unborn or newly born children. In developing countries, between 18% and 40% of infants born to HIV-1-infected women acquire HIV-1 infection, although the risk for HIV-2 transmission is much lower (Adjorlolo-Johnson et al., 1994; R. M. Anderson & May, 1992). The first cases of AIDS in children were reported in 1982, and AIDS is now among the top 10 leading causes of death in children older than 1 year (Rogers & Kilbourne, 1992). Infection from mother to offspring occurs by HIV crossing the placenta, usually during the second and third trimesters, and through contact with infected maternal blood and vaginal fluids during labor and delivery (Rogers & Kilbourne, 1992; Z. F. Rosenberg & Fauci, 1991; Ryder & Hassig, 1988). Studies have shown that newly infected women and women with advanced HIV infection are more likely to transmit HIV to the fetus than are women who are pregnant during times when HIV is less active (O'Brien et al., 1992). In addition, HIV is present in breast milk, making it possible for transmission to occur during breast feeding (Lifson, 1988;

Rogers & Kilbourne, 1992). Risk for perinatal HIV transmission is, however, reduced by maternal use of antiretroviral medications and other interventions (Baba, Sampson, Fratazzi, Greene, & Ruprecht, 1993; CDC, 1994f). The results of AIDS Clinical Trial Group Protocol 076 demonstrated that the antiretroviral drug zidovudine (AZT, ZDV) administered to a select group of pregnant women and their infants resulted in a two-thirds risk reduction for HIV transmission (CDC, 1994d; Connor et al., 1994), suggesting an effective means of preventing perinatal HIV transmission (Rogers & Jafffe, 1994).

An estimated 6,000 births to HIV-infected women occur each year in the U.S. (Gwinn et al., 1991; Rogers & Kilbourne, 1992). The majority of infants born to HIV-infected mothers test HIV antibody positive because maternal antibodies, although not necessarily the virus, cross the placental barrier during gestation. Actual HIV infection occurs in 20% to 40% of infants born to infected mothers (Potts et al., 1991; Rogers & Kilbourne, 1992). Conclusive testing for HIV antibodies in newborns can therefore only occur after maternal antibodies dissipate from the infant's bloodstream and are replaced with the infant's own HIV antibodies, if the infant has been infected. However, a test for the presence of HIV itself can be done earlier.

Each HIV-infected newborn represents a woman infected with HIV, and therefore, the characteristics of perinatally infected infants parallel those of women with AIDS (Gwinn et al., 1991). Mothers are most commonly infected through injection drug use (42%) and through heterosexual contact with a high-risk partner (32%; Rogers & Kilbourne, 1992). The greatest number of HIV-infected newborns are ethnic minorities, born in inner cities, and belong to low-income families (Rogers & Kilbourne, 1992). Infants born to injection-drug-using mothers may suffer additional health problems related to maternal use of drugs and impoverished living conditions. Thus, perinatally acquired HIV infection is a direct result of the HIV epidemic among women, and its prevention is tied to HIV prevention for women.

Injection Drug Use

Transmission of HIV occurs when needles, syringes, and other injection equipment is used by an infected person and shared with other injectors.

Residual blood contaminates the injection apparatus and can directly transmit HIV to a sharing partner (Chitwood et al., 1990). As many as 40% of injection drug users share needles and syringes (Magura et al., 1989), although the rate of infection has declined since the threat of contracting HIV through contaminated needles was first publicized (Des Jarlais, Freidman, & Casriel, 1990). Legal exchange of needles has the potential to prevent many HIV infections (Kaplan, Khoshnood, & Heimer, 1994). Unfortunately, public health benefits of needle exchange are often overshadowed by political issues surrounding substance abuse.

Sharing injection equipment occurs within the sociocultural and economic contexts of injected drug addictions. Users share equipment when learning how to inject, showing others how to inject, and sharing as a part of close and intimate relationships. Needle sharing can also occur because addicts are reluctant to carry clean needles and syringes with them because of the potential for criminal charges if caught (W. Booth, 1988). Addicts may support their drug addiction by renting or selling used needles and syringes (Booth, 1988). Used injection drug equipment is also obtained through "shooting galleries," places where injectors rent or otherwise obtain injection equipment and inject their drugs. Thus, HIV has been widely transmitted among injection drug users by way of injection equipment shared by a circle of friends as well as strangers. Once infected, injection drug users can transmit HIV to sexual partners, who may or may not also inject drugs (Des Jarlais et al. 1990).

Blood Transfusions and Recipients of Blood Products

Early in the U.S. AIDS epidemic, donated blood could not be tested for HIV antibodies, which were therefore unknowingly transmitted to transfusion recipients. Receiving a single unit of HIV-infected blood carries a 90% chance of HIV infection (Donegan et al., 1990). Persons at greatest risk for HIV infection through U.S. blood transfusions are those who received blood or blood products between 1978, when the U.S. HIV epidemic began, and 1984, when the HIV-antibody test became available and blood screening programs were initiated. Prior to blood screening, hemophiliacs were highly susceptible to HIV infection because of multiple blood transfusions and treatments with blood components combined from multiple donors. As a result of exposure to contaminated blood products in the early 1980s, 50% to 65% of U.S. hemophiliacs are HIV infected, and AIDS is the leading cause of death in this population (Dew, Ragni, & Nimorwicz, 1991). Furthermore, HIV-infected hemophiliacs unknowingly transmitted HIV to their sexual partners, and women infected with HIV through blood transfusions often infected their offspring (Chorba, Holman, & Evatt, 1993). However, blood-donor screening programs were implemented in March 1985 in the United States, the result of which has been to dramatically reduce HIV infection through blood transfusions. Unfortunately, most developing countries have not established widespread donor screening programs, making HIV transmission through blood transfusion a continued global problem (Mann et al., 1992).

HIV Transmission To and From
Health-Care Professionals

Invasive medical and dental procedures allow for bidirectional exposure to HIV. Health-care workers serving HIV-infected patients can become HIV infected when professionals have open wounds exposed to patient blood or when patient blood splashes on mucous membranes. HIV infection from contact with patient blood has occurred in several healthcare professions (CDC, 1992n; see Table 1.3). Among all occupationally infected health-care workers, 84% were exposed through percutaneous injury, such as a cut or needlestick puncture, and 13% through mucousmembrane exposure, such as through the mouth or eyes (CDC, 1992n). Still, the risk for occupational HIV infection is very low.

Among phlebotomists, professionals who draw blood samples, needlestick injuries are infrequent, with about one injury occurring for every 6,000 collected specimens. Among phlebotomists who experience needlestick injuries, less than 1% have become HIV infected (McGuff & Popovsky, 1989). Several prospective studies of other health care professions show similar low rates of occupationally acquired HIV infection. Among more than 4,000 heath-care workers, of whom half experienced percutaneous exposure to HIV-infected materials, there were minimal risks for infection (Gerberding, 1992). In one study, Hirsch et al. (1985) found no cases of occupational HIV transmission among hospital employees, including 33 with accidental needlestick injuries and other open wounds exposed to patient blood. Henderson et al. (1986) reported that

Table 1.3

Total Number of Possible Health-Care Occupationally Acquired HIV Infections in the United States (CDC, 1994a).

Occupation	Number of possible cases
Nurse	16
Laboratory technician	15
Health aide	14
Emergency medical technician/paramedic	9
Nonsurgical physician	9
Other health-care occupations	7
Dental worker	6
Embalmer/morgue technician	3
Surgical physician	2
Respiratory therapist	2
Surgical technician	1
Total	84

of 150 health-care workers with percutaneous or mucous-membrane exposure to HIV, none became HIV infected. Thus, although health-care occupational risk for HIV infection does exist, the overall rate of transmission has been extremely low for both percutaneous and mucous-membrane exposures to HIV (Gerberding, 1992).

HIV transmission can also occur from health-care workers to patients. Provider-to-patient transmission can result from direct exposure to an infected provider's blood during an invasive procedure or through the use of contaminated instruments (Gerberding, 1992). For example, two people in the United States and one in Europe have been infected with HIV as a result of invasive nuclear medicine procedures (CDC, 1992i). Although these incidents occurred out of 38 million annual procedures, they have prompted guidelines and recommendations to reduce procedure-related risks. The most widely discussed cases of provider-to-patient HIV transmission occurred when a Florida dentist apparently infected at least six patients with HIV (CDC, 1991e, 1992s; O'Brien et al., 1992). Genetic testing showed that all six patients were infected with a strain of HIV similar to that carried by the dentist, suggesting that the dentist was the origin of the patients' infections (O'Brien et al., 1992). It is believed that the infections occurred during procedures performed with instruments contaminated by previous use on the HIV-infected dentist himself (Gerberding, 1992), or through other means of improper infection control (CDC, 1993h). Although this case is considered unique, and risk of dentist-to-patient exposure is extremely low, HIV-infection control standards for dental practice have been established (CDC, 1992s).

On the basis of these and other cases, the American Medical Association has recommended that any "physician who knows that he or she has an infectious disease should not engage in any activity that creates risk of transmission of the disease to others" (Gerberding, Littell, Brown, & Schecter, 1990). For all health-care providers, infection-control guidelines, referred to as *universal precautions*, assure protection against exposure to HIV in either transmission direction (CDC, 1987b). Given concerns expressed by both patients and providers, some have called for mandatory testing of patients, and others have demanded that providers disclose their HIV status. However, such measures may infringe on privacy rights and will require careful examination of the relative costs and benefits before they are instituted (Brennan, 1991). Again, it is important to emphasize that transmission from HIV-infected providers to patients is extremely rare. Illustrating this is a study of 19,036 persons treated by 57 HIV-infected health-care workers that did not identify a single case of HIV transmission to patients (CDC, 1993h).

Transmission Through Casual Contact and Atypical Modes

There is conclusive evidence that HIV infection occurs as a result of direct exposure to the blood, semen, or vaginal fluids of an infected person. Direct contact with the blood or other body secretions of a person with AIDS can result in HIV transmission, but even cases of transmission after direct household exposure are rare (CDC, 1994c). However, a great deal of speculation and fear exists concerning HIV transmission through a variety of nonspecific, casual contacts with infected persons and through mediating mechanisms of transmission. There is, however, no evidence to support such claims. Numerous studies conducted with individuals who live with HIV-infected persons, who have daily household exposure to body fluids and who share eating utensils and bathroom facilities, have consistently shown that people who do not engage in sexual acts with infected persons do not become infected (Fischl, Dickenson, et al., 1987; Henderson et al., 1986; Hirsch et al., 1985; Lifson, 1988; Mann et al., 1986). In one investigation, Friedland et al. (1986) studied 68 children and 33 adults who shared close personal contact with 39 AIDS patients. The study failed to find any evidence of casual transmission of HIV. Likewise, no cases of HIV transmission have been known to occur in schools or day care-settings (Rogers & Kilbourne, 1992).

Because HIV has been isolated in body fluids other than blood, semen, and vaginal fluids, it is commonly believed that contact with these other fluids carries risk for HIV infection (Glasner & Kaslow, 1990). Although HIV can be in tears and urine, there is no evidence that contact with these fluids results in HIV infection. Even if infection from tears or urine were possible, it would require long and extensive exposure for transmission to occur (Lifson, 1988). Infection from saliva, on the other hand, has been more controversial, with studies yielding conflicting results. The consensus is that contact with the saliva of an infected person through kissing, cardiopulmonary resuscitation (CPR), or other such contacts carries no risk for infection (Lifson, 1988). Thus, aside from genital sexual contact and shared injection equipment, close contact poses no known risk for HIV transmission.

Other behaviors and mediating mechanisms once believed to present at least some risk for HIV infection have not been supported by epidemiological studies. For example, it was once believed that HIV could be transmitted by insects that first bite an infected person and then transmit the virus to subsequent bite recipients (Lifson, 1988). Studies have shown, however, that HIV does not replicate in arthropod cells, making insects an impossible host for HIV (Srinivasan, York, & Bohan, 1987). Furthermore, the amount of blood residue on an insect stinger would not be sufficient for HIV transmission because insects *ingest* blood; they do not *inject* it. Studies in areas with both high rates of AIDS cases and dense populations of mosquitos have shown that HIV infection is unrelated to mosquito exposure and that elderly persons and children do not show high rates of HIV infection despite multiple insect bites (Castro, Lifson, et al., 1988). Other theoretically possible modes of HIV transmission, such as tattooing, which involves needle puncture, and human bites have not demonstrated risk for HIV transmission (Castro, Lieb, et al., 1988; Lifson, 1988).

PATTERNS OF THE EPIDEMIC

Tracking the HIV–AIDS epidemic relies on two sets of data. First, local health departments, the CDC, and the World Health Organization closely monitor the number of people diagnosed with AIDS. Surveillance programs track persons infected with HIV who have progressed to AIDS. Thus, even the most accurate AIDS case monitoring only estimates the extent of the HIV epidemic as it existed about 10 years earlier (Mann et al., 1992).

A second set of data that tracks the epidemic is collected through HIV-antibody testing. The number of HIV-positive persons per population tested, or seroprevalence studies, yields the rate of HIV infection in specific populations. However, these studies provide only a snapshot of current infections because only certain subgroups in a given geographic area, such as homosexually active men, injection drug users, or medical patients, are included in any single study. Seroprevalence data that rely on testing volunteers underestimate the magnitude of the HIV epidemic because participants in these studies demonstrate substantially lower rates of HIV seroprevalence than do people who refuse to participate (Karon, Dondero, & Curran, 1988).

HIV–AIDS is a pandemic affecting all continents and virtually every country of the world (Mann et al., 1992). Mathematical models show that the AIDS pandemic has a continuous expansion (R. M. Anderson & May, 1992). It is estimated that 11.8 million adults and 1.1 million children in the world were infected with HIV by 1992 (Mann et al., 1992). The most heavily affected regions include sub-Saharan Africa, Latin America, the Caribbean Islands, and North America, with the highest prevalence occurring in developing countries (Mann et al., 1992). There are several explanations for the higher prevalence of AIDS in developing as compared with industrialized countries, including coepidemics of ulcerative sexually transmitted infections that facilitate HIV transmission, culturally related sexual practices such as prostitution, resistance to condom use, and sexual networks that span across high-risk groups (Potts et al., 1991).

Cases of AIDS in North America and the Caribbean have increased substantially each year since 1980 (CDC, 1991d). For example, the first case of AIDS reported in Canada occurred in 1982, and 5,246 cases of AIDS were reported as of 1991. In Canada, nearly 70% of all AIDS cases have occurred among homosexually active men (Mann et al., 1992). In contrast, HIV infection in Puerto Rico has primarily resulted from heterosexual contact. Puerto Rico represents the second highest rate of AIDS among U.S. cities and territories, with 99% of all AIDS cases from U.S. territories occurring in Puerto Rico (CDC, 1992b, 1992q). The number of U.S. AIDS cases increased 10% from 1990 to 1991 (CDC, 1992q), and over 48% from 1992 to 1993. Through 1993, there were over 361,000 cases of AIDS reported in the United States (CDC, 1994b). The annual rate of increase in AIDS cases is presented in Figure 1.4, showing that, whereas it took over 8 years for the first 100,000 cases of AIDS to occur in the United States, the second 100,000 accumulated in just 2 years, and the third 100,000 in less than 2 years. Because the number of AIDS cases includes people infected with HIV over 10 years ago, it is impossible to know exactly how many people are HIV infected at any given time. However, on the basis of the best available data, over one million adults in the United States were infected with HIV as of 1991, with an additional 40,000 to 80,000 new HIV infections occurring between 1991 and 1992 (Mann et al., 1992).

Seroprevalence studies show varying degrees of HIV infection across segments of the U.S. population. Studies of men who report having sex with other men consistently show that nearly 33% to 50% test positive for HIV antibodies (Chmiel et al., 1987; Mann et al., 1992; Quinn, Groseclose, Spence, Provost, & Hook, 1992). Seroprevalence among injection-drug-using adults in Houston is 11% (M. L. Williams, 1990), whereas seroprevalence for treatment-seeking injection drug users in New York City is as high as 60% (Stoneburner, Chiasson, Weisfuse, & Thomas, 1990). Seroprevalence among sexually transmitted disease (STD) clinic patients range between 2% and 15%, depending on geographic region and when the study was conducted (Mann et al., 1992; Quinn et al., 1988, 1992). Adolescent males with non-HIV sexually transmitted infections have a 1% HIV seroprevalence (Gayle & D'Angelo, 1991), and adults attending STD clinics in the Bronx, New York, have a 12% seroprevalence rate (Chiasson et al., 1991). As many as 70% of hemophiliacs who received blood components are HIV infected (Bartlett, 1993a). Other populations studied include homeless youth in New York City, of which 16% of 18- to 20-year-

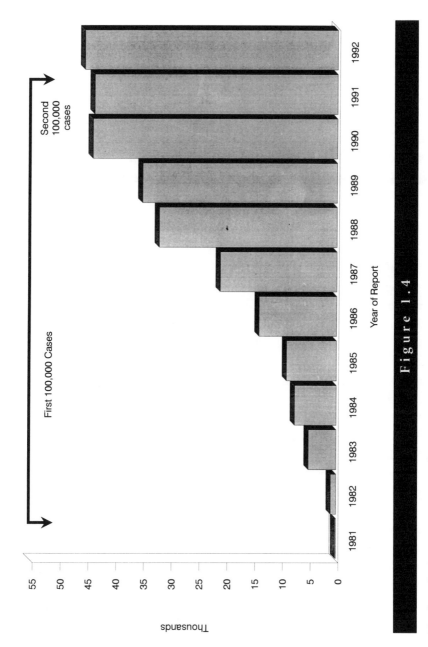

Figure 1.4

Number of U.S. AIDS cases reported since 1981.

olds were HIV infected (Hein, 1990), and runaway adolescents in New York City, with 5% HIV infected (Stricof, Kennedy, Nattell, Weisfuse, & Novick, 1991). Eleven percent of homeless adults in Miami are HIV-positive (CDC, 1991a), and between 6% and 19% of adults with psychiatric disorders living in New York City homeless shelters are HIV-positive (Empfield et al., 1993; Susser, Valencia, & Conover, 1993). High seroprevalence rates occur among prison inmates, 2% to 7%, and as many as 57% of female street prostitutes in some cities are HIV infected, with rates higher for minority than for nonminority prostitutes (CDC, 1987a; McKeganey, 1994; Vlahov et al., 1989). A study of women incarcerated in Quebec found that 7% were HIV-positive, with the highest rates occurring for women with injection-drug-using histories (Hankins et al., 1994). Finally, between 5% and 14% of chronic mentally ill adults in New York City test HIV-positive (Cournos et al., 1991; Cournos, Horwath, Guido, McKinnon, & Hopkins, 1994; Sacks, Dermatis, Looser-Ott, Burton, & Perry, 1992).

Regarding the public in general, blood samples obtained from pregnant women, umbilical cords, and newborns showed that between 1% and 2% of child-bearing women in New York City are HIV-positive (Novick et al., 1991; Stoneburner et al., 1990; Willoughby, 1989). Also in New York City, the seroprevalence among nearly 6,000 women receiving abortions between 1987 and 1989 indicated that 1 in 84 women seeking abortions in New York City during this 3-year period were HIV infected (Araneta, Weisfuse, Greenberg, Schultz, & Thomas, 1992). In a national study of residual blood specimens collected from metabolic tests of newborns, maternal HIV infection was as high as 6% in New York City, 5% in New Jersey, 5% in Florida, and 6% in Washington DC, with rates for women of color being 5 to 15 times higher than for nonminority women (Gwinn et al., 1991). Finally, blood samples collected from medical facilities showed that 1% of male cardiac-arrest patients in Seattle were HIV infected (CDC, 1992f), compared with 13% of emergency-room patients in the Bronx (Schoenbaum, Weber, Vermund, & Gayle, 1990). Thus, epidemiologic studies begin to piece together a picture of the U.S. epidemic that shows HIV infection occurring across diverse subgroups in varying degrees depending on geographic areas, HIV-risk behavior histories, and date of study.

AIDS cases have been reported in every state in the United States, with the greatest number in larger metropolitan areas (see Table 1.4). In 1992,

Table 1.4

AIDS Cases Reported in U.S. Cities: 1991, 1992, 1993 (CDC, 1994a).

City	1991 Number	1991 Rate	1992 Number	1992 Rate	1993 Number	1993 Rate	Total
Atlanta	1,107	37.9	1,351	43.0	1,391	43.0	7,215
Baltimore	579	24.0	767	31.5	1,780	72.7	5,032
Boston	685	18.2	735	13.0	2,441	42.9	7,084
Chicago	1,290	21.0	1,701	22.5	2,503	32.8	9,794
Dallas	706	26.9	696	24.9	1,879	65.8	6,105
Detroit	440	10.1	734	17.0	1,021	23.7	3,674
Fort Lauderdale	946	73.8	849	65.2	1,279	97.1	5,522
Houston	1,198	35.5	1,021	28.9	2,566	70.6	9,538
Los Angeles	1,642	29.3	4,113	45.4	5,193	57.2	22,803
Miami	2,023	102.6	1,217	60.6	3,511	172.8	10,920
Minneapolis–Saint Paul	189	7.5	189	7.2	578	21.7	1,700
Newark	937	51.5	803	41.8	2,132	110.4	8,248
New Orleans	478	38.6	549	42.1	613	46.9	3,161
New York	6,992	81.4	7,201	84.2	14,720	171.8	58,807
Oakland	439	20.7	546	25.4	1,288	59.5	4,318
Philadelphia	933	19.0	1,017	20.6	2,632	53.1	7,964
Phoenix	210	9.6	267	11.5	878	36.8	2,314
Portland	195	15.2	248	15.5	677	41.1	2,015
San Diego	621	24.2	684	26.3	1,693	64.3	5,302
San Francisco	1,968	121.8	2,119	130.3	4,669	287.5	18,135
San Juan	1,069	62.6	1,043	55.6	1,974	104.1	7,103
Seattle	408	20.0	430	20.2	1,011	46.8	3,718
Washington, DC	1,307	32.7	1,399	32.1	2,796	63.2	10,177

NOTE: The AIDS case definition was expanded in 1993, causing an apparent increase in diagnosed cases that does not reflect increases in HIV infection.
Rate = number of people per 100,000 population.

AIDS became the leading cause of death among men aged 35 to 44 in the United States and the second leading cause of death among young women. HIV is the leading cause of death among young men in 64 of 170 major U.S. cities, with AIDS accounting for 51% of deaths of young men in Ft. Lauderdale, 33% in New Haven, 29% in Minneapolis, 39% in Seattle, and 37% in San Diego. AIDS now ranks in the top three causes of death for young men in 21 U.S. states, with most deaths concentrated in metropolitan areas (Selik, Chu, & Buehler, 1993).

The disproportionate number of AIDS cases in urban centers has characterized the epidemic since its beginning (Quinn et al., 1992). For example, in New York state, AIDS is the leading cause of death among men 25 to 44 years old and among women 20 to 39 years old (P. F. Smith, Mikl, Hyde, & Morse, 1991), and the vast majority of deaths because of AIDS in New York state have occurred in New York City (Selik et al., 1993). Between 1990 and 1991, the number of AIDS cases increased 19% in Philadelphia, 11% in Chicago, 24% in Washington DC, and 22% in Miami (CDC, 1992a). Among U.S. cases of AIDS, 85% occur in metropolitan areas with populations greater than 500,000, compared with 9% of cases in cities with populations between 50,000 and 500,000 (CDC, 1994b). Thus, like previous epidemics dating back as early as the Black Plague (Ziegler, 1969), cities constitute the most heavily devastated geographic areas.

Inner cities, like underdeveloped countries, consist of highly mobile and rapidly changing populations, with a great deal of transience, poverty, social injustices, prostitution, and illegal drug use, all of which facilitate the spread of infectious diseases, particularly HIV (Morrow, Colebunders, & Chin, 1989). As HIV has spread, individuals have migrated to rural areas. Many towns have increased rates of AIDS that parallel patterns observed in U.S. epidemic centers a decade ago (Davis, Cameron, & Stapelton, 1992; Flemming, Cochi, Steece, & Hull, 1987; J. E. Smith, Landau, & Bahr, 1990).

The spread of infection in any given area is determined by three principal factors: First, rates of infection depend on the probability that an infected person will infect another person (R. M. Anderson & May, 1992). HIV infection occurs with greatest efficiency through anal and vaginal intercourse and sharing drug-injection equipment. Second, the number of partnerships an individual has with potentially infected persons determines the chances of infection. Finally, the length of time that an infected person can potentially infect others influences rates of spread. For HIV, individuals remain infectious for the remaining years of their life and are often unaware of being infected for the majority of that time (R. M. Anderson & May, 1992).

Links within and between sexual and drug-using networks determine the pattern and rate of the HIV epidemic (R. M. Anderson & May, 1992). For example, bisexual men who contract HIV from a male sexual partner may spread the virus to female partners. Injection drug users spread HIV to non-injection-drug-using sexual partners, and infected prostitutes infect their sexual trade customers. Thus, there are numerous subepidemics emerging across several subpopulations, both globally (Mann et al., 1992) and within the United States (Allen & Setlow, 1991; CDC, 1992q). Because HIV is spread within sexual and drug-injecting networks, individuals who engage in risk behaviors in areas with high rates of AIDS are characterized by relatively high levels of risk (Castro, Lifson et al., 1988; Fauci et al., 1984).

RISK CHARACTERISTICS OF HIGHLY AFFECTED SUBPOPULATIONS

Although HIV infection occurs across all geographic and demographic segments of the United States, several groups have been affected longest over the course of the epidemic. People at risk for HIV infection are defined on the basis of two necessary conditions for HIV infection. The first condition is the prevalence of HIV in a population, because this rate determines the probability that any given risk-related contact will result in HIV transmission. The greater the HIV seroprevalence in a subpopulation, the higher risk of infection. The second condition that determines infection is the frequency of behaviors that confer varying degrees of risk for HIV transmission. Table 1.5 summarizes the percentages of U.S. AIDS cases attributed to behavioral practices for men and women between 1989 and 1993. Individuals with HIV infection often report multiple modes of possible exposure, as shown in Table 1.6. Thus, although it has become less relevant to discuss traditional risk groups as the HIV epidemic has expanded, certain subpopulations continue to represent the highest rates of HIV infection and AIDS.

Table 1.5

AIDS Cases for Men and Women by Specific HIV-Exposure Categories

Exposure	Men					Women					Total
	1989	1990	1991	1992	1993	1989	1990	1991	1992	1993	
Men who have sex with men											
N	19,891	23,738	24,216	25,864	48,266	—	—	—	—	—	193,162
%	64	63	62	61	55	—	—	—	—	—	54
Injection drug use											
N	6,218	7,689	8,494	9,092	21,086	1,871	2,329	2,820	3,071	7,601	86,961
%	20	20	22	21	24	51	48	49	47	46	24
Men who have sex with men and inject drugs											
N	2,214	2,295	2,551	3,028	5,745	—	—	—	—	—	23,483
%	7	6	7	7	7	—	—	—	—	—	7
Heterosexual contact											
N	778	1,054	1,327	1,509	3,232	1,232	1,657	2,185	2,536	6,056	23,038
%	3	3	3	4	4	34	34	38	39	37	6
Recipients of blood transfusion											
N	469	501	442	405	701	308	365	253	305	518	6,304
%	2	1	1	1	1	8	7	4	5	3	2

Table 1.6

Cumulative Total of Categories of Multiple Modes of HIV
Transmission Through 1993

	AIDS cases	
Multiple modes of exposure	Number	Percent
Men who have sex with men and inject drugs	20,935	7
Injection drug user and heterosexual contact	12,093	3
Men who have sex with men and women	3,712	1
Men who have sex with men and a transfusion recipient	2,697	1
Men who have sex with men and women and use injected drugs	1,992	1

Homosexually and Bisexually Active Men

Because the first and greatest numbers of AIDS cases in the United States have occurred among homosexually active men, most attention regarding the AIDS epidemic has been given to this group. Although high HIV seroprevalence rates occur in gay communities, men who have sex with men are only at very high risk for HIV infection when they practice unprotected anal intercourse. In one study of over 2,000 men sampled from gay bars in 16 cities across the United States, Kelly et al. (1992) found that 31% of men reported engaging in anal intercourse without condoms. Men who engaged in unprotected anal intercourse were younger in age and were less likely to perceive safer sex as socially normative than men who did not engage in this highest-risk sexual behavior. Lemp et al. (1994) also found 33% of young gay men recently engaged in unprotected anal intercourse in the San Francisco Bay area. Condom use and safer sexual practices are less prevalent among homosexually active men who do not identify themselves as gay or bisexual (CDC, 1993a). Homosexually active adolescent males are less likely to identify with adult gay communities and are at particularly high risk for HIV infection (Ostrow & Wren, 1992). Still, there is considerable evidence that the HIV epidemic among homosexually active men in New York City has leveled off, that rates of HIV transmission among gay and bisexual men have decreased nationally since 1985 (Mann et al., 1992; P. F. Smith et al., 1991), that HIV infections in San Francisco have been reduced (Osmond, Page, et al., 1994), and that the number of AIDS cases among homosexual men has declined since 1991 (CDC, 1993f). Changes in behavior observed among homosexual and bisexual men account for these declines in HIV and AIDS, but similar changes have not occurred in other subpopulations.

Injection Drug Users

High rates of infection and sharing injection equipment account for HIV risk among persons who inject illicit drugs. Although actual rates of sharing practices are not known, more frequent injectors are likely to be HIV-positive (M. L. Williams, 1990). Younger male injectors are among the most likely to borrow needles and syringes, even when clean injection equipment is available (Hartgers, Buning, van Santen, Verster, & Coutinho, 1989). Needle sharing, like sexual behaviors, occurs within close, intimate, and private relationships as well as between anonymous partners (Magura et al., 1989). Sharing injection equipment is often an important aspect of social bonding among users. HIV transmission occurs when needles are shared within a network of users, where an infected person contaminates injection equipment that is subsequently used by others. Injection drug users often congregate in "shooting galleries," where injection equipment is loaned or rented. Shooting galleries are common in cities with a large number of injection drug users and where HIV seroprevalence rates are highest (Chitwood et al., 1990). Sharing needles, renting injection equipment, and other practices common to shooting galleries increases the risk for contracting HIV (Des Jarlais, Friedman, & Stoneburner, 1988). One study of injection needles collected from shooting galleries in a high-AIDS-incidence area found that 10% were contaminated with HIV infected-blood (Chitwood et al., 1990).

Patterns of HIV transmission among injection drug users are complicated by several sociocultural factors. First, people infected with HIV may infect their non-injecting sexual partners (W. Booth, 1988; Kane, 1991). Second, a close association exists between injection drug use and prostitution, with 30% of female injectors engaging in sexual commerce (Castro, Lifson, et al., 1988) and 76% of HIV-infected prostitutes using injection drugs

(CDC, 1987a). Third, noninjected drugs are also closely connected to sexually transmitted infections, particularly the use of cocaine (Chiasson et al., 1991). Injection drug users who smoke crack cocaine are at greater risk of contracting sexually transmitted HIV infection than are people who only inject drugs (Booth, Watters, & Chitwood, 1993). Finally, it is common for noninjected drugs, particularly crack cocaine, to be traded for sex and vice versa, further illustrating the complex link between drug use and HIV risk (CDC, 1991b; Chiasson et al., 1991; Schoenbaum et al., 1990).

Heterosexual Men and Women

Men and women who practice vaginal or anal intercourse constitute the most prevalent HIV-risk population in the world (Mann et al., 1992). Heterosexual transmission of HIV accounted for the largest jump in AIDS cases from 1991 to 1992 (CDC, 1993f). A study of singles-bar patrons in San Francisco found higher rates of HIV risk behaviors than in samples of men from San Francisco gay bars (Stall, Heurtin-Roberts, McKusick, Hoff, & Lang, 1990). Stall et al. found that heterosexuals at greatest risk were more concerned about AIDS, were more likely to have a history of other sexually transmitted infections, and showed a stronger tendency toward alcohol and drug use in conjunction with practicing risk-related sexual behaviors. People living in U.S. cities with greater numbers of sub-Saharan African and Caribbean immigrants, such as South Florida and New York City, may also be at higher risk for heterosexually transmitted HIV infection (Nwanyanwu et al., 1993).

Across geographic regions, heterosexuals in the United States demonstrate substantial rates of HIV-risk-related behaviors. In a random digit-dial telephone survey, Catania, Coates, et al., (1992) found that 15% to 31% of 10,630 adults were at behavioral risk for HIV infection. The study also found that 7% reported two or more sexual partners in the previous year. Ericksen and Trocki (1992) reported that 22% of a nationally representative sample reported two to four sexual partners in the previous five years. Other national surveys found similar rates of risk-related sexual behaviors practiced among heterosexuals (Billy et al., 1993; CDC, 1988). As HIV becomes more prevalent among heterosexuals in North America, substantial increases in HIV infection rates are expected (Poppen & Reisen, 1994).

Among heterosexuals, women are at particular risk for HIV infection. The number of women diagnosed with AIDS in the United States increased 15% between 1990 and 1991 (CDC, 1992q) and rose an additional 10% from 1991 to 1992 (CDC, 1993f), making AIDS the leading cause of death among young women in New York City (Mann et al., 1992) and in the top four leading causes of death among women nationally (Aral & Wasserheit, in press; Chu, Buehler, & Berkelman, 1990; Selik et al., 1993). The number of women with AIDS who were heterosexually infected surpassed the number infected by injecting drugs for the first time in 1992 (CDC, 1993f; see Figure 1.5).

AIDS has thus far occurred disproportionately among women of color and women living in U.S. inner cities (Hoff et al., 1988). Eighty-nine percent of HIV-infected newborns in New York City are born to women of color (Novick et al., 1991). HIV infection among women is frequently the result of injection drug use (approximately 50% of all cases) or having an injection-drug-using sexual partner (45% of heterosexually acquired cases). Women infected with HIV are also frequent users of noninjected

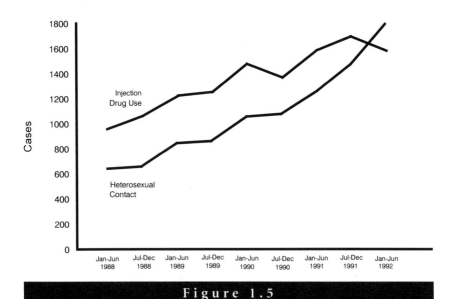

Figure 1.5

Changing trends in relative rates of U.S. AIDS cases among women due to injection drug use and heterosexual contact.

drugs. For example, Lindsay et al. (1992) found that 25% of HIV-infected women use crack cocaine, and cocaine use has been tied to elevated risk for HIV infection (R. E. Booth et al., 1993; Chiasson et al., 1991). There are other factors that place women at elevated risk for HIV infection, including the large number of infected men with whom women become sexually involved, the high efficiency of male-to-female HIV transmission, and the many inequalities in heterosexual relationships, where women may be disadvantaged in negotiating condom use with sex partners (Ickovics & Rodin, 1991; Stuntzner-Gibson, 1991).

Persons With Non-HIV Sexually Transmitted Diseases

Women and men who contract sexually transmitted infections other than HIV are at risk for HIV infection because the virus is transmitted through the same pathways as other sexually transmitted diseases (STDs) and because HIV and non-HIV infections frequently co-occur (Aral & Holmes, 1991; Mann et al., 1992; Onorato et al., 1990; Quinn et al., 1992). STD patients are likely to maintain high rates of sexual risk behaviors after STD treatment, increasing the chance of spreading HIV (Hutchinson et al., 1991; Quinn et al., 1988). A history of STDs is a strong independent predictor of HIV infection, particularly when non-HIV infections involve genital ulcerations, as is the case for nearly 25 million people with genital herpes in the United States (Aral & Holmes, 1991; Aral & Wasserheit, in press; Latif et al., 1989; Quinn et al., 1988; Schoenbaum et al., 1990). Chlamydia and gonorrhea infections also facilitate HIV transmission because of microscopic ulcerations from inflamed mucous membranes (Aral & Holmes, 1991). Nonulcerating diseases form a discharge that contains infected or susceptible cells (Aral & Wasserheit, in press). Among sexually transmitted infections, syphilis is the single best predictor of HIV infection (Castro, Lifson, et al., 1988; Quinn et al., 1988; Schoenbaum et al., 1990). Genital ulcers facilitate viral transmission because they provide an entry point for HIV infection and because they are likely to contain large amounts of HIV-infected (or infectable) immune cells (Levy, 1992). Open sores caused by a STD infection contain T-helper lymphocytes, which, when infected with HIV, carry a massive dose of virus when introduced to an uninfected person. Studies have shown that risk for HIV infection is increased between three and five times in the presence of other sexually transmitted diseases and that the risk increase is greater for women than for men (Aral & Wasserheit, in press).

Adolescents

Given that the average length of HIV latency between the point of infection and a diagnosis of AIDS spans several years, most of the 20- to 29-year-olds with AIDS, representing 19% of all AIDS cases, were likely infected during their teens (CDC, 1992k; Hein, 1990). Approximately 17,000 people between the ages of 13 and 19 were infected with HIV between 1981 and 1987 (Gayle & D'Angelo, 1991). Among women between 20 and 24 years old diagnosed with AIDS, 48% resulted from heterosexual contact, whereas 64% of male cases resulted from homosexual contact. Thirty-five percent of women and 12% of men with AIDS contracted HIV infection from injection drug use (CDC, 1994b). Risk among adolescents varies by gender, ethnic background, and geographic area, with males, ethnic minorities, and adolescents from inner cities being at greatest risk (Gayle & D'Angelo, 1991; Vermund et al., 1989).

National rates of other sexually transmitted diseases show that U.S. youth, 15 to 19 year olds, present the highest rates of gonorrhea of any age group (Gayle & D'Angelo, 1991). Ethnicity is also a factor, with 8% of African-American youth reporting previous sexually transmitted infections (CDC, 1992m). The prevalence of co-occurring sexual infections and increasing rates of HIV are particularly problematic given the frequency of sexual risk behaviors found among adolescents. National studies have shown that 54% of adolescents engage in sexual intercourse (CDC, 1992l) and that 19% have had four or more lifetime sexual partners, with those having more partners being the least likely to use condoms (CDC, 1992k; Tanfer et al., 1993). The average age of first sexual intercourse is approximately 16 years, with one third of male and 20% of female adolescents having their first intercourse experience before they are 15 years old (Billy et al., 1993; CDC, 1992k). Sexual activity, rates of sexually transmitted infections, and unintended pregnancies continue to escalate among adolescents (CDC, 1992l). Several factors indicate that HIV contracted during adolescence will continue increasing, including high rates of substance use in association with sexual behavior (Hein, 1990), high rates of HIV infection among inner-city disenfranchised youth (Stricof et al., 1991; Vermund et al., 1989), and prevalent misinformation regarding risk (Gayle & D'Angelo, 1991; Quadrel, Fischoff, & Davis, 1993).

Other Risk Groups

Several subpopulations that exhibit behavior patterns carrying significant risk for HIV transmission within closed sexual networks have been identified. Of particular interest are subgroups whose sexual behavior and relationships indicate that when HIV is introduced within a sexual network, the virus will rapidly spread. Individuals who exchange sex for money, drugs, or other material gain are at considerable risk for HIV infection because of the interrelationships among substance use, injection drug use, and multiple sexual contacts (CDC, 1987a). Sex workers are at particularly high risk, with 16% to 55% of street prostitutes in U.S. cities testing HIV-positive (Campbell, 1990). Prison inmates are also at elevated risk for HIV infection because of high rates of injection drug use (CDC, 1992e; Schilling et al., 1994; Vlahov et al. 1989) and the likelihood of homosexual activity within closed sexual networks. Nearly four million U.S. migrant and seasonal workers are at risk because of living in closed communities with HIV seroprevalence rates over 5% (CDC, 1992d). Chronic mentally ill adults engage in high rates of high-risk sexual practices. Psychiatric patients lack accurate information about HIV transmission and evidence high rates of HIV seroprevalence (Cournos et al., 1991; Kalichman, Kelly, Johnson, & Bulto, 1994; Sacks et al., 1992). Homeless adults with psychiatric disorders are also at substantial risk for HIV infection (CDC, 1991a; Empfield et al., 1993; Susser et al., 1993), with nearly 9% of San Francisco homeless adults testing HIV-positive (Zolopa et al., 1994).

In contrast, groups that are at low risk for HIV infection have also been identified. Although there are isolated case reports of sexual HIV transmission between women (Chu, Buehler, Fleming, & Berkelman, 1990; Chu, Conti, Schable, & Diaz, 1994; Marmor et al. 1986; Monzon & Capellan, 1987; Rich, Buck, Tuomala, & Kazanjian, 1993), a recent study of 960,000 female U.S. blood donors did not find a single case of HIV infection among women having exclusive sexual contact with other women (Peterson, Doll, White, Chu, and the HIV Blood Donor Study Group, 1992). These findings were supported by a study of over 1,000 women with HIV infection, among whom only one woman reported sexual contact with women as her only risk factor (Chu et al., 1994).[3] Although the elderly tend to be sexually active as a group, persons over the age of 55 who did not receive a blood transfusion prior to 1985 are also at low risk for HIV infection (Catania et al., 1989). Thus, as the HIV epidemic expands, people at highest risk remain those who engage in behaviors that afford efficient viral transmission within sexual and injection-drug-using networks with high rates of HIV infection.

GLOBAL PATTERNS OF HIV TRANSMISSION

The spread of HIV varies greatly by geographic regions of the world. The World Health Organization has estimated that over seven million Africans, one million North Americans, one million South Americans, and one million Asians are HIV infected. Differences in epidemiological patterns among continents are striking and lead to disparate rates of disease among men and women, heterosexuals and homosexuals, and infected children. In North America, Western Europe, Australia, New Zealand, and urban areas of Latin America, HIV has been primarily spread through male homosexual and bisexual contact and through contaminated injection equipment. On the basis of predominant transmission modes, these regions had been referred to as Pattern I countries of the HIV epidemic. In contrast, Pattern II regions, which included sub-Sahara Africa and some Caribbean Islands, were characterized by primarily heterosexual spread and transmission through contaminated blood products. Pattern III regions included North Africa, the Middle East, Eastern Europe, Asia, and the Pacific, characterized by infection introduced by travelers from Pattern I and Pattern II countries (S. A. Myers et al., 1993). New patterns emerge as the epidemic grows, and areas that were once one pattern may shift to other patterns. Therefore, this classification is not as useful as it was early in the

---

[3]HIV transmission routes are determined among infected persons through a hierarchical assessment procedure. Any given person may have a history of several possible routes of transmission, but the designated route is given to the behavior most probably linked to infection. Persons with more than one exposure category are classified in the one listed higher in the hierarchy, except men with a history of both homosexual contact and injection drug use, which makes up a separate category. Anal and vaginal intercourse occur higher in the hierarchy than oral–genital contact. Therefore, actual modes of contracting HIV can be masked by other risk behaviors assumed to be the means of infection among individuals who engage in multiple risk acts. This undoubtedly causes an underrepresentation of risk for some sexual behaviors. Therefore, woman-to-woman sexual contact may be the actual mode of transmission among some bisexual women with HIV infection.

epidemic. With changes in the epidemic come new waves of disease, diversifying the groups that constitute the AIDS crisis.

CONCLUSION

As noted, a small number of scientists believe that HIV is only related to AIDS, but not the cause of AIDS. These researchers argue that the link between HIV infection and AIDS-related illnesses hinges solely on correlational analyses, precluding causal conclusions. This position states that the illnesses that compose AIDS are determined by multiple factors and that HIV alone is insufficient, and even unnecessary, for the development of AIDS (Duesberg, 1988, 1989; Root-Bernstein, 1993). Alternative theoretical approaches to the etiology of AIDS remain controversial, but these views capture the attention of many AIDS activists, the news media, and individuals who question the legitimacy of traditional scientific establishments.

An overwhelming amount of evidence, however, shows that AIDS is the direct result of HIV infection (Gallo, 1988; Gallo & Montagnier, 1988; Maddox, 1993). Although there are several cases of HIV infection and AIDS that remain unclassified with respect to mode of viral transmission (Castro, Lifson et al., 1988), virtually all cases of AIDS are eventually linked to sexual behavior, injection drug use, or receiving blood or blood products. Despite the fact that HIV is controllable through behavior changes and that the vast majority of people at risk are aware of how HIV is contracted, the epidemic is expanding at dramatic rates. Thus far, projections of the number of AIDS cases have been accurate within margins of error (Karon et al., 1988; Morgan & Curran, 1986). Worldwide, the HIV epidemic doubles every 1 to 3 years among heterosexually active adults (Potts et al., 1991). It is predicted that 3.7 million people beyond those diagnosed as of 1991 will develop AIDS between 1992 and 1995 (Mann et al., 1992). By 1995, therefore, the cumulative total of adults infected with HIV will increase nearly 50%, and HIV infection among children will more than double (Mann et al., 1992).

Given the expansion of the AIDS epidemic, the rapid increase in the number of infected persons, and the fact that people with HIV infection are living longer with the disease, an increasing percentage of the population will be HIV infected in coming years. The number of persons with

HIV and AIDS who require mental health services will therefore also increase. Many of the psychological issues faced by HIV-infected people result from adjustment to a life-threatening illness. Aspects of the lengthy HIV infection process itself require substantial coping and adjustment. Thus, prior to discussing social and psychological dimensions of HIV infection and AIDS, I turn to the current state of knowledge about HIV disease processes.

2

Clinical Course and Manifestations

H IV infection emerged as a global health threat faster than any previous disease in history. AIDS is the first disease to establish itself as a leading cause of death within the same decade of its discovery (CDC, 1991d, 1992g) and is now the number one cause of death among men and women between the ages of 25 and 44. By 1986 AIDS was responsible for 38% of all deaths among San Francisco men ages 20 to 49 (Saunders, Rutherford, Lemp, & Barnhart, 1990), and this figure increased to 61% in 1990 (Selik et al., 1993). By the end of 1993, 220,871 people had died of an AIDS-related condition in the United States, 73% of whom were between 25 and 44 years old (CDC, 1994b). In contrast with other causes of death, AIDS has steadily increased each year over the past decade. The clinical course of HIV infection begins at the time of virus exposure and ends at the time of death from AIDS-related illnesses (Glasner & Kaslow, 1990). Because AIDS is a new disease, our knowledge of its mechanisms is still incomplete. Furthermore, most of what is currently known about HIV disease comes from studies of men who sexually contracted the virus from other men, people living in major urban centers who became infected through injection drug use, and individuals with blood clotting disorders (Minkoff & DeHovitz, 1991; A. R. Moss & Bacchetti, 1989).

Most information about the natural progression of HIV disease comes from the Multicenter AIDS Cohort Study (MACS), which enrolled 4,955 homosexual and bisexual men from four U.S. cities (Baltimore, Chicago, Los Angeles, and Pittsburgh), and followed them at 6-month assessment intervals (Kaslow, Ostrow, et al., 1987). The objective was to identify and study gay men who were HIV seropositive, men who became HIV infected during the study, and men who remained seronegative. MACS investigators sought information relevant to developing HIV prevention programs and early treatment strategies (Kaslow, Ostrow, et al., 1987). Information from a few similar cohorts supplements results reported from MACS, including the San Francisco City Cohort, San Francisco General Hospital Cohort, the Men's Health Study, and the Vancouver Lymphadenopathy–AIDS Study. Because these cohorts comprised gay and bisexual men, the generalization of results to women and ethnic minorities is highly limited.

HIV infection is silent for most of its duration, only becoming overtly symptomatic at its later stages. The natural history of HIV infection is highly variable and changes over the course of the epidemic. There is now considerable evidence that people infected with HIV will develop AIDS and will die of an AIDS-related illness (Schechter et al., 1990). The length of time from infection to an AIDS-related condition varies from as short as 1 year to 15 years or longer (Bartlett, 1993a; Friedman, Franklin, Freels, & Weil, 1991; Schechter et al., 1990). Studies have shown that 5% to 10% of HIV-infected people progress to AIDS within 4 years, and nearly 50% develop AIDS by 10 years after initial infection (Brettle & Leen, 1991; A. R. Moss & Bacchetti, 1989).

No single factor or combination of factors accounts for variability in HIV progression. Differences in rates of decline occur among individuals who contract HIV through different modes of transmission. For example, the San Francisco City Cohort Study, comprising primarily gay men, found that 54% of HIV-positive men progress to AIDS within 11 years of being infected, whereas 49% of people infected through blood transfusions develop AIDS within 7 years (Clement & Hollander, 1992). Other studies have not found survival differences across transmission groups (von Overbeck et al., 1994). Most studies have, however, found that the average duration from time of HIV infection to AIDS, in the absence of treatment, is between 7 and 10 years (Bartlett, 1993a; Friedman et al., 1991; Moss & Bacchetti, 1989; Schechter et al., 1990). The time between contracting HIV and developing AIDS is for the most part characterized by an absence of serious illness.

Several descriptive systems are available for staging HIV disease (Rabeneck & Wray, 1993). In an early classification scheme, the CDC had a four-stage progressive model that included an acute infection syndrome, a long period of asymptomatic infection, the development of persistent generalized lymphadenopathy (enlarged lymph nodes), and later disease manifestations. A second staging system developed by CDC included an expanded list of diseases associated with AIDS and an early symptomatic phase of disease referred to AIDS-related complex (ARC; CDC, 1987c). In the 1987 CDC system, stages I and II consist of asymptomatic periods, stage III is characterized by chronic lymphadenopathy, and the substages of stage IV represent later phases (see Table 2.1).

More recent staging systems rely on tracking the number of T-helper lymphocyte cells over the course of infection. For example, Bartlett's (1993a) system classifies people with T-helper cell counts greater than 500 cells/mm^3 as asymptomatic, those with cell counts between 500 and 200 cells/mm^3 as usually asymptomatic, and individuals with T-helper counts below 200 cells/mm^3 as vulnerable to major complications of AIDS, with most AIDS conditions occurring at or below 100 cells/mm^3. Similarly, Clement and Hollander (1992) offered a system with three stages of in-

Table 2.1

Centers for Disease Control (1987) Staging System for Human Immunodeficiency Virus Infection

Stage	Description
I	Acute HIV infection; asymptomatic or possible acute viral reaction
II	Latent infection
III	Chronic lymphadenopathy
IV-A	Constitutional symptoms: weight loss, fever, chronic diarrhea
IV-B	HIV-induced neuropathology: dementia, myelopathy, peripheral neuropathy
IV-C	Opportunistic infections
IV-D	HIV-associated tumors
IV-E	Other conditions

fection: early-stage disease defined by T-helper cell counts greater than 500 cells/mm^3; a middle stage with cell counts between 500 and 200 cells/mm^3; and later-stage disease defined by T-helper counts less than 200 cells/mm^3. Figure 2.1 summarizes the various staging systems using a time line of the natural history of HIV infection.

The course of HIV infection varies across subpopulations. For example, perinatally HIV-infected infants and children have shorter survival times compared with adolescents and adults. Although there are few significant differences between HIV-positive and -negative newborns at birth, HIV-positive infants become ill early, with a median onset of symptoms between 8 and 10 months of age and the majority of children becoming ill within one year (Johnson et al., 1989; Z. F. Rosenberg & Fauci, 1991). HIV-positive infants have higher rates of certain complications, such as neurological diseases, which occur in 30% to 60% of infected infants (Johnson et al., 1989; Z. F. Rosenberg & Fauci, 1991). Failure to thrive is also common (Johnson et al., 1989), as are delays in developmental milestones and the actual loss of milestones once achieved. HIV-positive infants are particularly susceptible to disease because HIV inhibits the development of the immature immune system, accelerating the course of HIV infection. The criteria for diagnosing AIDS in infants and children consist of the same AIDS-defining conditions that diagnose AIDS in adults, along with other specific and recurrent infections (CDC, 1987c, 1994g).

Unlike infants and young children, the clinical progression of AIDS for adolescents is more like that for adults (Gayle & D'Angelo, 1991). The following sections review HIV disease processes from the point of infection to later phases of illness.

PRIMARY HIV INFECTION

Following the introduction of HIV into the bloodstream, the body mounts an immune reaction that, unfortunately, is ineffective in stopping HIV infection (Gallo, 1987; Pantaleo et al., 1993). In response to HIV, the body may react with a brief period of acute infection symptoms. The usual time that lapses between exposure and acute illness is about two to four weeks, with the duration of symptoms lasting only one to two weeks (Tindall et al., 1992). Acute retroviral illness, when it does occur, is the earliest clini-

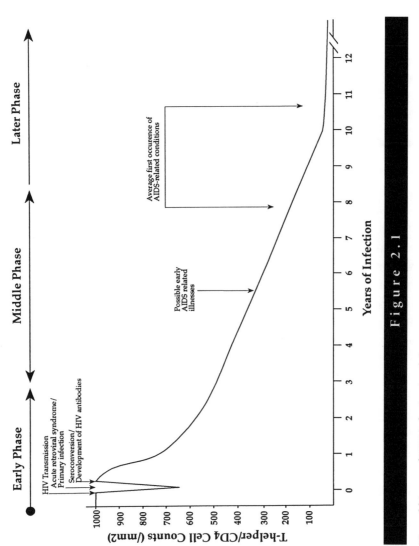

Figure 2.1

Natural history of HIV infection in adults.

cally recognizable event in the natural history of HIV infection (Glasner & Kaslow, 1990). Response to retroviral infection is similar to vague symptoms of mononucleosis (Bartlett, 1993a; CDC, 1986; Glasner & Kaslow, 1990; A. R. Moss & Bacchetti, 1989). However, retroviral infection actually consists of a distinct and recognizable clinical syndrome (Tindall et al., 1992). Most typically, acute HIV symptom illness, or primary HIV infection, presents with persistent fever, lethargy, malaise, muscle weakness, headache, pain in or around the eyes, sensitivity to bright light, sore throat, and skin rashes (Tindall, Carr, & Cooper, 1995). In most cases, primary HIV infection symptoms resolve themselves and usually do not recur (Tindall et al., 1995).

Not all people infected with HIV, however, develop symptoms of primary infection. Studies have found that between 40% and 90% of individuals experience an acute response to HIV infection (Moss & Bacchetti, 1989; Saag, 1992; Tindall et al., 1992). Symptoms occur among people infected through each major route of HIV transmission, and, at present, there is no conclusive evidence that any particular group is more likely to develop symptomatic acute illness (Tindall et al., 1992). In addition to the aforementioned early symptoms, HIV-positive persons may develop persistent generalized lymphadenopathy, defined by enlarged lymph nodes that are detectable by touch and remain enlarged for a minimum of three months (CDC, 1986). Swollen lymph nodes in the armpits, neck, or groin are common in HIV infection, as well as in other viral infections, with 70% of HIV-positive persons having swollen nodes within the first few weeks of infection (Kaslow, Phair, et al., 1987; Tindall et al., 1992). In the case of HIV infection, swollen lymph nodes are the result of disseminated HIV throughout the lymphatic system (Pantaleo et al., 1993). Most studies show that persistent lymphadenopathy does not have prognostic value for disease progression towards AIDS (Moss & Bacchetti, 1989; Schechter et al., 1990).

Following acute symptoms of HIV infection, although not dependent on the occurrence of such symptoms, antibodies are produced against HIV. Establishing HIV antibodies, or seroconversion to HIV, most likely results after a threshold of HIV replication has occurred and depends on the immune competency of the host to mount the antibody response (Imagawa et al., 1989). On average, HIV antibodies are detectable through serological testing slightly more than 2 months after viral transmission, and 95%

of HIV-infected individuals develop antibodies within 6 months of becoming infected (Saag, 1995). However, the incubation period for HIV may last longer than 6 months, and in rare cases incubation may last 2 to 3 years (Imagawa et al., 1989; Glasner & Kaslow, 1990). Variability in establishing HIV antibodies can come from numerous factors, including the virulence of viral strains, the dose of virus transmitted, the frequency of exposure, and an individual's immune response (Ranki et al., 1987). Once antibodies have developed, they are detectable through HIV testing.

HIV TESTING

Some diagnostic tests for HIV infection involve detecting HIV genetic material directly in blood cells or actually culturing the virus. However, the most widely used tests identify antibodies to the virus rather than the presence of HIV itself. Antibodies produced by the immune system provide immunologic "footprints" to viral infection (Saag, 1992). Antibody tests are safer for laboratories to perform than actual viral-detection procedures because antibody tests do not require direct contact with HIV (Saag, 1992). Antibody tests also tend to be less expensive than viral cultures and genetic testing (Glasner & Kaslow, 1990; Saag, 1992).

The standard procedures for HIV antibody testing involve providing written informed consent, pretest counseling for 30 to 90 minutes (including an explanation of the test), discussions of limited confidentiality when tests are not anonymous, personalized risk assessments, and exploration of individual concerns (Perry & Markowitz, 1988).[1] The test procedure itself involves drawing blood and sending samples for laboratory analysis. Posttest result notification and counseling usually occur about two weeks after the initial visit.

Blood collected for testing is first subjected to an *enzyme-linked immunosorbent assay* (ELISA) that tests for antibodies to HIV. ELISA tests are done first because they are highly sensitive to HIV antibodies. If an ELISA test is negative, it is highly improbable that the person is HIV infected. In other words, false negative results from an ELISA test are rare.

---

[1]Some places, such as street outreach programs, private clinics, and physicians' offices, may conduct HIV testing with minimal counseling and with little information about what test results mean (Henry, Maki, & Crossley, 1988). These situations may complicate the potential psychological distress associated with HIV testing.

However, positive ELISA tests must be repeated because the procedure is not specific to HIV antibodies. Thus, a greater likelihood exists that an ELISA result will be a false positive (Saag, 1992). For this reason, ELISA tests are used to screen blood samples for HIV antibodies. After a blood specimen receives a repeated positive ELISA, the test is confirmed using a *western blot procedure*. Like ELISA, western blot detects HIV antibodies, but western blot is highly specific because it determines the exact antigens toward which antibodies are directed (Saag, 1992). A positive western blot result means detection of two out of three precise antigen groups from components of HIV. This level of specificity reduces the chances of false positive results to an extremely low probability (Saag, 1992). Thus, both a positive repeated ELISA screening test and a positive western blot confirmatory test are required for diagnosis of HIV infection (Bartlett, 1993a).[2]

HIV antibody testing is now among the most accurate diagnostic tools in medicine (Bartlett, 1993a; Mortimer, 1988). In tests that indicate a false negative result (i.e., that the person is not found infected when he or she really is infected), the most common cause is that the blood sample was collected during the incubation window period before the presence of HIV antibodies (Bartlett, 1993a; Mortimer, 1988). A person cannot, therefore, know that they are HIV infected during the first month or two of infection, although HIV can be transmitted to others during this time. The potential for false negative tests requires that all persons who receive this result be tested again approximately 3 months later. People who test HIV-positive and have no identifiable risk history should also be retested, although false positive test results only occur because of laboratory errors (Bartlett, 1993a).

In addition to receiving either a positive or a negative result, a third possible outcome is an indeterminate result: neither conclusively positive nor negative. Indeterminate HIV test results usually occur when the ELISA test is positive and only one of the two required specific antigens is detected by western blot (Bartlett, 1993a). Ambiguous results occur with respect to both HIV-1 and HIV-2 antibody tests, and are most commonly found among individuals infected with HIV who are in the process of de-

---

[2]Persons who test negative for HIV antibodies should be retested at 6- to 12-month intervals if they continue to engage in HIV risk behaviors (Bartlett, 1993a).

veloping antibodies, and require that the test be repeated 2 to 6 months later (Bartlett, 1993a).

HIV testing is the only reliable means of determining HIV infection. Even after symptoms, many HIV-related illnesses can be caused by non-HIV immune-suppressing conditions (CDC, 1987c). Thus, individuals with symptoms should be tested for HIV antibodies rather than assuming that they are HIV infected on the basis of illness alone (Bartlett, 1993a).

ASYMPTOMATIC HIV INFECTION

During most of HIV infection, patients appear, feel, and are otherwise healthy. As much as 50% to 80% of the time that a person has HIV, they are symptom free. The virus is actively depleting T-helper lymphocytes during clinically asymptomatic phases, and HIV is also transmittible to others during this time. It was once thought that HIV replicated less during asymptomatic periods, primarily because of low concentrations of virus in the bloodstream. Although termed a *latency period*, asymptomatic HIV infection does not constitute a time of microbiological inactivity (Pantaleo et al., 1993). Recent studies have shown that HIV is productive in lymph nodes when patients are symptom free (Temin & Bolognesi, 1993). Following years of destruction, the immune system slowly degenerates, increasing vulnerability to illness.

The primary target of HIV, T-helper lymphocytes, is one of three types of thymus-originating cells (T-cells) of the immune system. These cells function to distinguish self from nonself and rid the body of foreign agents (Calabrese, Kling, & Gold, 1987). Cytotoxic T-cells identify and destroy infectious agents, suppressor T-cells reduce immune responses, and T-helper cells induce responses from several branches of the immune system. T-helper lymphocytes are the only of the three that express the CD_4 surface receptor, and HIV therefore binds with and infects these cells. T-helper lymphocytes have several functions, including the induction of non-T-helper cell activity. Cell-mediated immunity results from the production of cytokines that guide a number of immunologic responses. For example, T-helper lymphocytes mediate through cytokines the activity of natural killer cells, which in turn destroy viral-infected and certain cancerous cells (Hollerman, Bernstein, & Beute, 1987; O'Leary, 1990). Impaired natural killer-cell activity is an outcome of T-helper cell dysfunction. Cytokines also direct the proliferation and maturation of several other immune cells (see Figure 2.2).

Decreased numbers of T-helper lymphocytes were among the first immunologic abnormalities described in patients with AIDS (Hutchinson et

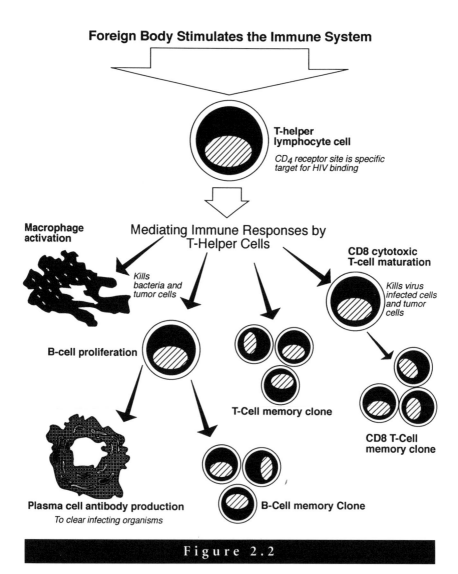

Figure 2.2

Functional roles of T-helper lymphocytes in the human immune system.

al., 1991). Over the course of HIV infection, the average decline in T-helper lymphocytes ranges from 50 to 80 cells/mm^3 per year (Bartlett, 1993a). At this rate, over a 10- year period, T-helper cell counts drop to between 200 and 0 cells/mm^3, increasing vulnerability to infections and malignancies (Bartlett, 1993a). The single best predictor of developing AIDS in HIV-positive gay men is the rate of T-helper cell decline and blood concentration of T-helpers relative to other immune cells (Saah et al., 1992).

Because the number of T-helper cells is inversely related to symptoms, low T-helper cell counts indicate impending illness (Hutchinson et al., 1991). During asymptomatic periods, T-helper cell counts are usually between 500 and 200 cells/mm^3 (Lifson, Hessol, Buchbinder, & Holmberg, 1991), although nearly half of individuals with counts below 200 cells/mm^3 are also asymptomatic at any given time (Hutchinson et al., 1991). T-helper cell counts are a marker for HIV disease progression, but they are limited by extreme fluctuations because of a number of factors, including variability in laboratory procedures and changes in cell concentrations over diurnal cycles. Changes in cell counts are also difficult to interpret because there are no normative data for HIV-infected patients and noninfected risk groups (Clement & Hollander, 1992). Despite their limitations, T-helper lymphocyte counts set guidelines for prognostic decisions, for initiating medications that suppress HIV production, and for determining when to initiate prophylaxis against opportunistic illnesses (Hutchinson et al., 1991). Thus, the risk for AIDS-related conditions increases over the course of HIV infection, and the most reliable marker for disease progression is the number of functional T-helper lymphocytes present in the immune system (Hutchinson et al., 1991; Polk et al., 1987).

Vulnerability to disease increases as the immune system loses T-helper cells and T-helper-cell-mediated immunity. Although immune-system suppression does not necessarily mean symptomatic illness, having an HIV-related illness does suggest severe immune suppression. Only 2% of cases progress to AIDS within 2 years of becoming infected, whereas as many as 10% progress to AIDS within 4 years (A. R. Moss & Bacchetti, 1989; J. M. Taylor, Schwartz, & Detels, 1986). The mean length of time between infection and developing AIDS is 8 to 10 years among homosexually active men, and it is considerably shorter for adults who contracted HIV through blood transfusions (Laurence, 1992; Lui, Darrow, & Rutherford, 1988). Evidence suggests, however, that the interval between infection and illness is lengthening as a result of advances in medical treatments (Fischl, 1995; M. G. Taylor, Huo, & Detels, 1991).

FACTORS ASSOCIATED WITH HIV PROGRESSION TO AIDS

The variable clinical manifestations of HIV infection have led to several hypotheses concerning factors that facilitate or inhibit the virus (Solomon, Kemeny, & Temoshok, 1991). There are several potential influences on the duration and course of most infectious diseases, including sociodemographic factors, general health status, nutrition, previous illness history, genetic immune factors, variations in viral strains, and seasons of the year (Cohen & Williamson, 1991; S. Solomon et al., 1991). Among sociodemographic characteristics, age is consistently associated with HIV progression, with older people having more rapid rates of immune suppression. Moss and Bacchetti (1989) found that people infected with HIV at ages over 40 years were more likely to become ill sooner than individuals infected at younger ages. Men who were infected after age 30 also have poorer survival than their younger-age counterparts (Hogg et al., 1994). Similarly, once diagnosed with AIDS, older adults die sooner than younger adults (Bacchetti, Osmond, Chaisson, Dritz, et al., 1988). For example, Clement and Hollander (1992) reported that being diagnosed with AIDS at age 35 and older is associated with a substantially poorer prognosis. Decreased survival time observed with advancing age is not, however, entirely understood. The accelerated rate of disease may involve a general decrease in ability to contend with opportunistic infections (Lemp, Payne, Neal, Temelso, & Rutherford, 1990).

Ethnic minorities demonstrate a more rapid decline in T-helper lymphocytes than do Whites (Munoz et al., 1988), and there are ethnic differences in the relative frequency of AIDS-related illnesses (Greenberg et al., 1992). Sex differences in prognosis have also been suggested; men live longer after an AIDS diagnosis than do women (e.g., Lemp et al., 1990; Melnick et al., 1994), aside from differences in lag time to diagnosis and inattention of the AIDS definition to variations among women (Murrain, 1993). Disease progression also varies by primary route of HIV transmission. Individuals who become infected through injection drug use survive longer compared with those infected through other modes of HIV transmission (Melnick et al., 1994), whereas contracting HIV by blood trans-fusion results in the most rapid death following an AIDS diagnosis (Lemp et al., 1990; S. A. Myers et al., 1993).

The route of contracting HIV is also related to relative frequencies of AIDS-related illnesses. Men who contract HIV sexually from other men are more likely to develop Kaposi's sarcoma, and injection drug users are more likely to develop *Pneumocystis carinii* pneumonia, recurrent bacterial pneumonia, and pulmonary tuberculosis (Greenberg et al., 1992). Differences in transmission routes may also account for most of the differences in opportunistic illnesses between men and women (Murrain, 1993). However, the associations between disease and HIV transmission routes are not well understood, with such factors as primary path of entry into the bloodstream, the volume of HIV transmitted, and number of exposures to the virus all potentially mediating HIV infection (Hamburg et al., 1990).

In addition to demographic and transmission-associated factors, an infected person's health status influences the course of HIV infection. For example, some studies show that pregnancy may accelerate the loss of T-helper lymphocytes among HIV-positive women (Biggar et al., 1989). However, other studies have failed to replicate these relationships, bringing the effects of pregnancy on HIV infection into question (Brettle & Leen, 1991; Carpenter et al., 1991). Cigarette smoking has also been associated with immune-system functioning (Royce & Winkelstein, 1990) and the progression of HIV infection to AIDS (Brettle & Leen, 1991). Ultraviolet light activates genetic expression of HIV (Morrey et al., 1991; Vogel, Cepeda, Tschachler, Napolitano, & Jay, 1992), suggesting that excessive exposure to the sun or tanning lights may promote HIV progression (Wallace & Lasker, 1992; Vogel et al., 1992). Exercise and nutrition, on the other hand, may slow HIV disease, although there is thus far little empirical support for direct relationships. There is also little evidence that alcohol and other psychoactive substance use play a significant role in HIV infection (Kaslow et al., 1989).

The most widely accepted cofactors for HIV infection, although not universally accepted (for a review, see Aral & Wasserheit, in press), have been infections with other pathogens. In particular, the interaction between HIV and other viruses (i.e., herpes viruses) has been considered important (Hirsch et al., 1984; Schoub, 1994). Sexually transmitted pathogens and infectious agents spread through nonsterile preparations of drug-injecting equipment trigger immune responses that can stimulate HIV (Des Jarlais et al., 1988) and activate HIV's replication cycle (Morrow et al., 1989). Co-infection with other immune-suppressing viruses can also facilitate the progression of HIV (Brettle & Leen, 1991; Tindall et al., 1995). Even worse, multiple infections are synergistic and make prognosis dependant on a chain of unpredictable biomedical events. Repeated exposures to HIV complicate the picture further by multiple strains of the virus with varied properties. Variation in viral strains occurs because of the drift in molecular composition demonstrated in HIV isolates within and between infected persons (Brettle & Leen, 1991). Although these and other factors appear related to HIV progression, no true cofactors for HIV disease have been conclusively established (Mulder & Antoni, 1992; Solomon et al., 1991).

Potential cofactors of HIV infection tend to co-occur and have inextricable effects. For example, studies that have found shorter survival times for women and ethnic minorities could be explained because women and people of color are often infected through injection drug use (Melnick et al., 1994; Murrain, 1993; Rothenberg, Woelfel, et al., 1987). In addition, exposure to infectious agents that may facilitate HIV disease occurs in different patterns among ethnic groups, sexes, and sexual-orientation subgroups (Greenberg et al., 1992). Therefore, associations between potential cofactors and disease progression are open to multiple interpretations, including bidirectional causes and unidentified third variables. For example, early in the HIV epidemic it was noted that men who sexually contracted HIV from other men and who had a history of using nitrite inhalers ("poppers") were at increased risk for developing Kaposi's sarcoma (e.g., Polk et al., 1987). Further support for linking nitrite inhaler use with HIV infection came from research showing short-term effects of nitrites on branches of the human immune system (Dax, Adler, Nagel, Lange, & Jaffe, 1991). Subsequent research, however, has shown that Kaposi's sarcoma in homosexual men is actually associated with sexual behaviors with direct human feces contact (Beral et al., 1992). In fact, the relationship between fecal contact and developing Kaposi's sarcoma is linear, with higher rates of oral–anal sexual contact related to increased risk for Kaposi's sarcoma. There is now good evidence that Kaposi's sarcoma is associated with a virus that is likely contracted through anal sex (Chang et al., 1994). Nitrite use, therefore, may be a frequent substance used by men who also engage in oral–anal sexual practices, which are in turn associated with Kaposi's sarcoma. This example illustrates the complex interplay among potential cofactors for HIV progression, AIDS-related conditions, and behavioral practices.

LATER-STAGE HIV INFECTION

Following long periods of asymptomatic infection, any number of general and nonspecific early symptoms may develop. Symptoms of HIV infection include chronic low-grade fever, persistent fatigue, diarrhea lasting at least 2 weeks, rashes or other skin conditions, unintentional weight loss of at least 10 pounds, night sweats, and mild infections of the mouth or throat. These symptoms were once referred to as ARC because it was thought that they signalled the imminent onset of AIDS. However, the term ARC has lost its clinical meaning because symptoms do not necessarily occur before AIDS. Rather, the same manifestations are referred to simply as early symptoms of HIV infection.

The later stages of HIV infection are characterized by severe depletion of T-helper lymphocytes and the onset of specific illnesses. Most clinical manifestations of HIV infection are evident relatively late in the course of disease, occurring only after significant immunologic impairment (MacDonell, Chmiel, Poggensee, Wu, & Phair, 1990). Illnesses that occur late in HIV infection reflect the defective-cell-mediated immunity caused by diminished numbers of T-helper lymphocytes. Similar immune dysfunction is common among cancer patients receiving chemotherapy, patients with certain lymphomas and other malignancies, and organ transplant recipients (Bartlett, 1993a). T-helper lymphocyte counts below 200 cells/mm^3 mark what otherwise would be unexplained significant weight loss, chronic diarrhea, new or persistent outbreaks of genital herpes, skin rashes, and infections of the mouth, esophagus, and vagina (Kaslow, Phair, et al., 1987; Lifson et al., 1991). Over 35% of all HIV-related hospitalizations, 29% of hospital costs, and over 35% of HIV-positive hospital inpatient deaths occur among people who become systemically ill but have not yet been diagnosed with AIDS (Andrulis, Weslowski, Hintz, & Spolarich, 1992).

Cohorts followed before the widespread availability of antiretroviral medications showed that most people survive between 11 and 12 months after receiving an AIDS diagnosis, less than 11% survive 3 years, and yet others are known to have a slow-progressing disease, surviving 15 years and beyond (Bacchetti, Osmond, Chaisson, Dritz, et al., 1988; Cao, Qin, Zhang, Safrit, & Ho, 1995; Glasner & Kaslow, 1990; Lemp et al., 1990; Pantaleo et al., 1995; Rothenberg, Woelfel, et al., 1987). T-helper cell counts below 200 cells/mm^3 substantially increase risk for developing AIDS-related conditions (Lifson et al., 1991; Masur et al., 1989; Phair et al., 1990), with 80% of people developing an AIDS-related illness within 3 years of T- helper cell counts dropping below 200/mm^3 (Chang, Katz, & Hernandez, 1992). The probability of serious illnesses increases as T-helper lymphocytes decline, with survival times for people with T-helper cell counts below 50 cells/mm^3 being generally less than 1 or 2 years (Clement & Hollander, 1992).

Several factors appear to predict length of life following AIDS-related symptoms. Studies have shown that the initial condition leading to an AIDS diagnosis strongly predicts survival (Lemp et al., 1990). Most consistently, individuals first diagnosed with Kaposi's sarcoma are more likely to survive longer than are people diagnosed with *Pneumocystis carinii* pneumonia, who in turn survive longer than those initially diagnosed with other AIDS-associated illnesses (Bacchetti, Osmond, Chaisson, Dritz, et al., 1988; Friedman et al., 1991). Rothenberg, Woelfel, et al. (1987) found that 72% of patients initially diagnosed with Kaposi's sarcoma survived 1 year and 30% survived 5 years, a substantially greater survival time than is associated with other AIDS-related illnesses. Friedman et al. (1991) concluded that the role of initial AIDS diagnosis in survival may be attributed to the organ systems involved, the degree of immune suppression that characterizes its onset, and the effectiveness of available treatments.

Survival time is also associated with characteristics of individuals, among which the sex of the infected person is the most controversial. Friedman et al. (1991) found that women who received an AIDS diagnosis survived for a significantly shorter time than men. However, subsequent research has failed to show that nongynecologic manifestations of HIV infection differ between men and women, and there are no known sex differences in AIDS prognosis or in the rate of disease progression from HIV infection to AIDS (Brettle & Leen, 1991; Kloser & Craig, 1994; Melnick et al., 1994; Minkoff & DeHovitz, 1991). Thus, although early explanations for findings of women surviving shorter periods of time tended to stress potential biological cofactors, such as genetics or hormones, sociocultural factors now offer the best explanation for women surviving with AIDS for a shorter time (Ickovics & Rodin, 1992). Men with HIV infection are diagnosed earlier, receive better medical care, and have stronger social support networks than do women, and those differences likely account for variations in survival (Carpenter et al., 1991; Melnick et al., 1994). A history of using injection drugs also contributes to an earlier death for women with AIDS (Melnick et al., 1994). Sex differences in survival also appear related to women historically having less access to adequate health care, including clinical trials for experimental treatments (Brettle & Leen, 1991; Carpenter et al., 1991; Ickovics & Rodin, 1992).

Ethnicity also predicts AIDS survival (e.g., Lagakos, Fischl, Stein, Lim, & Volberding, 1991; Rothenberg et al., 1987). African Americans survive a shorter time with AIDS than do their White counterparts. Ethnic differences in survival may be the result of several factors, including differences in immune functioning, prevalence of cofactors for disease progression, and differences in routes of contracting HIV. Ethnic differences in AIDS survival are, however, best accounted for by sociodemographic differences between African Americans and Whites found in study samples (Curtis & Patrick, 1993). For example, Hogg et al. (1994) found that like other diseases, AIDS morbidity and mortality is closely associated with income level.

Interpreting survival studies requires close attention to their methodological limitations. For example, early studies conducted in New York City demonstrated survival times substantially longer than those reported in San Francisco cohorts. It was at first thought that the difference reflected relative numbers of gay men versus injection drug users in the respective cohorts. Differences in survival, however, have been accounted for by data management strategies. The New York City studies, unlike those conducted in San Francisco, assumed that people who moved or could not be reached for follow-up were still alive, an assumption that would necessarily increase estimated survival (Bacchetti, Osmond, Chaisson, & Moss, 1988; Rothenberg et al., 1987). Studies of AIDS survival also differ across risk populations, with people who sexually contract HIV living longer than those infected through injection drug use. However, these findings are limited by numerous coexisting health and demographic factors associated with drug abuse. Finally, there are problems in trying to compare different survival studies, not only because AIDS has been defined differently over the course of the epidemic, but also because treatment has changed over time.

In summary, later stages of HIV infection are the result of a progressive depletion of the immune system. Loss of T-helper lymphocytes directly and indirectly impairs immune functioning over long clinically asymptomatic periods. Although studies show that some demographic and risk-related characteristics may be related to survival following an AIDS diagnosis, only initial AIDS-defining illnesses have reliably predicted prognosis. Most differences in survival are related to sociocultural factors, particularly access to medical care. Nearer the end of the disease process, people with HIV infection face an array of serious health threats as their immune system declines.

THE AIDS CASE DEFINITION

Clinical manifestations of HIV-related conditions fall within one of two general classes. Although most conditions result from a depleted immune system, others are a direct result of HIV infection itself, including HIV infection of the lymph nodes, brain, kidneys, abdominal cavity, and lungs (Bartlett, 1993a). Most AIDS-defining conditions, however, result from a deteriorating immune system, including the growth of malignant tumors and development of opportunistic infections that would otherwise be kept in check. Bartlett (1993a) identified the 10 most common clinical presentations of HIV infection: persistent lymphadenopathy; pulmonary symptoms suggestive of pneumonia; cytopenia (diminution of blood cells); fungal infections; constitutional symptoms including persistent fever and diarrhea; weight loss; bacterial infections; tuberculosis; persistent symptoms of sexually transmitted diseases; and nervous system disorders.

The first formal diagnostic criteria were established in 1982 as a result of early clinical experiences with men who contracted HIV infection through homosexual activity. The diagnosis was updated in 1985 and again in 1987 to include additional indicator diseases that characterized the diversity of HIV-infected persons (A. R. Moss & Bacchetti, 1989). The 1987 case definition for adults and adolescents consisted of 23 clinical diseases (CDC, 1987a). The case definition for children differed from adults by including recurrent bacterial infections and pulmonary problems among indicator diseases and by not considering children under 15 months old with HIV antibodies to be HIV infected because of passive perinatal transfer of maternal antibodies (CDC, 1987a).

The CDC AIDS case definition was once again expanded in 1993 (see Figure 2.3). In reference to the conditions included in the diagnosis of AIDS, the CDC stated that "the objectives of these changes are to simplify

AIDS-Defining Conditions
1993 Revision

* Candidiasis infection of bronchi, trachea, or lungs
* Candidiasis infection of esophagus
* Invasive cervical cancer
* Coccidioidoidomycosis, disseminated or extrapulmonary
* Cryptococcosis, extrapulmonary
* Cryptosporidiosis, intestinal, > 1 month
* Cytomegalovirus retinitis with loss of vision
* Cytomegalovirus disease
* HIV-related encephalopathy
* Herpes simplex infection, > 1 month
* Histoplasmosis, disseminated or extrapulmonary
* Isosporiasis, intestinal, > 1 month
* Kaposi's sarcoma
* Burkitt's lymphoma
* Immunoblastic lymphoma
* Primary lymphoma of brain
* *Mycobacterium* avium complex
* *Mycobacterium* tuberculosis
* *Myobacterium*, disseminated or extrapulmonary
* *Pneumocystis carinii* pneumonia
* Recurrent pneumonia
* Progressive multifocal leukoencephalopathy
* Recurrent salmonella septicemia
* Toxoplasmosis of the brain
* HIV wasting syndrome

Figure 2.3

Conditions included under the CDC AIDS case definition.

the classification of HIV infection, to reflect current standards of medical care for HIV infected persons, and to categorize more accurately HIV-related morbidity" (CDC, 1992h, p. 2). The revised case definition also addresses several criticisms of previous diagnostic criteria, such as failure to include manifestations of HIV common among women (Chang et al., 1992; Kloser & Craig, 1994)). The CDC case definition retains the 23 conditions included in the previous diagnosis and adds three new diseases: pulmonary tuberculosis, recurrent pneumonia, and invasive cervical cancer. Pulmonary tuberculosis (TB) was added because HIV-induced immune suppression increases the likelihood of activating latent TB (Buehler & Ward, 1993). Recurrent pneumonia was added to the case definition because of the prevalence of bacterial pneumonia, with as much as a five-fold increase among HIV-infected injection drug users compared with their non-HIV-infected counterparts (Selwyn et al., 1988). Finally, invasive cervical cancer was added to the revised case definition because as many as 22% of HIV-infected women present signs of early cervical disease (CDC, 1992h).

The major change in the 1993 AIDS case definition was the inclusion of immunologic diagnostic criteria. Unlike previous AIDS diagnoses, the definition specifies that individuals who are asymptomatic but receive an accurate, although not necessarily most recent, T-helper lymphocyte cell count below 200 cells/mm^3 in conjunction with HIV infection meet the criteria for diagnosis with AIDS (Buehler & Ward, 1993; CDC, 1992h). Immune dysfunction is included in the new case definition because immunologic markers are associated with disease progression and used as clinical prognostic indicators (CDC, 1992h, 1992p, 1992r; MacDonell et al., 1990; Saag, 1992). Another reason for including an immunologic marker independent of specific illnesses is that T-helper cell counts carry similar meaning among subgroups of infected persons who may vary in illness presented, some of which may not yet be listed in the case definition. Finally, people with suppressed immune systems who did not yet have a case-defining illness became eligible for disability benefits.

A substantial increase in the number of diagnosed AIDS cases occurred as a result of the expanded 1993 definition. The increase was due to the sudden inclusion of individuals with T-helper counts below 200 cells/mm^3 among persons living with AIDS. Figure 2.4 shows the first quarter of 1993 increase in AIDS due to the new definition over and

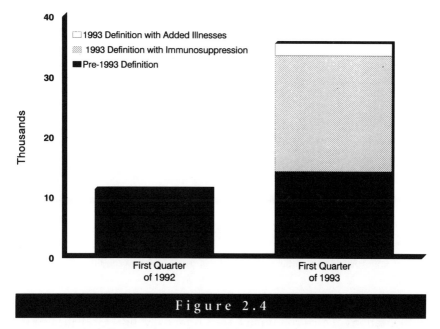

Figure 2.4

Reported cases of AIDS among adolescents and adults following implementation of the expanded AIDS case definition, 1993.

above the cases reported on the basis of the 1987 definition. Of the 35,779 AIDS cases reported in the first quarter of 1993, 60% were based on criteria from the expanded definition, with the majority resulting from criteria related to suppressed T-helper lymphocyte counts (CDC, 1993b). Nearly half of all AIDS cases in 1993 were attributed to the T-helper cell criteria (CDC, 1994e). According to the CDC (1992h), if all of the estimated one million HIV-infected persons in the United States were to obtain T-helper cell counts, as many as 120,000 to 190,000 would have less than 200 cell/mm^3 but would not yet have had an AIDS-defining illness (CDC, 1992h).

Each AIDS-defining condition entails its own disease processes and implications for prognosis. Figure 2.5 presents the proportion of adolescent and adult AIDS cases initially diagnosed with various conditions. The majority of AIDS cases have been initially diagnosed with *Pneumocystis carinii* pneumonia. Numerous other AIDS-defining conditions are rare and do not typically occur as initial diagnoses. The signs, symptoms, and

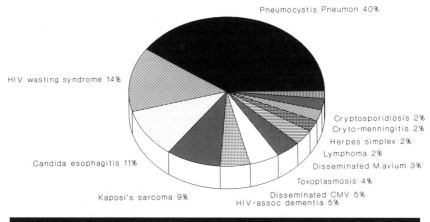

Pneumocystis Pneumon 40%

HIV wasting syndrome 14%

Cryptosporidiosis 2%
Cryto-menningitis 2%
Herpes simplex 2%
Lymphoma 2%
Disseminated M.avium 3%

Toxoplasmosis 4%

Candida esophagitis 11%

Kaposi's sarcoma 9%

Disseminated CMV 5%
HIV-assoc dementia 5%

Figure 2.5

Proportion of AIDS cases initially diagnosed with AIDS-defining conditions.

complications of each condition pose substantially different challenges for people living with AIDS.

Immune suppression can mean multiple, simultaneous illnesses. The manifestations of HIV infection represent a wide spectrum of diseases and a multitude of problems for infected persons. Mental health professionals, of course, are not in a position or role to diagnose or treat these ailments. However, professionals who provide services to clients with HIV infection should be aware of the symptoms, course, and potential outcomes of each illness. Below is a brief description of the AIDS-case-defining conditions and other diseases that commonly confront people living with HIV infection. Greater detail concerning the diagnostic, disease process, and therapeutic aspects of AIDS-related conditions is provided by Broder, Merigan, and Bolognesi (1994); Sande and Volberding (1992, 1995); and Wormser (1992).

Clinical Conditions Caused Directly by HIV

HIV-Related Wasting Syndrome

Although several disease processes affect the gastrointestinal system and cause chronic, persistent, disabling loss of weight and body mass, HIV itself can directly cause these symptoms. HIV wasting syndrome is an AIDS-defining condition. Diagnosis is determined by involuntary loss of at least 10% of body weight along with either chronic diarrhea or chronic weakness and fever over the course of 30 days, in the absence of other illnesses that could otherwise explain these symptoms (CDC, 1992h). In association with severe weight loss are symptoms of fatigue, lethargy, and physical weakness.

HIV-Related Neurological Disease

Mild to moderate cognitive, affective, and motor dysfunctions can occur in HIV infection, with individuals at later stages of AIDS more often experiencing such symptoms (McCutchan, 1990; Worley & Price, 1992). Subtle signs of dysfunction, however, can appear earlier in the course of HIV infection (Koppel, 1992). Early signs of HIV-related neurological disease include difficulty maintaining concentration, memory problems, and motor disturbances, including slowing of arm, leg, and eye movements (R. W. Price & Sidtis 1992). HIV-related neurological disease is usually diagnosed when symptoms become moderate to severe and disrupt occupational, basic self-care, intellectual, social, or motor functioning. HIV-related neurological disease is caused by the toxic effects of HIV infection of the brain. Clinical symptoms are almost always caused by diffuse brain damage (Fauci, 1988). Neurological effects of HIV infection occur in as many as 90% of HIV-infected individuals, although functional impairment ranges from none to profound (Koppel, 1992).

Viral Infections

Cytomegalovirus (CMV)

Cytomegalovirus is a herpes virus and is a very common cause of disease in HIV infection, with a majority of people with AIDS developing some form of active CMV infection (Drew, Buhles, & Erlich, 1992). Cytomegalovirus can cause pneumonia (Hollerman et al., 1987), vaginal infection (Shah & Barton, 1993), hepatitis, encephalitis, and colitis (Drew et al., 1992). However, the most common manifestations are CMV retinitis, CMV esophagitis, and CMV colitis. Among the most distressing manifestations of CMV infection is retinitis, which threatens the vision of a significant number of people with AIDS (Yarrish, 1992). Irreversible loss of visual acuity and blindness often result from untreated CMV retinitis (Drew et al., 1992). Almost all patients who develop CMV retinitis have

T-helper lymphocyte counts below 50 cells/mm^3 (Drew et al., 1992), making it a later manifestation of HIV infection. In addition to symptomatic illness, CMV also has immune-suppressing effects of its own, potentially complicating the course of HIV infection (Yarrish, 1992). Although CMV infection is difficult to treat, advances in antiviral medications have been effective in managing this condition (Yarrish, 1992).

Herpes Simplex Virus Infection

Because more than 25 million people in the United States are believed to be infected with herpes simplex virus (Aral & Holmes, 1991), and because HIV infection is often associated with other sexually transmitted diseases, people with HIV infection are frequently co-infected with herpes simplex virus. Studies have found that as many as 95% of gay men with AIDS were previously infected with herpes simplex virus (Drew et al., 1992). Symptoms of herpes simplex infection include small, painful, erupting blisters. When outbreaks of herpes lesions are persistent for at least 1 month, they constitute an AIDS-defining condition. Herpes simplex virus causes ulcerations of the oral, genital, and anal mucous lining (Finley, Joshi, & Neill, 1992). In non-immune-suppressed persons, herpes blisters heal within 3 to 4 weeks of their onset. People with compromised immune systems, however, may have chronic prolonged lesions lasting months if untreated or unresponsive to treatment (Drew et al., 1992; Minkoff & DeHovitz, 1991). Herpes simplex lesions may occur in the esophagus, causing pain and possibly interfering with swallowing. Pneumonitis, pulmonary infection, and encephalitis are also possible manifestations. Finally, like cytomegalovirus, herpes simplex virus is a potential cofactor in the progression of HIV infection (Brettle & Leen, 1991).

Epstein–Barr Virus and Hairy Leukoplakia

Epstein–Barr virus is associated with infectious mononucleosis. Among people with HIV infection, Epstein–Barr virus infection also involves hairy leukoplakia, an AIDS-defining condition the symptoms of which include white lesions on the tongue and other areas of the oral cavity (Greenspan & Greenspan, 1992; Greenspan, Greenspan, & Winkler, 1992). Hairy leukoplakia occurs in 19% of individuals with otherwise asymptomatic HIV infection, and more frequently among people with advanced immune suppression (Greenspan & Greenspan, 1992). Although hairy leukoplakia may resolve on its own, symptoms are relieved by a number of treatments, including antiviral medications (Greenspan & Greenspan, 1992).

Progressive Multifocal Leukoencephalopathy (PML)

Caused by a human papovavirus, progressive multifocal leukoencephalopathy occurs in approximately 2% to 4% of AIDS cases (Bacellar et al., 1994; Worley & Price, 1992). The papovavirus infects the oligodendrocytes of the brain, cells responsible for producing the myelin sheath that coats and insulates neurons (Krupp, Belman, & Shneidman, 1992). The neurologic symptoms of PML are usually rapid, progressive, and fatal, with the majority of afflicted persons dying within months of symptomatic disease (Krupp et al., 1992). Symptoms of PML include changes in mental status, memory, and language; headache; seizures; loss of coordinated movements; and other motor disturbances (Krupp et al., 1992; Worley & Price, 1992). Neurological deficits are focal, affecting specific functions, in contrast with the diffuse and generalized symptoms of HIV encephalopathy (Worley & Price, 1992).

Fungal Infections

Candidiasis

Candida is a fungus that normally exists in the mouth and esophagus (Finley et al., 1992). With immune suppression, however, candida often progresses to an active disease. Oral infection with candidiasis is commonly called *thrush*, usually forming removable white plaques on the surface of the tongue and oral cavity (Greenspan et al., 1992). Plaques may be small or widespread and can alternatively appear as small red areas rather than white patches. Thrush is found in later stages of HIV disease and was described in the first U.S. cases of AIDS (Greenspan et al., 1992). Localized candida infection is related to declining numbers of T-helper lymphocytes and is often the first indicator of advanced immune suppression (Bartlett, 1993a; Finley et al., 1992; Greenspan et al., 1992; Kaslow, Phair, et al., 1987). Although for an AIDS diagnosis, candidiasis must involve the esophagus, bronchi, trachea, or lungs, infection may also occur in other organ systems, including the gastrointestinal system (Finley et al., 1992) and the female genital tract (Bartlett, 1993a). Vaginal candidiasis is among the earliest signs of immune suppression for women with HIV infection, often occurring when T-helper cell counts are still relatively high (Wofsy, 1992) and causing discomfort and possibly discharge (Kloser & Craig, 1994). Vaginal candidiasis, however, is related to HIV progression toward AIDS in women (Bartlett, 1993a; Carpenter et al., 1991; Imam et al., 1990; Rhoads, Wright, Redfield, & Burke, 1987).

Coccidioidomycosis

An infection that occurs after fungus particles are inhaled into the lungs (Sarosi, 1992), coccidioidomycosis is among the least frequent AIDS-defining conditions (CDC, 1994b). Dysfunctional T-helper lymphocyte mediated immunity allows active and progressive coccidioidomycosis of both the inside and outside lung (Sarosi, 1992). Risk for coccidioidomy-cosis is greatest in areas where the fungus is endemic, including the south-western United States (Sarosi, 1992). Risk increases in direct proportion to declining T-helper lymphocytes, particularly when cell counts drop be-low 250 cells/mm^3. There are two general forms of coccidioidomycosis, primary and chronic. The primary form is an acute self-limiting condi-tion involving only the respiratory system. In contrast, the chronic form of the disease may involve several organ systems (C. L. Thomas, 1977). People with severely impaired immune systems are most likely to develop pulmonary disease followed by widespread dissemination (Finley et al., 1992). For coccidioidomycosis to allow an AIDS diagnosis, the disease must become disseminated to nonpulmonary organs (CDC, 1992h).

Cryptococcoses

Advanced HIV infection increases susceptibility to cryptococcal infections, affecting as many as 6% to 9% of people with AIDS (Masci, Poon, Wormser, & Bottone, 1992). Cryptococcal infection tends to occur with severe immune suppression (Stansell & Sande, 1992). Although the dis-ease may occur in any organ system and often affects the respiratory sys-tem, the most common form of infection is Cryptococcal meningitis (Bartlett, 1993a), presenting with headache, stiff neck, nausea, vomiting, malaise, and possible seizures (Stansell & Sande, 1992). Other common symptoms include hypersensitivity to light and marked changes in men-tal status (Masci et al., 1992; Stansell & Sande, 1992).

Histoplasmosis

Like other fungal infections, histoplasmosis first occurs through inhaling fungus particles, with infection potentially disseminating to other organ systems. Clinical manifestations of infection include fever, skin rashes, anemia, lymphadenopathy, and involvement of vital organs (Finley et al., 1992). Histoplasmosis occurs at varying rates across regions of North America, with the central and south-central United States and Ontario and Quebec Canadian provinces having the most concentrated number of cases (Sarosi, 1992). As many as 27% of AIDS patients in these areas develop histoplasmosis, as compared with other regions, where infection is virtually nonexistent (Finley et al., 1992).

Pneumocystis carinii *pneumonia (PCP)*

Pneumocystis carinii pneumonia is the most frequently occurring AIDS-defining condition in the U.S. epidemic. Prior to the wide-scale use of prophylaxis, active PCP occurred in as many as 80% of advanced HIV disease cases (Bartlett, 1993a). First classified as a protozoan (e.g., Hollerman et al., 1987), most authorities now agree that *Pneumocystis carinii* is a fungus (Hopewell, 1992; Martinez, Suffredini, & Masur, 1992), although this is not conclusive and the taxonomy remains debated. *Pneumocystis carinii* exists in the environment and is believed to be universally contracted at young ages through inhalation of fungus particles (Hopewell, 1992). However, *Pneumocystis carinii* is only clinically expressed under severe immune suppression, particularly when T-helper lymphocyte cell counts fall below 200 cells/mm^3. However, children infected with HIV develop PCP at earlier stages of infection. Thus, because almost everyone is exposed to *Pneumocystis carinii*, and because the fungus is suppressed by cellular immunity mediated by T-helper lymphocytes, it has been the predominant manifestation of AIDS in the United States and the most frequent identifiable cause of AIDS-related death (Bartlett, 1993a; Rothenberg, Woelfel, et al., 1987).

Pneumocystis carinii pneumonia can present with early and diffuse symptoms, including mild tightness of the chest, chronic fever, fatigue, and weight loss. Respiratory symptoms usually include dry/nonproductive cough and progressive shortness of breath (Hopewell, 1992). As the pneumonia progresses, tasks with even limited demands become taxing and exhaustive. *Pneumocystis carinii* can, although rarely, infect the skin, central nervous system, eyes, abdominal walls, lymph nodes, kidneys, liver, and several other organ systems. Thus, although *Pneumocystis carinii* is usually limited to the respiratory system, it can become widely disseminated. Recent declines have been observed in the number of people with AIDS developing PCP because of widespread use of prophylaxis medications (Ong, 1993).

Protozoan Infections

Cryptosporidiosis

Infection with Cryptosporidiosis occurs after spores of the microorganism are either inhaled or ingested (Naficy & Soave, 1992). Cryptosporidia causes chronic diarrhea and is responsible for about 4% of all diarrhea-related illnesses in U.S. AIDS cases (Finley et al., 1992). Infection can involve any area of the gastrointestinal tract, but the usual site is the small intestine. The AIDS case definition requires that symptoms of chronic diarrhea caused by cryptosporidia persist for a minimum of one month (CDC, 1992h). Cryptosporidiosis also causes gallbladder disease in up to 10% of U.S. AIDS cases (Finley et al., 1992). Treatment for this infection is extremely limited, and symptoms, therefore, are chronic, debilitating, and often lethal (Naficy & Soave, 1992). Outbreaks in cities where drinking water and swimming pools have been contaminated by Cryptosporidiosis have resulted in several deaths among people with suppressed immune systems (CDC, 1994a). People with HIV infection are therefore advised to routinely boil their drinking water or use bottled water.

Isosporiasis

Isosporiasis has been reported in less than 1% of U.S. AIDS cases but in more than 15% of people with AIDS in Haiti (Naficy & Soave, 1992). Like cryptosporidiosis, this infection strikes the gastrointestinal tract, causing diarrhea, abdominal cramping, and weight loss (Naficy & Soave, 1992). However, unlike other protozoan infections, effective treatments are available for Isosporiasis (Cello, 1992).

Toxoplasmosis

The intracellular protozoan *Toxoplasma gondii* is the cause of toxoplasmosis, the most common infection of the human central nervous system (Mariuz & Luft, 1992; Wong, Israelski, & Remington, 1995). Exposure to *Toxoplasma gondii* occurs principally through contact with cat feces (Mariuz & Luft, 1992). Immune suppression allows for toxoplasmosis infection because of defective cellular immunity (Israelski & Remington, 1992). Between 20% and 47% of people with AIDS who carry *Toxoplasma gondii* eventually develop toxoplasmosis encephalitis (Israelski & Remington, 1992). Manifestations are often insidious and usually include a mixture of focal and generalized neurological symptoms, including disturbances in thought processes, lethargy, confusion, memory and language deficits, and motor disturbances. Although *Toxoplasma gondii* can infect vital organ systems outside of the central nervous system, a disseminated course of infection is atypical even among HIV-infected persons (Mariuz & Luft, 1992).

Malignancies

Invasive Cervical Cancer

Cervical abnormalities, or cervical dysplasia, are a common precursor to cervical cancer. Several studies have shown that HIV-infected women frequently develop cervical dysplasia, with prevalence rates as high as ten times greater than those found in non-HIV-infected women (CDC, 1992h). The occurrence of cervical dysplasia in women with HIV infection is related to increased immune suppression (CDC, 1992h). Studies of women who receive organ transplants, however, suggest that progression to cervical cancer may require prolonged periods of immune suppression (Kaplan & Northfelt, 1992). Therefore, relatively few cases of invasive cervical cancer have been reported among HIV-infected women (Kaplan & Northfelt, 1992). Because invasive cervical cancer usually occurs late in HIV infection, and because it has been reported in some HIV-infected women, it was added to the 1993 AIDS case definition following controversy about previous exclusion of conditions related to AIDS in women (Buehler & Ward, 1993). Inclusion of invasive cervical cancer as an AIDS-defining condition was also meant to emphasize "the importance of integrating gynecologic care into medical services for HIV infected women" (CDC, 1992h, p. 8). Early detection of cervical cancer is possible with pap smears, which should be a regular part of health care for HIV-positive women.

HIV-Related Lymphomas

Non-Hodgkin's-disease lymphomas were among the earliest recognized manifestations of HIV infection. Unlike other lymphomas, those related to HIV infection tend to progress rapidly and have extremely poor prognoses (Naficy & Soave, 1992). Although most non-HIV-infected lymphomas involve disease contained to the lymph nodes, HIV lymphomas are distinguished by their widespread involvement of vital organs (Kaplan & Northfelt, 1992). Approximately 26% of HIV-related lymphomas involve the gastrointestinal system, 25% bone marrow, 12% liver, 9% kidneys, and 9% lungs (Naficy & Soave, 1992). Most common, however, is central nervous system involvement, occurring in 25% to 32% of HIV-related cases of lymphoma and only rarely in non-HIV lymphomas (Herndier, Kaplan, & McGrath, 1994; Naficy & Soave, 1992). Symptoms of central nervous system lymphoma include seizures, localized neurologic dysfunction, and headache (Naficy & Soave, 1992). HIV-related lymphoma usually occurs late in infection, after other AIDS-related conditions have occurred and when T-helper lymphocyte counts drop below 50 cells/mm^3 (Kaplan & Northfelt, 1992).

Kaposi's Sarcoma

Although rare before the HIV epidemic, Kaposi's sarcoma has been the most common malignancy among people with AIDS, with the majority of cases occurring among men who sexually contracted HIV from other men. Homosexually infected men are 20,000 to 40,000 times more likely to develop Kaposi's sarcoma than same-age HIV-negative men (Mann et al., 1992). Relatively few cases of Kaposi's sarcoma have occurred among injection drug users, and only 2% of cases have an initial diagnosis of Kaposi's sarcoma (Kaplan & Northfelt, 1992; Wofsy, 1992). Kaposi's sarcoma typically develops as a mass on the skin, mucous membranes, or internal organs. The disease is usually first noted by skin lesions that appear as dark red-to-violet-colored areas on light-skinned persons, and black or brown lesions on dark-skinned persons (Bartlett, 1993a). Lesions commonly first occur near the head and neck, as well as on the inside of the mouth (Kaplan & Northfelt, 1992). It is also common for Kaposi's sarcoma to afflict internal organs, with 20% to 50% of cases involving the lungs (A. Levine, Gill, & Salahuddin, 1992). Thus, the lethality of Kaposi's sarcoma is entirely dependant on the site of disease. In most cases, however, Kaposi's sarcoma has an aggressive and unpredictable course (Kaplan & Northfelt, 1992).

The exact etiological agent of Kaposi's sarcoma remains unknown, although, as discussed earlier, there is evidence that a pathogen causing the disease, possibly a virus, is transmitted through contact with human feces (Beral et al., 1992; Chang et al., 1994). When Kaposi's sarcoma develops in the absence of other HIV-related diseases, it usually occurs early in immune suppression. People who have Kaposi's sarcoma are likely to later develop opportunistic infections and other malignancies. There has, however, been a steady decline in the number of Kaposi's sarcoma cases observed in recent years among people with AIDS (M.G. Taylor et al., 1991).

In addition to being an AIDS-defining condition and a life-threatening malignancy, Kaposi's sarcoma carries additional psychological burden because of its skin lesions. Symptoms of Kaposi's sarcoma are disfiguring, and their appearance will frequently mark a person as being seriously ill and can lead to identifying a person as having AIDS. The result of Kaposi's sarcoma's symptoms, therefore, can interfere with rights to privacy and add a stigmatizing dimension to an already stigmatized disease (Kaplan & Northfelt, 1992).

Bacterial Infections

Mycobacterium Diseases

Mycobacterial infections include mycobacterium TB, mycobacterium avium complex, and other disseminated mycobacteria. Following a long period of decline in incidence, mycobacterium TB has reclaimed its place among global health threats (Mann et al., 1992; Raviglione, Snider, & Kochi, 1995) and as a major U.S. epidemic (Pitchenik & Fertel, 1992). It is estimated that between 4% and 40% of people with AIDS in the United States have active TB and that up to 40% of individuals with active TB are HIV infected (Bartlett, 1993a). The scenario is even worse in developing counties, with the number of cases of TB in sub-Saharan Africa doubling in recent years (Mann et al., 1992). In some South African countries, nearly one third of HIV infections present clinically with TB as their first manifestation (Pitchenik & Fertel, 1992). Mycobacterial TB is contracted person-to-person through respiratory routes of transmission, posing a highly alarming chance for spread. Active mycobacterial TB occurs relatively early in HIV infection, usually with T-helper lymphocyte cell counts between 500 and 200 cells/mm^3.

Tuberculosis can become disseminated to a number of organ systems, with less than half of all TB cases in AIDS being confined to the respiratory system (Jacobson, 1992). The course of TB in people with AIDS is typically aggressive, particularly when it remains untreated. Symptoms may include fever, night sweats, fatigue, malaise, and weight loss. When TB is pulmonary, symptoms will usually include persistent cough, production of sputum, and chest pain (Pitchenik & Fertel, 1992). Pulmonary disease occurs in 70% to 90% of HIV-infected individuals with TB (Pitchenik & Fertel, 1992). However, antituberculosis drugs are highly effective when used properly (Jacobson, 1992). Unfortunately, as the TB epidemic has escalated, several multiple-drug-resistant strains of mycobacterium TB have emerged (Bartlett, 1993a). Thus, HIV infection and TB reciprocally complicate each other's disease processes: Persons with HIV are at greater risk of developing TB, standard medical interventions for TB are less effective in HIV-infected persons, and TB may be more infectious in persons with HIV infection (Mann et al., 1992).

In addition to mycobacterium TB, mycobacterium avium complex (MAC) is common in HIV infection (Hawkins et al., 1986). Although discussed as a single disease, MAC consists of two closely related organisms, mycobacterium avium and mycobacterium intracellular, with mycobacterium avium being the more frequently occurring. These mycobacterium are contracted through contaminated soil, food, water, and air-borne water droplets. Although occurring in as many as 40% of AIDS cases in the United States (CDC, 1993d), disseminated MAC infection is virtually nonexistent in non-HIV-infected persons (Pitchenik & Fertel, 1992). Cases of MAC have increased each year of the HIV epidemic (Horsburgh, 1991). Disseminated MAC infection usually occurs late in HIV infection, typically with T-helper lymphocyte counts below 100 cells/mm^3 (Jacobson, 1992). Clinically, MAC presents as diffuse symptoms of infection that include fever, weight loss, malaise, severe anemia, anorexia, and a number of possible gastrointestinal symptoms, including chronic diarrhea, abdominal pain, and malabsorption (CDC, 1993d; Horsburgh, 1991; Jacobson, 1992). Disseminated MAC infection is often lethal among people with AIDS (Jacobson, Hopewell, et al., 1991). Because MAC occurs late in HIV infection, other opportunistic illnesses commonly precede MAC (Pitchenik & Fertel, 1992; Horsburgh, 1991). Unfortunately, there are few effective treatments available for MAC infections (Pitchenik & Fertel, 1992), although there have been many advances in preventive and therapeutic medications (CDC, 1993d).

Recurrent Bacterial Pneumonia

Pneumonia caused by any one of nine different bacteria are frequently seen in people with HIV infection (Chaisson, 1992; Greenberg et al., 1992). Bacterial pneumonia was observed early in the HIV epidemic, and pulmonary infections have contributed substantially to HIV-related deaths (Buehler & Ward, 1993; Carpenter et al., 1991), with as many as 10% of pneumonias in AIDS patients the result of community-acquired bacterial infections (Polsky et al., 1986). The onset of bacterial pneumonia is typically abrupt, and the duration can last several days, making it distinguishable from the insidious onset and persistent symptoms of *Pneumocystis carinii* pneumonia (Chaisson, 1992).

Pneumonia caused by bacteria in HIV-infected persons has a course of disease similar to that found among immune-competent individuals, including persistent fever, productive cough, dyspnea (labored or difficult breathing), and chest pain (Chaisson, 1992; Schrager 1988). However, unlike people with functional immune systems, symptoms of pneumonia in HIV infection persist for long periods of time. Recurrent bacterial pneumonia is now an AIDS-defining condition.

Non-Pneumonia-Causing Bacterial Infections

Compromised immune systems increase susceptibility to a wide range of bacterial infections. The most common infections associated with HIV involve the gastrointestinal system, skin, meninges, and sinuses (Chaisson, 1992). Bacterial infections tend to occur early in immune suppression, reflecting the aggressive disease-causing capabilities of bacteria in even relatively healthy people (Bartlett, 1993a).

Recurrent salmonella infection occurs frequently and early in HIV infection and is an AIDS-defining condition (Simberkoff & Leaf, 1992). More than 50% of cases of salmonella infection cause severe diarrhea (Scrager, 1988), and nearly half involve febrile illness: high fevers that may result in seizures (Chaisson, 1992). Salmonella infection in HIV infection is most likely to recur because of incomplete elimination of the disease during what would usually be adequate treatment (Chaisson, 1992; Schrager, 1988). The bacteria are also likely to become resistant to treatments following recurrent use (Chaisson, 1992).

Sinusitis is another common bacterial infection that is persistent when it occurs among HIV-infected persons. Caused by as many as four different bacteria, symptoms of sinusitis include fever, headache, and upper respiratory distress (Schrager, 1988). Symptoms are most chronic among people with T-helper lymphocyte counts below 200 cells/mm^3 (Chaisson, 1992). Additional bacterial infections common to HIV infection include oral infections such as gingivitis and periodontitis, both of which can be progressive and painful (Schrager, 1988).

Other frequent bacterial infections are sexually transmitted diseases (Bartlett, 1993a). Pelvic inflammatory disease resulting from gonorrheal infection becomes persistent and aggressive in HIV-infected women (Minkoff & DeHovitz, 1991). Syphilis also takes an aggressive course in HIV infection and includes an increased risk of neurosyphilis (Minkoff & DeHovitz, 1991; Schrager, 1988). HIV infection further complicates syphilis by speeding up its course and reducing the effectiveness of antibiotic treatments (Bolan, 1992). Thus, similar to other bacterial infections, co-infection of HIV and sexually transmitted bacteria poses specific problems not encountered when bacterial infections occur in people with functional immune systems.

Other Conditions Not Yet Included in the AIDS Case Definition

Virtually any infection or malignancy that is normally suppressed by immune responses can become a complication of HIV infection. For example, although only three cancers are included as AIDS case-defining conditions (non-Hodgkin's lymphoma, Kaposi's sarcoma, and invasive cervical cancer), HIV infection is associated with Hodgkin's disease, melanoma, and cancers of the colon, lung, and testes (Kaplan & Northfelt, 1992; Mann et al., 1992). Numerous viral, protozoan, fungal, and bacterial infections that are usually managed by immune responses frequently cause serious illness. For example, varicella-zoster virus causes chicken pox in childhood and usually remains inactive throughout adulthood. When reactivated in adulthood, varicella-zoster virus is the cause of shingles, painful skin eruptions in association with nerve endings. However, shingles are common to early and late HIV infection and usually take a severe and aggressive course (Cockerell, 1992).

In summary, manifestations of HIV infection result from interactions among several defects in the protective immune system resulting from interference with and destruction of T-helper lymphocytes (Bollinger & Siliciano, 1992). Thus, as HIV infection progresses, disease-causing agents that are usually either completely suppressed or easily managed by immunity become potentially life threatening. Serious immune suppression is also likely to result in simultaneous infections and malignancies that require multiple medical interventions. For these reasons, medical treatments that slow the loss of T-helper lymphocytes, prevent malignancies, or protect against opportunistic infections have been the principal means of combating HIV infection.

BIOMEDICAL INTERVENTIONS

People with HIV infection live longer today than at any other time in the history of the HIV epidemic and can expect to live even longer in the future. Advances in the medical management of HIV disease are constantly emerging. Treatments for HIV infection and its associated complications generally fall into three categories: interventions directed at impeding the progress of HIV, prevention and treatment of opportunistic illnesses, and complementary treatments.

Antiretroviral Therapies

For most viral infections, immune system responses are intact and antiviral medications synergize with the body's immune system to effectively suppress infection. However, because HIV selectively eliminates the branch of the immune system that recognizes antigens and coordinates immune responses, antiretroviral treatments act entirely on their own to suppress HIV (Fauci, 1986). HIV's cycle provides points of potential attack on HIV (McCutchan, 1990). For example, *tat*, one of HIV's regulatory genes, is essential for the synthesis of proteins used for HIV production. A drug that inhibits the activity of the *tat* gene disrupts the HIV replication cycle and stops production of HIV in chronically infected as well as newly infected cells. Several *tat* inhibitors have demonstrated some effectiveness in clinical trials and show promise as a future treatment (James, 1994). Drugs that inhibit reverse transcriptase, the enzyme necessary for HIV activation, interfere with the transcription phases of virus production (Fauci, 1986). Reverse transcriptase inhibitors have been the most widely developed and studied antiretroviral medications (S. A. Myers et al., 1993).

Reverse transcriptase is necessary for the replication of HIV and is not found in non-HIV-infected cells (McCutchan, 1990). Thus, inhibiting reverse transcriptase does not interfere with normal cell functioning. Viral replication is interrupted by the drug when RNA is transcribed to DNA. A nucleic acid from the antiretroviral drug is incorporated into the RNA–DNA transcription process, causing a termination in the chain of nucleic acids. Reverse transcriptase inhibitors, however, only suppress HIV replication in newly infected cells. Once HIV is established in a cell, the effects of reverse transcriptase inhibitors become limited.

The first approved and most widely used reverse transcriptase inhibitor is zidovudine (AZT), a drug first developed in the 1960s to treat murine retroviruses (Schooley, 1992). Numerous studies have shown that zidovudine is effective in slowing HIV progression for most people treated. Effects of zidovudine treatment include increased numbers of T-helper lymphocytes (Fischl, Richman et al., 1987), decreased HIV activity, reduced frequency and severity of opportunistic illnesses, and improved general health status (Bartlett, 1993a; Fischl, 1992). There is also evidence that AIDS is delayed by zidovudine (Fischl, Richman, et al., 1987; Schecter et al., 1990). Zidovudine appears to extend survival for some people with AIDS (Creagh et al., 1988; Volberding et al., 1994). For example, Lemp et al. (1990) found that patients receiving zidovudine had increased survival times across subgroups of people infected through various modes of HIV transmission. In addition, Moore, Hidalgo, Sugland, and Chaisson (1991) showed that survival with AIDS has increased substantially since 1987, and zidovudine therapy was attributed with much of the improvement. People with AIDS treated with zidovudine demonstrate greater longevity than those who, for what ever reason, did not receive treatment. Zidovudine has its greatest effects when started within 1 year of receiving an AIDS diagnosis (Cooper, 1994; Lundgren et al., 1994).

Zidovudine is typically initiated when T-helper lymphocyte counts fall between 200 and 500 cells/mm^3 (Saag, 1992; Sande, Carpenter, Cobbs, Holmes, & Sanford, 1993; Schooley, 1992). Early use of zidovudine, before the onset of overt immune suppression or opportunistic illnesses, has been recommended but controversial. Some patients treated before the onset of AIDS survive longer after an AIDS diagnosis when compared with people not treated early in the course of infection (Graham et al., 1992). Antiretroviral therapy is tolerated best when a person is generally healthy, because zidovudine is highly toxic for people with advanced immune suppression (Clement & Hollander, 1992). However, results from clinical trials show that the maximum benefits of zidovudine are time limited, and there is disagreement about exactly when treatment should be initiated (Bartlett, 1993b; Hirsch & D'Aquila, 1993; Volberding et al., 1994). It is generally recommended that antiretrovirals be started when T-helper counts drop below 200 cells/mm^3.

There are a number of limitations associated with zidovudine therapy. Zidovudine may slow down the replication of HIV, but it will not prevent persistent infection (Tindall et al., 1992). People treated with zidovudine, particularly at high doses, are vulnerable to early side effects that result from its toxicity, including headache, insomnia, nausea, vomiting, abdominal pain, diarrhea, fatigue, rashes, muscle pain, and fever (Fischl, 1992). However, most side effects resolve within 8 weeks (Bartlett, 1993a). The most threatening adverse effect of zidovudine is bone marrow suppression, causing anemia and other potentially serious conditions (Bartlett, 1993a). Bone marrow suppression therefore leads to immediate discontinuation of zidovudine treatment.

Prolonged use of zidovudine, particularly when started early in HIV infection, can result in long-term, often irreversible side-effects (Clement & Hollander, 1992). Zidovudine toxicity is directly related to dose, and adjustments often relieve adverse symptoms. Also related to toxicity are the possible teratogenic effects on pregnancy, although they have not yet been fully determined (Bartlett, 1993a; CDC, 1994f). Expectations of potential adverse effects of zidovudine are among the most common reasons for refusing treatment.

Three additional reverse-transcriptase-inhibiting drugs have been developed and tested: Dideoxycytidine (ddC), Dideoxyinosine (ddI), and 3'-Deoxythmidine-2'-ene (d4T). Each functions similarly to zidovudine by inhibiting the action of reverse transcriptase and therefore interfering with HIV replication. The antiretroviral actions of ddC are increased when taken in combination with zidovudine (Bartlett, 1993a; Schooley, 1992). Unfortunately, ddC also has toxic side effects, including peripheral neuropathy (numbness, tingling, or pain in the hands and feet), oral ulcerations, and skin rashes. Similarly, ddI presents problems with peripheral neuropathy, diarrhea, and pancreatitis (Bartlett, 1993a; Schooley, 1992). Although d4T has not been as fully tested, it has shown promise as an antiretroviral treatment, although it too has potential adverse effects (James, 1994). Other antiretroviral treatments are under development and may effectively inhibit reverse transcription with lower levels of toxicity (Schooley, 1992). For example, phosphonosformate (foscarnet) is an effective antiviral drug used to treat herpes viruses, particularly cytomegalovirus, that also has antiretroviral properties (Schooley, 1992). Foscarnet exerts an inhibitory effect against viral enzymes that are important in HIV replication, without interfering with normal cell enzymes. Foscarnet, however, requires intravenous administration and can have many toxic effects (S. A. Myers et al., 1993).

Advances in antiretroviral medications have been most promising in the area of combination therapies. Concurrent use of two or more treatments, or convergent combination therapy, may increase effectiveness and prohibit HIV resistance to these medications (Chow et al., 1993; S. A. Myers et al., 1993; Schooley, 1992). For example, synergistic reverse transcriptase inhibitory effects of zidovudine and ddI have been well established (Bartlett, 1993a; Fischl, 1992; Schooley, 1992). Zidovudine in combination with ddC has also shown promise in slowing HIV infection (Schooley, 1992), and 3TC (lamivudine), another antiretroviral, has also shown promise when combined with zidovudine (Mascolini, 1994). Certain antiretroviral drugs used in combination with other treatments have also been effective. For example, zidovudine in combination with prophylactic treatments against *Pneumocystis carinii* pneumonia increase survival times for people with AIDS (Friedman et al., 1991). Combination therapies have potential for future developments in treating AIDS because new drugs are constantly appearing in clinical trials and because when given in the right combination, they may create an effect greater than any single drug.

Treatments targeted to other points of the HIV replication cycle have, unfortunately, been less successful at slowing down HIV infection. One avenue has been to interfere with HIV's binding with CD_4 receptor molecules (S. A. Myers et al., 1993). Receptor-based therapy is geared toward blocking HIV from attaching to the surface of and entering T-helper lymphocytes. Because HIV has such a strong affinity for CD_4 surface molecules, infusion of soluble CD_4 molecules into the bloodstream of infected persons could allow HIV to bind directly with free CD_4 molecules, preventing the virus from subsequently binding with T-helper lymphocyte cells

(McCutchan, 1990). Unfortunately, HIV is substantially less sensitive to recombinant, or free, CD_4 than to CD_4 surface receptors (Schooley, 1992).

Other treatments include drugs that inhibit proteins necessary for the production of regulatory genes specific to HIV and drugs that inhibit cellular enzymes important in HIV production (Schooley, 1992). For example, a new group of drugs that inhibit protease, an enzyme that is essential for HIV replication, has shown efficacy in clinical trials. These drugs bind with the protease enzyme, interfering with its usual functions. It appears that protease inhibitors can effectively slow HIV progression with few toxic side effects, and may synergize with zidovudine, ddI, ddC, or d4T (James, 1994; Loftus & Gold, 1995). Promising HIV treatments like protease inhibitors have accelerated government approval procedures for life-threatening illnesses and reach the stage of clinical trials much more rapidly than almost any other treatment in medical history. At any given time, there are hundreds of investigational drug trials for HIV infection and AIDS (Bartlett, 1993a). Information about clinical trials is available from several AIDS-related service organizations, some of which are listed in Appendix B. Still, the success of treatments for HIV infection has thus far been limited.

Prophylaxis and Treatments for Opportunistic Illnesses

Most manifestations of HIV infection involve opportunistic infections and malignancies that are usually protected against by T-helper lymphocyte-mediated immunity. Prevention of opportunistic illnesses results in sustained illness-free periods for people with HIV infection. Because many opportunistic illnesses were rare before the HIV epidemic, there has been a rush to establish prophylactic and treatment guidelines (Bagdades, 1991; Sweeney, Peters, & Main, 1991). For example, guidelines for prophylaxis against *Pneumocystis carinii* pneumonia (PCP) include actions to prevent an initial episode of pneumonia, primary prophylaxis, where individuals with T-helper lymphocyte cell counts below 200 cells/mm^3 routinely begin treatment with anti-PCP drugs (CDC, 1992k). Dapsone, bactrim, and aerosolized pentamidine are effective in preventing primary and secondary episodes of PCP (Bartlett, 1993a; Ong, 1993). Prophylaxis is credited with reductions of PCP ranging from 62% in 1988 to 46% in 1990 (CDC, 1992q). Prophylactic treatments against PCP have also extended the longevity of HIV-infected individuals (Friedman et al., 1991; Hoover et al., 1993; Osmond, Charlebois, Lang, Shiboski, & Moss, 1994; Rothenberg et al., 1987).

Prophylaxis has also been established for toxoplasmosis encephalitis and mycobacterial infections. Antiviral drugs are widely used to control recurrent symptoms of herpes viruses and members of other virus families (Bartlett, 1993a). Interferons have been effective in treating Kaposi's sarcoma (Lane, 1994). Additional advantages are offered by some prophylactic agents because they frequently guard against multiple opportunistic illness. For example, TMP-SMX, used as a PCP preventive, also helps protect against other diseases, including toxoplasmosis (Bartlett, 1993a). Standards of care are also in place for preventing HIV-related malignancies (Kaplan & Northfelt, 1992).

In addition to prevention, treatments are available to manage several opportunistic illnesses. Most treatments effective in dealing with diseases in the context of a functional immune system do so in conjunction with cell-mediated immunity. Unfortunately, as the immune system deteriorates the effectiveness of opportunistic-illness interventions requires greater doses and more time to achieve equal effectiveness. This is problematic in and of itself because many treatments have adverse side effects with prolonged use, particularly in immune-compromised individuals. Another limitation is the potential for resistance to treatments over time, as has been the case with some strains of HIV and several bacteria.

It is important to note that advances in the treatment of HIV-related diseases develop rapidly. New treatments are the product of converging areas of medicine including, but not limited to, infectious diseases, immunology, oncology, hematology, neurology, and pharmacology. For example, oncology has shown that bone marrow transplantation has promise in treating non-Hodgkin's lymphomas in AIDS patients (H. K. Holland et al., 1989). Similarly, clinical immunology has experimented with transplanting thymus gland tissue in AIDS patients, also suggesting limited results that warranted further testing (Dwyer, Wood, McNamara, & Kinder, 1987). As treatment approaches from different disciplines emerge, they will likely be combined into promising new therapeutic avenues.

Complementary Treatments

Treatments for HIV infection and related illnesses that have not yet gone through rigorous approval processes are often sought by HIV-infected people. Searching for unconventional treatments when faced with a chronic, life-threatening disease is often an outgrowth of disillusionments and frustrations with traditional medicine (Abrams, 1992). Although initially considered alternatives to standard medical care, unapproved treatments are now referred to as *complementary* therapies because they are not necessarily replacements as much as they are adjuncts to mainstream treatments.

Complementary therapies have become part of a social activist movement within communities heavily affected by AIDS. People who seek out complementary treatments are likely to reestablish a sense of personal control over their health and therefore increase their attempts to deal with illnesses. Underground organizations have established routes for disseminating information and complementary therapies, including "buyers' clubs" that serve as distribution centers for otherwise unavailable treatments (Abrams, 1992). Several newsletters inform people of the progress and development of traditional and complementary treatments (see Appendix B). The demand and accessibility of complementary therapies has increased to where many primary care physicians routinely discuss these options with their patients (Abrams, 1992). For example, a study of mostly homosexually HIV-infected men receiving treatment from an AIDS clinic in San Francisco found that 40% had received a prescription medication from someone other than their primary care provider and that 11% received treatment from an unorthodox provider (Greenblatt, Hollander, McMaster, & Henke, 1991).

Complementary therapies intervene at different points along the HIV replication cycle. Among those that are more commonly used are megadoses of vitamin C, which have been shown to have antiretroviral activity against human retroviruses in laboratory studies (Abrams, 1992). Also used is AL-721, a mixture of lipids believed to alter the membrane of T-helper lymphocytes and viral protective envelope proteins, in an effort to disrupt virus-to-cell binding properties (Greenblatt et al., 1991). Other presumed antiretroviral agents include Compound Q (a purified root of a Chinese cucumber), hypericin (an herbal tea), and several preparations related to proteins necessary for HIV biosynthesis (Abrams, 1992). In addition to antiretrovirals, several complementary therapies may act as modulators of the immune system (e.g., naltrexone and disulfiram). Most of these agents showed early promise but have not stood up to rigorous scientific testing. Other treatment modalities have been suggested, such as chiropractic methods, acupuncture, herbal remedies, multiple vitamins, and mental imagery. These treatments are acceptable to traditionalists only to the extent that they do not interfere with standard medical care (Abrams, 1992).

Although complementary treatments can involve holistic and naturalistic approaches, there are invasive procedures that have not yet demonstrated effectiveness but are nonetheless undertaken by many HIV-infected patients. Two examples are passive hyperimmune therapy and ozone treatments. In passive hyperimmune therapy, or passive immunotherapy, HIV-positive people who are unusually healthy are sought to donate blood plasma, which is pooled for antibodies against multiple strains of HIV and treated to clear disease-causing microbes. The treated plasma is transfused into an HIV-infected recipient, usually with advanced HIV disease or AIDS. The idea behind the treatment is that antibodies from healthy patients may suppress HIV. The process is similar to that used in intravenous immunoglobulin treatment, which is a general approach to building immunities in immune-suppressed patients. Passive hyperimmune therapy for HIV infection differs because it attempts to concentrate antibodies against HIV (Jackson et al., 1988). Passive immunotherapy is highly controversial for treating HIV–AIDS, and rigorous clinical testing has been limited.

Ozone therapy is another unorthodox technique for treating HIV infection that involves removing the blood of an HIV-infected person over a series of transfusions, treating it with heat and exposing it to ultraviolet light, ozone, or both. The entire process is intended to inactivate HIV. The treated blood is then replaced into the original patient. Unfortunately, there is little support for ozone therapies and some evidence against their effectiveness (Garber, Cameron, Hawley-Foss, Greenway, & Shannon, 1991).

There are several potential risks associated with complementary therapies. First, many complementary approaches have serious adverse effects, such as AL-721, which can cause abdominal pain, nausea, and increased cholesterol (Abrams, 1992). Second, it is likely that many of these agents result in immune stimulation or immune suppression, either of which can interact in unpredictable and dangerous ways with HIV infection and traditional medications. Finally, the use of complementary therapies may prohibit individuals from participating in standard medical care and AIDS clinical trials (Abrams, 1992). People with HIV infection who are considering complementary treatments should be advised by a physician about their use.

CONCLUSION

The costs of AIDS in terms of lives and human resources are immeasurable. The majority of people with AIDS are in the most productive years of their lives. Potential years of life lost because of AIDS is disproportionate among subgroups, particularly ethnic minorities. As early as 1987, AIDS deaths in New York and New Jersey among African American women were comparable to rates reported for women in South Africa (Chu, Buehler, & Berkelman, 1990). HIV infection has widened the mortality gap observed among ethnic groups in the United States, further decreasing the life expectancies for ethnic minorities (CDC, 1992g).

HIV infection also directly strains the infrastructure of cities because of health care costs, demands on social services, lost work force, and so forth. From AIDS diagnosis to death, the cost of care falls between $62,000 and $73,000, and the estimated lifetime cost of HIV infection to death is $119,000 per person (Hellinger, 1993). On the basis of length of hospital stays, outpatient treatments, and commonly used medications, the cumulative cost of treating all people in the United States diagnosed with AIDS was expected to reach $7.8 billion in 1993 (Hellinger, 1990). Broadened criteria for an AIDS diagnosis place an even greater burden on service delivery systems. For example, in San Francisco the cost of care for HIV infection increased $5.8 million per year because of the new AIDS case definition (Chang et al., 1992). Thus, inner cities hit hardest by AIDS are even further depleted of their health and social service resources (Ozawa, Auslander, & Slonim-Nevo, 1993).

Individually, the cost of care for HIV infection is catastrophic. Using 15 months as a typical survival time following an AIDS diagnosis, the lifetime cost of the drug zidovudine is over $2,200. Aerosol pentamidine, a prophylactic against *Pneumocystis carinii* pneumonia, costs over $2,000 per year (Hellinger, 1990). Thus, the cost of medical care for an AIDS patient is estimated as high as $147,000 (Ozawa et al., 1993). Although some people with HIV infection have private health insurance, the majority rely on public assistance. People with HIV infection will increasingly need public funds as insurance companies require HIV testing prior to accepting new

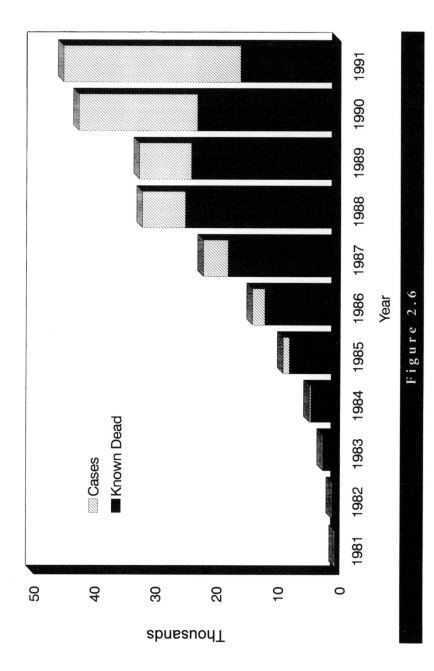

Figure 2.6

U.S. AIDS cases and deaths due to AIDS, 1981 to 1991.

policies. As the number of HIV infections increases, and as people with HIV continue to live longer, there will be increasingly more HIV-positive patients in need of care. These two patterns, more people becoming HIV infected and infected individuals living longer, promise to continue over the next several years. As shown in Figure 2.6, new cases of AIDS have increased each year of the U.S. epidemic, whereas the number of deaths because of AIDS has decreased.

There is great potential for people with AIDS to become burdened by treatment needs. Growing numbers of people with HIV infection live in poverty. Inner-city minorities are less likely to receive early interventions than are their nonminority counterparts (Piette, Mor, Mayer, Zierler, & Wachtel, 1993) and have less access to standard medical treatments for HIV, such as zidovudine and prophylaxis against *Pneumocystis carinii* pneumonia (Piette et al., 1993). Furthermore, minorities and women have historically lacked access to AIDS clinical trials, and expansions of medical treatment options available to infected people will continue to be accompanied by cost escalations.

3

Illness-Related and Environmental Stressors

The context of the HIV epidemic plays a direct role in the psychological adjustment of people who test HIV positive. Physical deterioration and uncertainties about the future make the psychological adjustment to HIV infection similar to reactions to other chronic illnesses such as cancer and heart disease. HIV infection does, however, have aspects that do not overlap with other life-threatening diseases. For example, HIV infection is the result of an identified virus that is contracted by socially stigmatized behaviors. Unlike other illnesses, groups in the United States most affected by AIDS have thus far been sexual and ethnic minorities, the socially disadvantaged, and people living near or in poverty. In addition, AIDS is a chronic disease of the young, causing physical decline and social losses that are usually not encountered until older ages. Thus, HIV-infection-related stressors come from three primary sources: the physically debilitating effects of the disease, social losses and limitations, and preexisting problems in groups most affected by AIDS (Forstein, 1984). Figure 3.1 illustrates that HIV risk and disease occur in a context of losses that are due to AIDS as well as mental health issues that exist prior to HIV infection. Yet an even broader context is set by the social problems that coexist with AIDS.

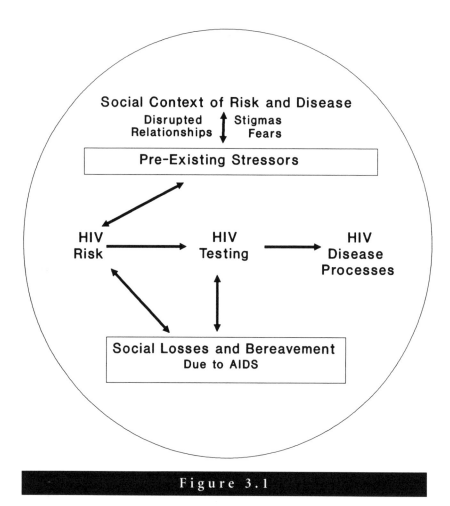

Figure 3.1

Conceptual framework of stressors related to HIV and AIDS.

This chapter overviews the stressors associated with HIV infection and AIDS. Here *stressors* refer to environmental events, situations, and circumstances that commonly result in psychological distress. Although my focus is on distress-producing situations, these events are confounded by an individual's stressful reactions (S. Cohen & Williamson, 1991), the subject of a later section. Adverse events are linked to negative emotions, perceptions, and interpretations. Consequently, psychological adjustment to HIV infection consists of complex interactions among events, interpretations, reactions, and coping resources. The focus of this chapter is on three aspects of stress: HIV-related stressors, social pressures, and potential adverse effects of stress on health.

HIV-RELATED STRESSORS

Psychosocial stressors associated with HIV infection can include a history of engaging in stigmatized behavior, long periods of asymptomatic illness, and loss of physical functioning at a young age. HIV-related stressors change over HIV infection and include HIV risk, HIV antibody testing, receiving positive antibody test results, asymptomatic HIV infection, early symptoms of illness, and developing AIDS. Each of these areas will be discussed in detail.

Risk Perceptions and Related Stressors

People living in areas with high rates of AIDS experience epidemic-related stressors. Personal perceptions of risk and vulnerability are influenced by the likelihood of knowing someone with AIDS, mass media messages, and the ongoing spread of HIV. People who engage in risk behaviors in cities with high rates of AIDS can excessively worry and even become preoccupied with physical sensations perceived as symptoms. When healthy people become concerned over risk for HIV infection on the basis of their previous sexual and drug use behaviors, they can be characterized as the "worried well" (Faulstich, 1987). At its most serious level, worry persists despite repeated negative HIV antibody tests and other medical evaluations (Catalan, 1988; Cochran & Mays, 1988; D. Miller & Riccio, 1990). The stress can become severe enough to cause persistent panic symptoms (Soni & Windgassen, 1991; E. V. Valdiserri, 1986).

Past experiences unrelated to actual risk can lead to irrational or even phobic responses. AIDS phobia occurs most frequently among people who lack accurate information about HIV transmission and overestimate their personal risk. For example, learning that one's employee is HIV positive, getting a tattoo, or discovering that a friend has AIDS can cause unnecessary worry about having contracted HIV infection. Overestimating personal risk for low-probability threats is a well-known phenomenon in the risk perception literature (Slovic, Fischhoff, & Lichtenstein, 1982). Increased vividness of low-probability events makes them more imaginable and salient and therefore increases their perceived threat (Slovic et al.,

1982). For this reason, rare circumstances of HIV transmission that are widely publicized, such as contracting HIV from a dentist, are often perceived as high risk.

Misinformation that was prevalent early in the HIV epidemic persists in the public's AIDS knowledge base. Media coverage and popular books based on inaccurate information have reinforced the perception that HIV is a gay disease and that HIV can be contracted through casual contacts. Dispelling myths over the course of the epidemic has taken place slowly, but some segments of the U.S. population remain unaware of basic facts about HIV and AIDS (e.g., CDC 1991c; Kappel, Vogt, Brozicevic, & Kutzko, 1989; LeBlanc, 1993).

People with established risk behavior histories do not necessarily perceive themselves at risk for HIV infection and therefore do not experience their behavior as a stressor. The relationship among past behavior, risk perceptions, and sense of personal threat interacts with certain life circumstances. Personal risk perceptions are also based on identification with a known risk group as well as having engaged in risk behaviors. For example, a survey in Chicago showed that women of color at high behavioral risk for HIV infection expressed relatively little concern over personal risk for HIV infection (Kalichman et al., 1992). That ethnic minority women at high behavioral risk are not overly concerned about AIDS and misperceive personal risk is particularly alarming because of the disproportionately high rates of AIDS among women of color. Thus, perceived threat of HIV infection is not a simple function of risk awareness but, rather, the product of complex interactions among perceptions and factors associated with the social context of AIDS.

A particularly important social dimension known to affect risk perceptions is having personally known an HIV-positive person (Gerbert, Sumser, & Maguire, 1991). Identification with a person who has HIV infection brings close to home the possibility of risk. In fact, identification with an HIV-infected person increases perceptions of personal risk and vulnerability. This was illustrated by the disclosure of HIV infection by basketball star Earvin "Magic" Johnson, which had an immediate and substantial impact on HIV risk perceptions among several populations, but particularly among African American men (Kalichman, 1994). The effects of Magic Johnson's announcement on risk perceptions were, however, relatively short-lived, with changes in perceptions running parallel to the amount of mass media coverage of the event (Kalichman, 1994). Importantly, there were virtually no effects of the announcement among men who previously knew a person with HIV infection. That African American men were more affected by the announcement than were White men suggests that identification with the infected person plays a key role in influencing personal risk perceptions. For some people who did not already have a close experience with AIDS, Magic Johnson seemed to form a personal connection to the epidemic.

Risk-related stressors influence continued risk behaviors. People living under stressful conditions engage in an array of poor health practices that ultimately result in increased risk for disease (S. Cohen & Williamson, 1991). Of particular relevance to AIDS is how stressful situations may increase rates of sexual behavior and drug use (S. Cohen & Williamson, 1991). Perceived threat of social stressors, including crime, drug abuse, and discrimination, is associated with increased frequencies of HIV risk behaviors among men and women (Kalichman, Adair, Somlai, & Weir, in press). J. Joseph et al. (1987) found that homosexual and bisexual men with greater self-perceived risk for infection reported fewer reductions in high-risk sexual practices. Similarly, McKusick, Horstman, and Coates (1985) found that gay men reported unsafe sexual practices with multiple partners as a means of reducing tension. Thus, high-risk sexual practices can serve as coping responses in a similar manner as does smoking, alcohol and drug use, and overeating (Folkman, Chesney, Pollack, & Phillips, 1992). Substance use to alleviate stress can also influence high-risk sexual practices (Ostrow, 1990). However, unlike other health-related behaviors, sexual relations are uniquely tied to self-worth, self-esteem, love, affection, and intimacy.

Personal efforts to reduce risk for HIV infection can become stressful in and of themselves. Pressure to initiate and maintain safer sexual and drug-use behaviors, and doubts that such efforts are effective, can become stressful (Tross & Hirsch, 1988). D. Martin (1993) found that perceptions of threat, to oneself or to others, increase efforts among gay men to reduce their risk. Similarly, uncertainty about having contracted HIV motivates some people to seek HIV antibody testing (CDC, 1992c; Perry, Jacobsberg, Fishman, Frances, et al., 1990; Siegel, Levine, Brooks, & Kern, 1989). People who believe they are not HIV infected before seeking testing, and who in fact do test negative, experience substantial relief after receiving test results (Perry, Jacobsberg, Fishman, Weiler et al., 1990; Siegel et al., 1989). People who do not seek testing until they have symptoms of infection, which may constitute as many as 40% of individuals who test HIV antibody positive (McCann & Wadsworth, 1991), also experience a sense of relief following the knowledge of their positive HIV status. As is the case for other life-threatening diseases (Mastromauro, Myers, & Berkman, 1987), seeking presymptomatic testing will, if nothing else, end the stress caused by uncertainties. Although some concerns about being HIV positive are relieved by obtaining an HIV antibody test, the experience of testing itself can be a stressor.

HIV Antibody Testing

More than two million U.S. HIV antibody tests were performed in 1991 (CDC, 1993a), and the number of tests continues to increase each year (CDC, 1992j). Testing for HIV antibodies involves the possibility of learning that one has a chronic, incurable, life-threatening illness. Huggins, Elman, Baker, Forrester, and Lyter (1991) pointed out the importance of a self-assessment of personal risk for HIV infection as a part of HIV-testing decisions. Self-assessments of HIV risk, however, are meaningless unless conducted with accurate knowledge about HIV transmission. For example, a man with numerous heterosexual partners may wrongly believe he is not at risk for infection if he has never had a homosexual experience, and a person may incorrectly believe he or she is at risk of infection from an HIV-positive dentist. After an informed and complete risk assessment, a person should identify their coping resources, social supports, and relative coping strengths and weaknesses and develop a coping plan should their HIV antibody test result be positive (Huggins et al., 1991). Seeking HIV testing should also be an informed decision as to the different testing options available, namely private or public and confidential or anonymous.

HIV testing is offered by private physicians and medical clinics, public health clinics, and community-based organizations. Testing by private providers and many public testing programs is usually confidential. Confidential testing, however, is very different from anonymous HIV testing. In confidential testing, identifying information is obtained and kept as part of a medical record, whereas in anonymous testing, names and other identifying information are not recorded and test results are obtained through a randomly assigned numbering system. Laws regulating HIV testing vary among states. Some states require people who test HIV positive be reported to health officials, whereas others do not require reporting and still others have anonymous testing.

Receiving a positive HIV test result can lead to adverse social consequences, so anonymous testing offers a number of advantages. Concerns that HIV testing is not truly anonymous are a common reason for individuals at risk to avoid testing (T. Myers, Orr, Locker, & Jackson, 1993). Despite the important distinction between confidential and anonymous testing, one study found that more than half of patients of a public sexually transmitted disease clinic did not know the difference between testing options (Kalichman, Adair, et al., in press).

There are several reasons that people who perceive themselves to be at high risk for HIV infection seek testing, and there are as many reasons why testing is avoided. Siegel et al. (1989) interviewed 120 gay men and found that HIV testing was believed to provide access to medical treatments effective in combating HIV infection. Siegel et al. also found that men believed testing would motivate them to make positive health and life-style changes, such as reducing substance use and increasing health consciousness. Similarly, many of the men in this study reported that testing for HIV would allow them to make more informed decisions regarding sexual relationships. Some men were motivated to get tested in order to diagnose the origin of an ambiguous health condition that they feared could be related to HIV infection. Finally, Siegel et al. found that a substantial number of gay men got tested to relieve the psychological tension caused by not knowing their HIV antibody status. These results, however, may not generalize to women, and similar studies with women have not been conducted.

Heterosexual men and women surveyed at a sexually transmitted disease clinic and gay and bisexual men surveyed in Canada appeared to engage in a cost–benefit analysis in their HIV-test decision making (Kalichman, Adair, et al., in press; Myers, Orr, et al., 1993). Potential for health care and relief of tension were among the most important benefits associated with HIV testing, and fear of not being able to cope with a positive test result was among the most salient costs.

Because of the potential benefits of testing and the emphasis on social responsibility, HIV antibody testing has become the norm in many areas with high rates of AIDS. Most high-HIV areas have accepted that testing is the healthy, ethical, and informed course of action. People who do not feel psychologically prepared to get tested, or for whatever other reason do not seek testing, may therefore be pressured to get tested. Such expectations may result in strained relationships, misunderstandings with medical professionals, psychologically premature decisions to get tested, and pressure to lie about having been tested.

The potential benefits of HIV testing, although accepted by many, can be offset by perceived costs. Even with anonymous testing, unwanted disclosure of HIV test results is a pervasive concern among individuals who have been at risk for HIV infection (Cassens, 1985). Studies have shown that a sizable number of people at risk for HIV infection have not been tested, including nearly one third of gay men surveyed in national studies (Kelly et al., 1992; National Task Force on AIDS Prevention, 1990) and a majority of people with diverse risk histories (Hardy & Dawson, 1990; Kalichman & Hunter, 1993). A study conducted in Los Angeles county found that 37% of individuals at risk for HIV infection either had not been tested or did not return for their test results (CDC, 1993e). Similarly, a national survey found that 40% of homosexually active men, 54% of injection drug users, and 67% of heterosexuals at risk for HIV infection had not been tested (Berrios et al., 1993). Perceptions of personal risk, fears of not being able to cope with infection, and concerns about being socially sanctioned for testing HIV positive all exert chilling effects on testing decisions.

HIV testing shares several features in common with medical screening for other life-threatening illness. For example, Huntington's disease, an inherited neurodegenerative illness that becomes symptomatic during adulthood, is inherited and therefore poses risks for people with a family history (Mastromauro et al., 1987). Like HIV infection, Huntington's disease occurs in early and middle adulthood. Also like HIV infection, there is no cure for Huntington's disease, but there is a test that detects its presence with 95% accuracy (S. Kessler, 1987). Because of the stress of testing positive for the gene that causes Huntington's disease, nearly one third of people at risk refuse to get screened (S. Kessler, 1987; S. Kessler, Field, Worth, & Mosbarger, 1987; Mastromauro et al., 1987). Similarly, one third of women afforded the opportunity to receive free breast cancer screening decline (Fink, Shapiro, & Lewison, 1968). It is also common for people with cancer symptoms to delay seeking medical evaluation and testing (S. Fisher, 1967). Although the exact mechanisms involved may vary, avoidance of screening and early diagnostic testing for life-threatening diseases is not unique to HIV infection.

For people who perceive themselves at risk for HIV infection, there are many fears that inhibit getting tested. Seeking HIV testing, regardless of the result, can affiliate a person with a risk group and have adverse social consequences. Another stressor associated with testing is the waiting period for test results, which lasts about 2 to 3 weeks. Worries and concerns escalate during the wait for test results (McCann & Wadsworth, 1991). Biological factors associated with stress, such as hormonal reactions, occur in response to anticipating the results of serological testing among gay men who subsequently receive HIV-negative test results (Antoni, Schneiderman, et al., 1991; Antoni, August, et al., 1990). Negative HIV test results usually bring relief, but they can also have adverse reactions. Individuals who test HIV negative experience pressures to modify risk behaviors (Perry et al., 1993). There may also be guilt associated with having been at high risk and "gotten away with it." The potential for testing positive carries additional fears of stigmatization, discrimination, and disruption to social relationships (Siegel et al., 1989). Finally, the perceived threat of AIDS and the lack of effective treatments cause stress among persons at risk even after testing HIV negative (Lyter, Valdiserri, Kingsley, Amoroso, & Rinaldo, 1987; Ostrow, 1988; Siegel et al., 1989).

Receiving a Positive HIV Test Result

Initial reactions to receiving positive HIV test results can be characterized by shock and denial (D. Grant & Anns, 1988; D. Miller, 1990). Receiving an HIV-positive result makes it nearly impossible for people to retain information provided to them during posttest counseling (Grant & Anns, 1988; Perry & Markowitz, 1988; Perry et al. 1993). This too parallels experiences of receiving diagnoses of other life-threatening illnesses (J. Holland, 1982). HIV-positive women who have children also become immediately concerned about the possibility of their children being infected (Kloser & Craig, 1994). Shortly after the immediate shock, a series of negative emotional states follow, including anger (D. Grant & Anns, 1988; Mc-

Cusker et al., 1988), anxiety (Coates, Moore, & McKusick, 1987; D. Grant & Anns, 1988; Huggins et al., 1991; Ostrow, Monjan, et al., 1989), and reactive depression (Coates et al., 1987; Ostrow, Monjan, et al., 1989). Preoccupations with one's own mortality are also common among people who test HIV positive, further increasing their sense of vulnerability to disease and death (Tross & Hirsch, 1988). Receiving HIV-positive test results can lead to obsessive and compulsive health concerns (Ostrow, Monjan, et al., 1989), as well as anxiety specifically related to developing AIDS (Huggins et al. 1991). Changes in risky sexual practices occur to protect sexual partners as well as because of declines in sexual interest (D. Grant & Anns, 1988). However, sexual behavior changes are not universal among people who test HIV positive (Huggins et al., 1991; Ickovics, Morrill, Beren, Walsh, & Rodin, 1994).

Although fear of progressing to AIDS can occur over long periods of time following receipt of positive test results (e.g., Huggins et al., 1991), some HIV-positive persons quickly adjust. Strategies for coping are often effective following a brief period of immediate psychological distress (Perry & Markowitz, 1988). In a prospective study of people at risk for HIV infection, Perry, Jacobsberg, Fishman, Weiler, et al. (1990) assessed psychological distress before, immediately after, and at 2 weeks and 10 weeks following receipt of test results. Using visual analogue scales of affective disturbance where participants reported anxiety and fears along a continuum, the study showed that people who tested HIV positive were distressed immediately before and immediately after receiving their test results. However, distress levels significantly decreased 2 weeks and 10 weeks later. Concerns of having infected others with HIV and fears of developing AIDS, which were also high when receiving test results, decreased at the follow-up assessments. Ironson et al. (1990) reported similar findings in a prospective study of gay men who suffered substantial psychological distress upon learning they were HIV positive but returned to baseline levels within 5 weeks after notification. Psychological adjustment has been reported among women who tested HIV positive while in the U.S. Air Force (Brown & Rundell, 1990). These women were, however, not representative of women with HIV infection because they did not reside in an inner city and were of middle income. In summary, people experience psychological distress following learning they are HIV positive, and psychological adjustment usually occurs within weeks following notification of a positive test. The traumatic impact of a life-threatening medical diagnosis is often followed by an existential plight that has subtle psychological affects (Tross & Hirsch, 1988).

Reactions to a positive test are influenced by the manner in which results are delivered. One study found that 23% of people who test HIV positive view the delivery of results as unclear, insensitive, and unkind (McCann & Wadsworth, 1991). Adverse responses to the quality of communication during test notification are directly related to psychological distress (Jacobsen, Perry, & Hirsch, 1990). The psychological effects of HIV-positive results also depend on where a person is in the HIV disease spectrum. People who test HIV positive early in the disease and in the absence of clinical symptoms become concerned about the possibility of developing symptoms and of someday having AIDS. The situation, however, is quite different for people who wait to get tested until symptoms occur. Beevor and Catalan (1993) found that although women who test HIV negative are most likely motivated to get tested by their past behaviors, women who test positive are motivated by HIV-related symptoms. News of being infected with HIV when already symptomatic shortens the time line for developing AIDS, and in some cases notification of HIV infection occurs simultaneously with an AIDS diagnosis. Thus, delay of testing until symptoms develop complicates coping because the disease has progressed toward its later stages.

Illness-Related Stressors

HIV infection is a lifelong condition that results in physical decline and a very high mortality rate (Chuang, Devins, Hunsley, & Gill, 1989). People must face threats to long-term survival, the necessity of immediate lifestyle changes, fears of potentially infecting others (Christ, Wiener, & Moynihan, 1986), health concerns, changes in appearance, and declining quality of life (Donlou, Wolcott, Gottlieb, & Landsverk, 1985; Sadovsky, 1991). HIV infection invariably involves a pervasive uncertainty about when HIV-related illnesses will occur (Dilley, Ochitill, Perl, & Volberding, 1985). Uncertainty is exacerbated by long asymptomatic periods permeated by illnesses. Symptoms appear and disappear, keeping patients on constant watch. Coupled with uncertainties about disease progression is the loss of control over directing one's own future. People who test HIV positive know that a debilitating and life-threatening illness may strike at any time, causing the stress of a "walking time bomb" (Tross, & Hirsch, 1988).

Long asymptomatic periods are eventually followed by symptomatic illnesses. During symptomatic HIV infection, almost any sign of illness can elevate anxiety. Distress, however, depends on where an individual is located on the spectrum of HIV disease (Kelly, 1992). Close monitoring of fluctuations in T-helper lymphocytes often follows awareness of being HIV positive. Early symptoms serve as a reminder that HIV disease is degrading the immune system and that the virus is becoming increasingly threatening (Chuang et al., 1989). For women with children, symptoms have the added burden of demanding assistance with child care.

The onset of AIDS-related conditions causes acute distress and preoccupations with illness (Tross & Hirsch, 1988). In a study of HIV-positive gay men who were asymptomatic, had early symptoms, or had been diagnosed with AIDS, Chuang et al. (1989) found that all three groups demonstrated substantial distress. A 7-year longitudinal study of gay and bisexual men in New York City found that knowledge of HIV seropositivity and symptoms were consistently related to psychological distress, including depression, traumatic stress reactions, suicidal ideations, and increased use of sedatives (J. L. Martin & Dean, 1993b). These results suggest that illnesses contribute to maladjustment, leading to depression, anxiety, and preoccupations with AIDS (Mulder & Antoni, 1992).

HIV-related psychological distress also occurs in response to concerns over medical treatments aimed at controlling HIV infection. Multiple hospitalizations, intrusive treatments, the threat of side effects, and uncertainty over treatment effectiveness are also common occurrences (Solomon et al., 1991). The need for medications, usually in large amounts taken several times a day, can continually disrupt attempts to cope with HIV infection (D. Miller & Pinching, 1989). Contributing further to distress associated with treatments is that they are taken without the potential for a cure.

AIDS is like cancer with respect to its life-threatening nature, lifelong duration, illness concerns, and existential issues (Chuang et al., 1989; Faulstich, 1987). Like cancer, HIV infection is related to physical decline, bodily disfigurement, loss of physical functioning, emotional anguish, financial crisis, pain, and death. Both diseases are also catastrophic (Mc-

Corkle & Quint-Benoliel, 1983). People with HIV infection can therefore have psychological reactions characteristic of stress responses (Faulstich, 1987). The course of cancer and other life-threatening diseases, however, includes the availability of multiple curative treatments. J. Holland (1982) discussed four possible clinical courses of cancer: (a) a successful curative attempt that results in no recurrent disease, (b) a curative attempt with response but with later recurrence of disease, (c) a curative attempt and no effective response, and (d) no curative attempt (see Figure 3.2). The chance for a cure in three of the four courses offers hope and may culti-vate the spirit to keep fighting. Thus, psychological adjustment to a life-threatening disease relies heavily on the degree to which there are real pos-sibilities for cure.

In contrast with cancer, it is not possible to offer curative attempts for HIV infection. The clinical course of HIV infection is therefore sig-nificantly different from that of other diseases. Although HIV-related illnesses are treated, and lives are extended, illness signifies the under-lying disease. Symptomatic illness can be treated until, ultimately, there are no treatment responses and death ensues (see Figure 3.3). The

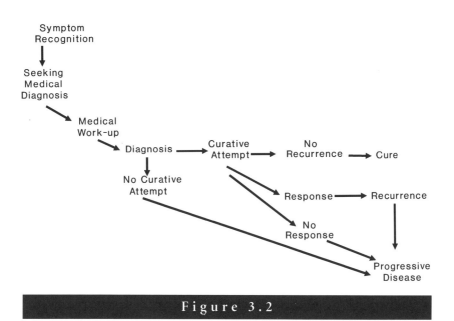

Figure 3.2

J. Holland's (1982) descriptive model of possible clinical courses of cancer.

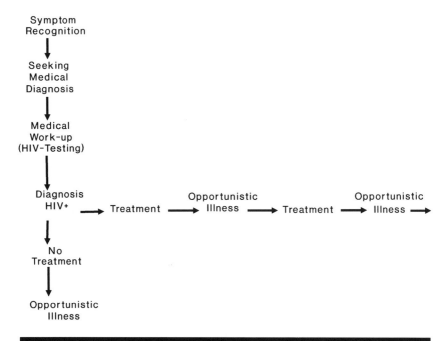

Figure 3.3

Descriptive model of possible courses of HIV infection adapted from J. Holland (1982).

prospect of persistent opportunistic illnesses in the midst of a degenerating immune system therefore poses a relentless succession of psychological challenges.

SOCIAL STRESSORS

Knowledge that one has HIV infection necessarily alters the nature of close interpersonal relationships. Being HIV positive can bring about fears of abandonment by friends and family, rejection from coworkers, and loss of employment. Losses associated with AIDS can be particularly devastating because they occur out of synch with developmental expectations (Dilley, Faltz, Macks, & Madover, 1986). Because HIV infection first appeared in North America, the epidemic has hit hardest among the socially disadvantaged. Social problems of relevance to the HIV epidemic create a context of preexisting stressors that interact with the psychological manifestations of HIV infection.

Social Losses

A positive HIV antibody test result can lead to loss of employment, the threat of eviction, denial of health and life insurance, refusal of professional services, and denial of health and dental care (Tross & Hirsch, 1988). Exhibit 3.1 summarizes the potential sources of social loss associated with HIV infection. People with HIV often suffer disruptions to their partnered

---

Exhibit 3.1

Losses Associated With HIV Infection–AIDS and Their Causes

- *Employment:* due to infection status or disability

- *Family:* fears and stigmas or inability to cope

- *Friends:* fears and stigmas, inability to cope, or friends dying of AIDS

- *Health care:* inability to obtain insurance benefits

- *Financial:* health-care costs coupled with diminished employment

- *Social supports:* fears and stigmas or inability to cope

- *Self-esteem and pride:* self-blame for the epidemic and personal infection

- *Physical/affectionate contact:* irrational fears of casual transmission

- *Future goals and aspirations:* facing a chronic life-threatening illness

- *Sexual partners:* fears or inability to cope

- *Physical functioning:* disease progression

- *Pets:* potential to carry pathogens

- *Life-style changes:* potential ill effects on health, such as smoking and alcohol

---

or intimate relationships. Sexual practices must be limited to protect sexual partners from infection, as well as to protect people with HIV from reinfection and exposure to other sexually transmitted diseases. These issues are magnified for women with HIV involved in power-imbalanced relationships where control in changing sexual practices is minimal. Disclosure of HIV infection to a partner for his or her protection may even place women at risk for violent repercussions. Individuals with HIV infection must decide how and when to disclose their HIV status to sexual partners (D. Grant & Anns, 1988). Disclosure of HIV-positive status to sexual partners can lead to rejection because of fears, inability to cope, not being able to deal with the potential loss of a partner, and dissatisfaction with new limitations placed on the relationship. Fears of losing a partner at a time when support is most needed may inhibit disclosing serostatus altogether.

Disclosure of HIV infection is usually a selective process. Huggins et al. (1991) showed that HIV-infected gay men tend to disclose their serostatus to sexual partners they felt emotionally invested in, as opposed to more casual sexual partners. The study found that 96% of men told exclusive and long-term sexual partners that they were HIV-positive, whereas only 44% disclosed to regular but not exclusive partners, and none disclosed to casual and anonymous sexual partners. Selective disclosure was also demonstrated in a study of HIV-positive Hispanic men, where intimate partners were frequently informed of the HIV infection (Marks, Bundek, et al., 1992). Similarly, the majority of gay men sampled from four U.S. cities informed their regular partners of their HIV serostatus, and their relationships tended to last longer than those of men who did not disclose (Schnell et al., 1992). It should be noted, however, that people who do not disclose their positive serostatus to sexual partners do not necessarily put their partners at risk, because they may alter their behavior to protect them. Issues of informing sexual partners can be circumvented by effectively removing risks for HIV transmission. Taking responsibility to protect sexual partners from HIV infection, whether disclosure of a positive serostatus occurs or not, weighs heavily on people living with HIV. Not surprisingly, people who learn they are HIV-positive often experience conflicts and break-ups in their intimate relationships (Coates et al., 1987).

Bereavement

The most common source of loss for many HIV-positive people is the death of partners and friends because of AIDS. Studies have found complex interactions among cognitive, affective, and behavioral reactions to the loss of someone to AIDS (Calabrese, Kling, & Gold, 1987; J. L. Martin, 1988; Neugebauer et al., 1992). Cities with high AIDS prevalence rates lose many young citizens. Thus far, multiple bereavements resulting from AIDS-related deaths have been recognized mostly among gay men. In a large Chicago cohort studied relatively early in the epidemic, 45% of gay men reported knowing someone with AIDS, and 35% knew someone who had died of AIDS (R. C. Kessler et al., 1988). In a cohort of over 700 gay men in New York City who were asymptomatic for HIV-related illnesses, 27% had lost a sexual partner or close friend to AIDS (J. L. Martin, 1988). Among those classified as bereaved, 18% lost two and 15% lost three or more persons to AIDS. When Martin included men who lost any friends to AIDS, 52% of the cohort was considered bereaved. Perry, Fishman, Jacobsberg, and Frances (1992) also found 55% of people with HIV infection in New York City to have suffered the death of someone because of AIDS. Similarly, a study of 207 gay and bisexual men in New York City found that 51% lost one close friend to AIDS, 11% reported two such losses, and 18% had lost three or more close friends (Neugebauer et al., 1992). Although multiple losses occur frequently in high-AIDS-incidence areas, men who are HIV infected themselves suffer the greatest number of AIDS-related losses (R. C. Kessler et al., 1991). HIV-positive social networks often originate in clinics, service organizations, social activities, and supportive services. The fact that HIV is spread most rapidly within social–sexual networks also increases the likelihood of social connections among HIV-positive persons (Gupta, Anderson, & May, 1989).

Bereavement is a well-known, multidimensional source of stress, and multiple losses have additive effects. J. L. Martin (1988) described a close response relationship between the number of bereavements from AIDS a person suffers and the degree to which they experience psychological trauma. Martin observed demoralization, sleep disruptions, affective disturbances, intrusive thoughts, and illicit and prescription drug use that increased proportionally with the number of AIDS-related deaths. Following the same cohort studied by J. L. Martin (1988), J. L. Martin and Dean (1992b) identified persistent psychological distress among both HIV-positive and HIV-negative gay men. Men who lost someone to AIDS at any point in the 7-year study showed the greatest traumatic stress, and distress symptoms increased in conjunction with the number of losses suffered. Similar results were reported by Neugebauer et al. (1992), finding an increased number of bereavement symptoms, such as preoccupation with and searching for the deceased person, with increased numbers of deaths from AIDS.

Bereavement from AIDS prompts a sense of AIDS vulnerability and increases the likelihood of seeking psychological assistance to cope with AIDS-related concerns (J. L. Martin, 1988). In J. L. Martin and Dean's (1993b) longitudinal study, men who both were HIV positive themselves and lost someone to AIDS invariably demonstrated the most psychological distress on all measures used across all 7 years of the study. AIDS-related bereavement in HIV-positive persons has several qualitatively different dimensions. Bereaved persons with HIV are likely to self-identify with the deceased person in terms of their own mortality (Mulder & Antoni, 1992), and each death from AIDS exacerbates fears of developing AIDS (Solomon et al., 1991).

Women with HIV infection are likely to suffer additional stress. Women must often contend with their own HIV infection while serving as the primary caregiver for their HIV-positive partner (not unique to women with HIV), as well as caring for their children. Obviously, having an HIV-positive child further contributes to stress levels. A qualitative study of HIV-positive women found that caring for their children and concerns about who will care for them if she should become ill is the single most significant stressor for these women (Hackl, Kalichman, & Somlai, 1995). Pregnancy for HIV-positive women requires anguishing over decisions about terminating or carrying the pregnancy to term and about whether to use antiretroviral medication that may significantly reduce the risk for perinatal transmission but with unknown side effects. Issues are often complicated by conflicting advice from family, clergy, physicians, and friends. Thus, HIV-positive women, because of their dual role as patient and caregiver, face added stress in an already difficult situation (Hackl et al., 1995; Kloser & Craig, 1994).

In summary, HIV-related stress develops out of fears of contracting

HIV, worries about one's own behavioral risk history, knowledge of being HIV infected, waiting and worrying through asymptomatic infection, and the onset of HIV-related symptoms and illnesses. Women face added stress mostly related to issues of caregiving and caring for their children. Surrounding HIV stressors is a second layer of pressure that exists in the immediate social context. Misinformation, fear, and worry among close friends and family, as well as employers and health-care providers, can serve as sources of stress. Finally, the attenuation of social networks because of AIDS-related deaths causes people with HIV infection to confront the ultimate outcome of AIDS. Beyond disease-related and relationship stressors, a third dimension of AIDS-related stress involves preexisting characteristics of subgroups most affected by AIDS.

PREEXISTING SOCIAL STRESSORS

AIDS has affected people from diverse ethnic, socioeconomic, and sociocultural backgrounds. It is therefore less meaningful today to discuss HIV-risk groups because any person engaging in high-risk sexual or drug use behavior is at potential risk of infection. However, because HIV spreads most rapidly within social, sexual, and drug-injecting networks, particularly early in the course of an epidemic (Gupta et al., 1989), communities with high rates of HIV seroprevalence are at greatest risk for spread. HIV infection has thus far been concentrated among gay and bisexual men and people living in large cities. Thus, gay men, injection drug users, ethnic minorities, and other socially disadvantaged groups have been hit hardest by AIDS, and these persons face other multiple life stressors (Chuang et al., 1989). Social problems surrounding groups affected most by AIDS serve as preexisting stressors, potentially complicating HIV infection and exacerbating distress (Christ & Wiener, 1985). The sections below review the preexisting social problems relevant to homosexually active men, persons living in inner cities where injection drug use is prevalent, hemophiliacs, and adults with chronic mental illness.

Gay and Bisexual Men

Gay and bisexual men have long been recognized as a socially stigmatized sexual minority (Solomon et al., 1991). It is common for families to reject homosexual members and for gay men to be victims of harassment and violence. Prejudice against gay and bisexual men has subsequently been amplified by the AIDS crisis, both from outside and within gay communities. Social isolation of gay men now results from both homophobia and AIDS phobia. Among themselves, gay men commonly assume personal responsibility for AIDS. However, communities can splinter on the basis of beliefs about risk behaviors, such as labeling people as hustlers, cruisers, and tricks and blaming them for the spread of HIV. Thus, blaming gay men for AIDS originates from outsiders (Moulton, Sweet, Temoshok, & Mandel, 1987) and can become internalized.

Stress within gay communities is further potentiated by high-risk sexual practices. Although longitudinal cohort studies show substantial reductions in high-risk sexual behaviors among gay men over the course of the HIV epidemic (Becker & Joseph, 1988; Fox, Odaka, Brookmeyer, & Polk, 1987; J. L. Martin, 1988; McKusick et al., 1985), cross-sectional surveys outside of AIDS epidemic centers have shown higher rates of risk behaviors (Kelly et al., 1992). Continued risky sexual practices result in personal distress for many gay men (Joseph et al., 1987; Ostrow, 1988). Feelings of not being able to change also leads to heightened distress (Ostrow, 1988). Gay men who engage in HIV risk behaviors often become ostracized and labeled uncaring and irresponsible.

Independent of their risk behavior, HIV has emerged as a major source of stress for gay men living in most urban areas (D. Martin, 1993; Noh, Chandarana, Field, & Posthuma, 1990). Folkman et al. (1992) found that the top five most stressful life domains for homosexual and bisexual men included illness of close friends and monitoring personal health. In a large study of self-identified gay men, D. Martin (1993) also identified five dimensions using a factor analysis of a threat-perception questionnaire: threats to personal goals and aspirations for the future; personal appearance; integrity; health; and the health of friends and partners. Although many sources of stress identified by Folkman et al. and Martin are not caused directly by HIV, the epidemic has contributed new dimensions of stress (Kemeny, in press; Kemeny et al., 1994).

Cultural and ethnic differences within gay communities may lead to additional stress for gay men of color. Homophobic reactions are more open among ethnic minorities, allowing overt rejection (Ceballos-Capitaine et al., 1990; J. Peterson & Marin, 1988). It is therefore common for ethnic minority homosexual men to report stress related to accepting their own sexual orientation (Ceballos-Capitaine et al., 1990). A large number of ethnic minority homosexual men do not label themselves as gay and thereby remain disconnected from gay social networks (Peterson & Marin, 1988). Ethnic minority men are less likely to access information available through gay newspapers, brochures, and outreach to gay bars and organizations (Peterson & Marin, 1988). Cultural differences, prejudices, and an absence of well-organized ethnic minority gay communities leads to the social isolation of gay men of color, who tend to be more misinformed about HIV transmission and AIDS than their nonminority counterparts. Social isolation of ethnic minority gay men is also apparent in longitudinal and cross-sectional studies, which have included less than 10% ethnic minorities.

Urban Communities and the Inner City

More than 52% of all U.S. AIDS cases have originated from 16 cities (CDC, 1994b). That urban areas are most affected by HIV is not unique to this epidemic. Congested living conditions, poor health resources, poverty, and relatively closed social and sexual networks all increase the potential for rapid spread of disease. Inner cities have been particularly vulnerable to AIDS because injection drug use and gay men are concentrated in urban centers. Thus, a combination of factors have brought HIV to its present level of crisis in urban centers.

People with injection-drug-using addictions are well recognized as a socially disadvantaged group. Injection drug users are generally rejected and mistrusted on the basis of their drug use alone (Des Jarlais et al., 1988). Stress results from socioeconomic stressors that coexist with injection drug use, social stigmas associated with drug addiction, and addiction to drugs itself (Des Jarlais et al., 1990; D. Miller & Pinching, 1989). Because injecting drugs is illegal, it also requires the evasion of law enforcement, another potential chronic stressor. As a group, injection drug users lack social cohesion and live generally chaotic, impoverished lives (D. Miller & Pinching, 1989). Drug use is often a means of psychological escape from the inner city and poverty. Drug dependence is therefore commonly related to coping deficits for managing serious life stressors. Therefore, adjustment to HIV infection may be complicated for injection drug users because of vulnerability to social and personal stressors (Tross & Hirsch, 1988).

Women living in inner cities constitute another special population within the epidemic. Among women with AIDS, 49% were infected by injection drug use and 20% through sexual behavior with an injection-drug-using partner (CDC, 1994b). Inner-city women infected with HIV are predominantly ethnic minorities and therefore face prejudices and discriminations placed on members of all three subgroups: minorities, women, and people with HIV (Minkoff & DeHovitz, 1991). Women may encounter verbal and physical abuse as a result of initiating safer sexual practices to protect their partners (Mays & Cochran, 1988). HIV-positive women may have limited access to health care and may be unable to obtain treatment for HIV infection in a timely manner (Ickovics & Rodin, 1992). Another major source of stress among HIV-infected women is the possibility of becoming pregnant after infection or dealing with an existing pregnancy. For many women, the connection between HIV infection and pregnancy is immediate because prenatal clinics routinely conduct HIV screening.

Women are unlikely to have prior experience discussing HIV testing with a health-care provider and may be offered testing only after they are already pregnant (Minkoff & DeHovitz, 1991). Women who learn they are HIV positive early in a pregnancy must decide whether they should terminate the pregnancy. HIV-positive women are prone to feeling guilty because of the potential harm caused to their unborn. Thus, the usual sources of stress that accompany a normal pregnancy are overshadowed by the burden of deciding whether to terminate the pregnancy, all in addition to dealing with one's own HIV infection.

Women with HIV infection who already have families face similar stressful decisions. Studies of families with injection drug users have shown that women are most often primary caregivers (Carr, 1975; Michaels & Levine, 1992). Women may be caregivers in families where their spouse is also HIV positive, and they may have an HIV-positive child, making it necessary for women to balance their own care with the needs of their family (Minkoff & DeHovitz, 1991). HIV-positive women with uninfected partners may be rejected, emotionally isolated, and financially disconnected. Women with children are burdened with finding care for their children as they anticipate becoming ill. Many women with HIV infection are single parents and must plan for the long-term safety, shelter, and care of their children. The number of children and adolescents orphaned by AIDS is growing at a rapid pace, with 18,500 children orphaned by AIDS at the end of 1991 and 45,700 orphans expected by the end of 1995 (Michaels & Levine, 1992). Children who become motherless to AIDS are, of course, concentrated in the inner cities, where they face social stigmas of having had a parent who died of AIDS. Concerns for the future of their children are the most pressing issues for HIV-positive mothers (Hackl et al., 1995).

Women and men living in inner cities often lack access to resources that facilitate coping with HIV infection (Jillson-Boostrom, 1992). People with late-stage infection tend to be unemployed and without health insurance (Hutchinson et al., 1991). Even when it is available, the inner-city poor and ethnic minorities may not access health care because of a social history of discrimination. Sociopolitical abuses of the recent past have erected barriers for many disadvantaged groups. For example, the Tuskegee Syphilis Study, funded by the U.S. federal government to observe the natural history of untreated syphilis, followed a cohort of African American men in the 1930s to 1972. In this study, syphilis was allowed to progress and partners became infected without intervention. The Tuskegee study formed the basis of an understandable distrust of public health agencies among African Americans (S. Thomas & Quinn, 1991). These barriers pose obvious problems for managing HIV infection and act as additional stressors for ethnic minorities. Moreover, because of such events as the Tuskegee Study, ethnic minorities frequently express the belief that HIV is a means of oppression, as well as a form of genocide (S. Thomas & Quinn, 1991).

The social context of AIDS, particularly in urban areas, forms a complex hierarchy of competing life stressors and survival needs, of which AIDS is one of several. In a study of women living in Chicago, Kalichman et al. (1992) examined the relationships among stress-related social problems facing urban women. The study found several life stressors perceived as more immediately pressing than AIDS, including employment, child care, and crime. Kalichman et al. (1992) also found that each social problem was perceived as a more serious concern for ethnic minorities than for nonminorities.

In a follow-up study, Kalichman, Somlai, et al. (in press) conducted a similar survey of male and female patients of a sexually transmitted disease clinic, 78% of whom were African American and 74% of whom were living in poverty. Because the sample was drawn from a clinic, it was thought that the participants would be more sensitized to AIDS than a general community sample. Men and women rated 11 social problems along dimensions of perceived seriousness. Results replicated Kalichman et al.'s (1992) findings by showing that AIDS was perceived as a greater concern than housing, alcoholism, and child care, but less of a problem than employment, crime, discrimination, drug abuse, and teen pregnancy (see Figure 3.4).

People With Blood-Clotting Disorders

Hemophilia is a relatively rare disorder caused by a deficiency in blood-clotting factors. Hemophiliacs bleed from even the slightest injury. There-fore, activity is often restricted because small injuries can cause severe bleeding. Blood-clotting disorders are life-long, chronic, disabling, and in-volve pain and suffering. These disorders are themselves highly stressful (Solomon et al., 1991; Wicklund & Jackson, 1992).

Hemophiliacs with HIV infection have typically been infected through clotting factors, aggregated across multiple donors. Fortunately, the abil-ity to screen blood and blood parts for HIV antibodies has substantially reduced the number of HIV infections among hemophiliacs. Those who are HIV infected face a number of medical complications, added expenses, and the compounded stress of two life-threatening illnesses (Wicklund & Jackson, 1992). HIV-positive hemophiliacs are at risk of infecting their sexual partners (Chorba et al., 1993). Hemophiliacs infected with HIV typ-ically express anger at an unknown donor and feel they have been vic-timized (Wicklund & Jackson, 1992).

Preexisting Mental Health Problems

In a prospective study conducted among persons at risk for HIV infec-tion, Perry, Jacobsberg, Fishman, Frances et al. (1990) found high preva-lence rates of psychological disturbances among HIV risk groups prior to receiving their HIV test results. Lifetime rates of psychiatric syndromes were roughly two times that of epidemiologic studies; 60% of men and 72% of women receiving HIV testing had a history of psychological dis-turbances. Among those who tested HIV positive, the rates were nearly seven times as high as epidemiologic studies. High rates of psychological problems suggest substantial vulnerability to psychological distress and

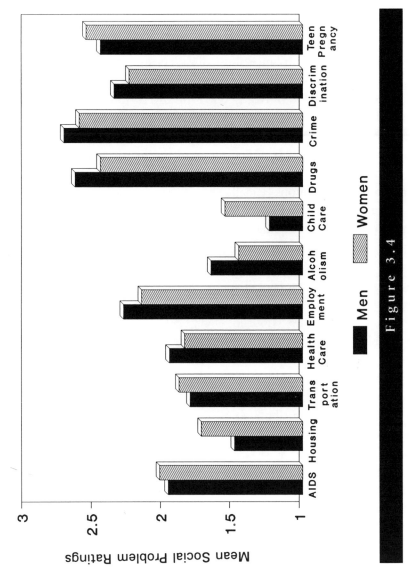

Figure 3.4

AIDS as a relative social problem as perceived by clinic patients with sexually transmitted infections.

maladjustment for many people with HIV infection (Perry, Jacobsberg, Fishman, Frances, et al., 1990).

There is also considerable overlap between characteristics of some HIV-risk groups and psychological disturbances. In particular, injection drug use is closely associated with antisocial personality disorder (Brooner, Greenfield, Schmidt, & Bigelow, 1993). Studies also suggest higher rates of bipolar affective and substance-abuse disorders among homosexually active men at risk for HIV infection (Perry, Jacobsberg, Fishman, Frances, et al., 1990; Pillard, 1988). Nearly one third of HIV-positive gay men in one study had a personality disorder diagnosis, a significantly higher rate than that found among HIV-negative gay men (Perkins, Davidson, Leserman, Liao, & Evans, 1993). Comorbidity of psychiatric history and HIV infection can complicate the course of illness by disrupting treatment and increasing hospitalizations (Uldall et al., 1994).

Recent research has focused on the HIV risk of chronic mentally ill adults. A majority of psychiatric patients are sexually active, frequently contract sexually transmitted infections, and often exhibit other HIV risk behaviors (Cournos et al., 1991; Kalichman et al., 1994). Patterns of HIV risk among chronic mentally ill adults are particularly alarming because they occur in the context of high rates of HIV infection, with HIV seroprevalence as high as 6% (Cournos et al., 1991) or 7% (Sacks et al., 1992) for psychiatric inpatients, between 6% (Empfield et al., 1993) and 19% (Susser et al., 1993) among homeless adults with psychiatric disorders, and 10% among alcohol-rehabilitation patients (Mahler et al., 1994), rates which exceed those found in many sexually transmitted disease clinics.

Several factors contribute to HIV risk among chronic mentally ill adults, including a lack of accurate information about HIV transmission, misperceptions of personal risk, failure to recognize risk-producing situations, and difficulty communicating assertively in sexual relationships (Hanson et al., 1992). In addition, psychiatric patients may be particularly vulnerable to contracting HIV infection because of impulsive sexual behaviors, relationships characterized by turmoil and transiency, and the overlap among risk taking, psychopathology, and cognitive disturbances that leads to poor judgment (Carmen & Brady, 1990; Lyketsos, Hanson, et al., 1993). In summary, a large number of people at risk for HIV infection have preexisting mental health problems, and many of the stressors known to exist in inner cities, including poverty, substance abuse, and multiple competing survival needs, apply to chronic mentally ill adults. However, limited cognitive functions and coping resources among people with histories of chronic mental illness will exacerbate the stress of HIV infection.

STRESS AND HEALTH

The multiple and competing pressures and demands in the lives of HIV-positive persons interfere with their quality of life. The relationship between stress and physical health among persons with HIV infection is, however, less clear. Psychoneuroimmunology, the study of central nervous system and immune system interactions, has extensively investigated the mechanisms underlying psychological influences on immune diseases (Solomon et al., 1991).

There is a substantial body of evidence that shows that both acute and chronic stressful life events affect several branches of the immune system (for reviews, see S. Cohen & Williamson, 1991; Herbert & Cohen, 1993; Jemmott & Locke, 1984; O'Leary, 1990). Negative life events and lack of social supports also increase the likelihood of illness (Sarason, Sarason, Potter, & Antoni, 1985). The persistent stress of caring for a person with a chronic illness suppresses immune responses, including declines in the number of T-helper lymphocytes and natural killer cell responses (Esterling, Kiecolt-Glaser, Bodnar, & Glaser, 1994; Kiecolt-Glaser, Fisher, et al., 1987). Chronic stress associated with living through an environmental catastrophe also adversely affects immune functioning (Schaeffer & Baum, 1984). Minor and acute life stressors can have important effects on the immune system in healthy and resourceful populations, such as the observed effects of exams on the immune functioning of medical students (Kiecolt-Glaser et al., 1984). Minor stressful life events may accumulate over time and act as chronic stressors, with similar effects on the immune system (Kiecolt-Glaser et al., 1984). The immune system reacts to chronic stress with long-term suppressed responses (O'Leary, 1990). The effects of stress on the immune system have therefore been widely observed, but it has not been determined if the nature and magnitude of such changes alter susceptibility to disease (S. Cohen & Williamson, 1991).

Several studies have reported links among depression, immune functioning, and disease, but the findings have not been conclusive (Schleifer, Keller, Bond, Cohen, & Stein, 1989; Schleifer, Keller, Siris, Davis, & Stein,

1985; Stein, Miller, & Trestman, 1991; Zonderman, Costa, & McCrae, 1989). Depression that lasts days, however, can alter several branches of the immune system (Kiecolt-Glaser & Glaser, 1988b). Suppressed immune activity occurs as a direct result of bereavement following the death of a spouse, independent of the stress effects of caregiving (Bartrop, Luckhurst, Lazarus, Kiloh, & Penny, 1977; Schleifer, Keller, Camerino, Thornton, & Stein, 1983). Similar changes occur among people with poor marital satisfaction and those who experience a marital separation (Kiecolt-Glaser, Fisher, et al., 1987; Kiecolt-Glaser et al., 1988). Immune disruptions are therefore observed among people who are stressed, depressed, and bereaved (Calabrese et al., 1987).

The immune system is affected by stress through complex interactions among the central nervous and endocrine systems. Laboratory experiments have shown that changes in the immune system occur within 15 minutes after exposure to a mild stressor and that changes can persist for long periods of time (Zakowski, McAllister, Deal, & Baum, 1992). Perceptions of threatening situations activate the sympathetic branch of the autonomic nervous system to invoke a "flight or fight" response. Activation of the sympathetic nervous system may directly affect the immune system through innervation of the hypothalamus and immune system organs (S. Cohen & Williamson, 1991; O'Leary, 1990). Hormones released during stress mediate central nervous system and immune system activities (Calabrese et al., 1987; S. Cohen & Williamson, 1991; Kiecolt-Glaser & Glaser, 1988a; Schleifer et al., 1983). For example, cortisol is released under stress, during depression, and following periods of social deprivation. Cortisol also suppresses immune system responses, particularly with regard to reducing counts of T-helper lymphocytes (Kemeny, 1991; O'Leary, 1990).

Retrospective and prospective studies have reported relationships among stressful life events, psychological distress, upper-respiratory illnesses, and a number of bacterial infections (S. Cohen & Williamson, 1991). Stress is also involved in the progression of viral infections. In addition, stress affects the course of latent viral infections such as herpes simplex viruses, cytomegalovirus, and Epstein–Barr virus. Stressful events can down-regulate immune mechanisms that normally maintain control over latent viruses (R. Glaser & Kiecolt-Glaser, 1987). Stress increases herpes virus antibodies and the onset of clinical symptoms of herpes infection (S. Cohen &

Williamson, 1991; R. Glaser, Kiecolt-Glaser, Speicher, & Holliday, 1985; Kemeny, 1991; Kemeny, Cohen, Zegans, & Conant, 1989). Substantial evidence therefore shows that stress can modulate immune processes involved in controlling infections. Because these processes are directly related to cell-mediated immunity and activate latent viruses, it is reasonable to propose stress as a cofactor in the progression of HIV infection.

There are two potential mechanisms by which stress can complicate the course of HIV infection. First, stressful events, as they have an impact on the central nervous and endocrine systems, may directly affect branches of the immune system of relevance to HIV infection. Cortisol is of particular importance because it affects the blood concentration and functions of T-helper lymphocytes (Fauci & Dale, 1975; O'Leary, 1990). The second potential role that stress may play in HIV progression involves the activation of HIV itself. For example, Markham, Salahuddin, Veren, Orndorff, and Gallo (1986) found that corticosteroids and other stress-related hormones enhance the expression and release of HIV. Thus, people with already lowered immune defenses because of HIV infection may be more vulnerable to the immune-suppressing effects of stress (Kiecolt-Glaser & Glaser, 1988a).

Despite the evidence that stress has immunologic effects, the likelihood that stress-related reactions interact with the expression of infectious disease, and the logical formulation of hypotheses that stress reactions interact with HIV disease (e.g., Gorman & Kertzner, 1990; Kiecolt-Glaser & Glaser, 1988b; Solomon & Temoshok, 1987; Temoshok, 1988), research has not confirmed these relationships. For example, a study of asymptomatic men with HIV infection did not find bereavement or clinical depression to significantly predict any of several markers of immune functioning (Kemeny et al., 1994). However, this study did report that for men who were not bereaved, depressive mood, although not clinical depression, was correlated with immune markers relevant to HIV disease. The authors acknowledged that these relationships may have been mediated by awareness of physical decline that may accompany both decreased immune function and depressed mood. In another study, researchers failed to identify relationships among measures of psychological distress and immune functions in HIV infection, although an active coping style did correlate with some immune markers (Goodkin et al., 1992). Thus, some studies have suggested relationships among psychological factors and immune functions in HIV infection, but there has not been a consistent pattern of results (Kemeny et al., 1994).

Research has more often failed to identify any stress–immune system relationships of clinical relevance in HIV infection. In one study, stress-induced activation of the sympathetic nervous system did not result in loss of T-helper lymphocytes beyond that already seen in the early phases of HIV infection (Gorman et al., 1991). A follow-up study of this sample also failed to identify relationships among distress, levels of cortisol, and markers of immune system functioning (Kertzner et al., 1993). In addition, widely accepted effects of depression on immune system functioning (Herbert & Cohen, 1993; Weisse, 1992) are not observed among HIV-infected individuals (Rabkin et al., 1991; Sahs et al., 1994). Highly stressful life events do not predict the onset of HIV-related symptoms among gay men (R. C. Kessler et al., 1991). Cross-sectional analyses by J. B. W. Williams, Rabkin, Remien, Gorman, and Ehrhardt (1991) failed to find relationships between measures of psychological distress with markers of immune functioning in HIV-positive gay men. In a prospective study of 221 people with HIV infection not diagnosed with AIDS, Perry, Ryan, Ashman, and Jacobsberg (1992) found that psychological distress was not associated with immune markers, in both concurrent and prospective analyses. Thus, several immune system responses to stress seen in HIV-negative populations have not been observed in similar studies of HIV-positive people (Antoni et al., 1991). Also contrary to theoretical predictions, stress-reduction interventions designed for HIV-infected individuals have not successfully demonstrated stabilization or reversal of immune suppression (Coates, McKusick, Kuno, & Stites, 1989; Esterling et al., 1992).

The most compelling evidence against effects of emotional distress on HIV disease progression comes from two longitudinal studies, the MACS (Lyketsos, Hoover, et al., 1993), and the San Francisco Men's Health Study (Burrack et al., 1993). Both studies reported several years of prospective data on large samples of gay and bisexual men. In both studies, cohort members were assessed using the Center for Epidemiological Studies Depression Scale at study entry, before the HIV-antibody test was available. Blood samples were stored and later evaluated after the HIV test was developed. Baseline levels of depression, which would not have been affected by knowledge of HIV status, although potentially affected by the onset of HIV symptoms, were used to predict declines in T-helper lymphocyte counts, the onset of AIDS, and death. For both studies, multivariate statistical techniques and survival analyses failed to demonstrate depression as a significant predictor of AIDS or death. Although Burrack et al. found a statistically significant relationship between baseline depression and T-helper cell counts, the degree of association was small and of questionable clinical significance (Perry & Fishman, 1993). Data from these two studies therefore suggest that effects of negative emotions on the clinical status of HIV infection is negligible.

Failure to consistently identify associations between emotional reactions to stress and immune system response among people with HIV infection may be due to the pervasive damage caused by HIV. That is, immune responses in the context of HIV infection are likely different from normal immune responses (Coates et al., 1989; Ironson et al., 1990; Mulder & Antoni, 1992; O'Leary, 1990). Even if stress does affect immune system functioning in HIV-positive persons, the stress–immune relationships will likely differ at various phases of HIV disease (Kiecolt-Glaser & Glaser, 1988b; O'Leary, 1990), making any such relationships far more complex than they are in normal cases. In summary, although proposed relationships between stress and HIV disease progression are based on studies of stress–immune interactions in the psychoneuroimmunology literature, the relatively small number of studies, their methodological limitations, underrepresentation of women and ethnic minorities, and lack of positive findings precludes conclusions of stress–immune relationships in HIV infection (Mulder & Antoni, 1992; Perry & Fishman, 1993). Thus, although stress seriously affects the quality of life for persons with HIV infection, it is not clear whether stress affects HIV disease progression.

CONCLUSION

The HIV epidemic is actually composed of multiple smaller epidemics, unfolding at various rates and patterns within subpopulations. Characteristics of the disease are distinctively different across geographic regions and subgroups (Mann et al., 1992). Social processes related to HIV infection result in psychological distress and potential maladjustment. Figure 3.5 summarizes the dimensions of the HIV epidemic that directly relate to psychosocial stress across the HIV disease spectrum.

The myriad of medical and social stressors of HIV infection often de-

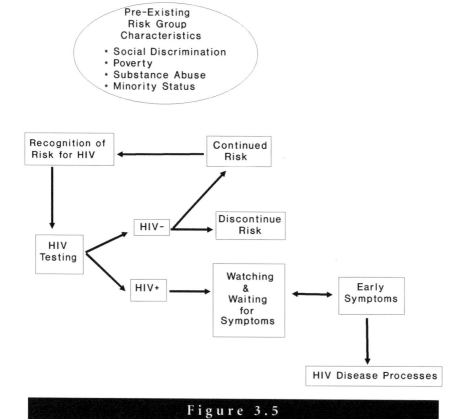

Figure 3.5

Stress-related events of HIV infection.

mand multidisciplinary and integrated treatment approaches. It is obvious that no single service provider can possibly meet the needs of people with HIV infection and address the diversity of issues facing them. Medical services, which themselves are usually multidisciplinary, are supplemented and often coordinated by case management within social service agencies and community-based AIDS service organizations. Case management coordinates access to services and provides supportive functions, but caseworkers do not usually have the training or time to provide counseling and psychotherapy. Mental health professionals therefore offer an added and needed dimension to the care of people with HIV infection by addressing the psychological distress and maladjustment that often accompanies HIV infection.

PART TWO

Psychological, Neuropsychological, and Social Sequelae

Ivan Ilyich saw that he was dying, and he was in a constant state of despair. In the depth of his heart he knew he was dying, but not only was he unaccustomed to such an idea, he simply could not grasp it at all.

(Leo Tolstoy, *1886/1981, p. 93*)

4

Psychological Sequelae

The threats of HIV infection to mental health, social relationships, and quality of life were recognized early in the AIDS epidemic (Coates, Temoshok, & Mandel, 1984; Morin & Batchelor, 1984). The first studies of psychological adjustment to HIV infection found significant distress and maladjustment among infected individuals (e.g., Dilley, Ochitill, et al., 1985; Donlou et al., 1985; Perry & Tross, 1984). The psychological aftermath of HIV infection, however, has a range as broad as the HIV disease process itself and is as diverse as the individuals affected. Factors such as psychological disturbances predating HIV infection (Atkinson et al., 1988; O'Dowd, Biderman, & McKegney, 1993; Perry et al., 1993), comorbid substance abuse, and social disenfranchisement increase the psychological vulnerability that usually occurs with life-threatening illnesses (Ostrow, 1990). Acute psychotic reactions are even observed in some instances among HIV-positive people not known to be substance abusers and who did not present with central nervous system disease (Halstead, Riccio, Harlow, Oretti, & Thompson, 1988; Sewell et al., 1994).

This chapter focuses on emotional reactions and behavioral responses common to HIV infection. First, to clarify study findings, methodological issues in this literature are reviewed. Second, factors that interact with or exacerbate psychological reactions to HIV infection are discussed. Third, emotional reactions related to HIV infection are reviewed in terms of their prevalence, severity, and symptom presentation. Finally, the psychological sequelae of HIV infection are placed in the context of the natural history of HIV disease progression.

METHODOLOGICAL ISSUES

Before discussing psychological reactions to HIV infection, there are several methodological constraints commonly found in this literature that should be addressed (for a further discussion of these issues see Kalichman & Sikkema, 1994). AIDS first emerged as a world health crisis in the absence of theory, prior research, and understanding of the disease. A lack of theoretical models of human sexuality and the political issues surrounding research on sexual and drug-using behaviors further stifled systematic investigations (Gardner & Wilcox, 1993; Kelly & Kalichman, 1995). Because studies were initiated in response to the crisis of a new epidemic, it was impossible for research to benefit from prior empirical findings. As the epidemic emerged, little was known about the people most affected. Years of neglect in psychological research of the urban poor, gay and bisexual men, ethnic minorities, and injection drug users created a vacuum for research on AIDS. For these reasons, the context of HIV-related emotional distress is not well understood. The first several years of psychological and social research on HIV–AIDS were therefore atheoretical, exploratory, descriptive, and methodologically limited. Three major methodological issues are discussed in this chapter: changes in context over the epidemic, sample selection, and measurement.

Variations Over the Course of the Epidemic

Changes in medical terminology, advances in diagnostic procedures, scientific discoveries, and new treatments continuously shape the HIV epidemic. For example, updated case definitions of AIDS, which occurred in 1985, 1987, and 1993, have affected personal perceptions of health and illness. Changes in the 1993 AIDS case definition brought many HIV-positive asymptomatic patients to be diagnosed with AIDS on the basis of impaired immunologic functioning. Many study findings prior to 1993 now provide little understanding of the experience of being diagnosed with AIDS, because the physical condition and medical status of people with AIDS has changed. This is particularly true for studies that compared groups of asymptomatic patients with those experiencing early symptoms and those diagnosed with AIDS. It is impossible to know from the pre-1993 literature whether people given an AIDS diagnosis were responding to serious illness or to the news that they had a terminal illness, whereas today serious illness and an AIDS diagnosis can be independent events. Studies published prior to 1987 were generally conducted before 1985, before the HIV antibody test became available. Therefore, early studies are necessarily limited to symptomatic patients. Thus, the point in the epidemic when a study was conducted must be considered when interpreting its findings.

Similarly, the availability of antiretroviral therapy and medical prophylaxis has rapidly changed, and with it expectations for survival, quality of life, and optimism. For example, zidovudine at first raised hope for significantly increasing the length of survival with HIV infection. However, since then widespread use and scientific study have found that antiretroviral drugs have only limited effects, and hope has subsequently diminished.

Study designs also affect interpretations of findings. Results from cross-sectional designs are influenced by changes in understanding of the disease, treatments, and social climate. On the other hand, longitudinal cohort designs involve highly selective samples that are sensitized to measures and repeatedly exposed to diagnostic evaluations, treatment opportunities, and other aspects of long-term study participation. Another methodological issue in this literature is that, with few exceptions (e.g., Perry, Jacobsberg, Fishman, Weiler, et al., 1990), studies have not assessed the prevalence of psychological distress and maladjustment prior to HIV antibody testing (Kessler et al., 1988). Subpopulations with high base rates of psychological disturbances may present as psychologically distressed upon testing HIV-positive, whereas those who are well adjusted before getting tested may adjust better.

Sampling Issues

The majority of studies of psychological adjustment to HIV infection have oversampled gay men, most of whom were White, well-educated, and of middle to upper incomes. Although representative of the early U.S. epidemiology of HIV infection, these findings may not generalize to other subpopulations affected by HIV and AIDS, particularly women and ethnic minorities. Recent studies from outside of the centers of the HIV epidemic have been somewhat more diverse in sampling gender and ethnicity. Still, there have been few studies of psychological sequelae among HIV-positive women, adolescents, and heterosexual non-injection-drug-using men.

Measurement Issues

Studies of the psychological sequelae of HIV infection contain a number of measurement problems. Like most areas of applied clinical research, studies have relied on self-report measures of psychological distress and on in-depth diagnostic interviews. However, the clinical course and symptoms of HIV disease are confounded with indicators of depression and anxiety tapped by self-report assessments and interview-based diagnostic systems (Belkin, Fleishman, Stein, Piette, & Mor, 1992). Many constitutional symptoms of depression, including fatigue, night sweats, gastrointestinal disturbances, loss of appetite, poor concentration, and unintentional weight loss, overlap with HIV-related illnesses (Belkin et al., 1992; Burgess, Irving, & Riccio, 1993; Ostrow, 1990). Distress measures and illness symptoms overlap most during the early symptomatic phases of HIV infection (Kalichman, Sikkema, & Somlai, 1995). Signs of encephalopathy, including forgetfulness, poor concentration, confusion, irritability, psychomotor retardation, decreased alertness, apathy, withdrawal, and diminished interest in pleasurable activities, also occur during early HIV symptomatic phases. Neuropsychological symptoms can mimic the clinical picture of depression and confound assessments of depression (J. C. Holland & Tross, 1985). Unfortunately, the degree to which symptoms result in misdiagnoses of psychiatric or physical illness is not known.

The comorbidity of disease and distress may explain why different clinical indexes yield different rates of depression among HIV-positive individuals. For example, Bornstein et al. (1993) found that clinical diagnoses using the Diagnostic and Statistical Manual of the American Psychiatric Association (*DSM-III-R*; American Psychiatric Association, 1987) resulted in 19% of people with HIV infection being classified as depressed, compared with 29% of the same patients scoring over the clinical cutoff on the Beck Depression Inventory, and 27% meeting a cutoff score on the Hamilton Depression Rating Scale. Each of these clinical instruments reflects behavioral and physical symptoms of depression that overlap with HIV symptoms.[1] The effects of overlapping depression and illness symptoms on assessment instruments have been widely demonstrated. In the Edinburgh cohort study of injection-drug-using adults, people at later stages of HIV infection scored higher on the Beck Depression Inventory than those at earlier stages. However, the difference between later and earlier phases of infection was substantially reduced when the test was rescored with the somatic items omitted (Egan, Brettle, & Goodwin, 1992). Furthermore, Krikorian and Worbel (1991) found that people with symptomatic HIV infection and people with AIDS had significantly higher scores on the somatic items of the Beck Depression Inventory but less magnified scores on the affective and cognitive component. Additional research has confirmed that somatic depression items disproportionately increase depression scores among persons with HIV infection to such a degree that false positives are likely (Drebing et al., 1994: Harker et al., 1993; Kalichman et al., 1995).

The extent to which symptoms of HIV infection confound estimates of depression among HIV-positive samples is further illustrated by two longitudinal cohort studies. First, Burrack et al. (1993) found that nearly 20% of HIV-positive men could be classified as depressed on the Center for Epidemiological Studies Depression Scale (CESD) using a standard clinical cutoff score. However, when five somatic items were omitted, 16% of the men were classified as depressed, showing that a portion of the sample was identified as depressed because of physical symptoms. In addition, men who indicated depression on the CESD reported significantly greater frequencies of persistent fatigue, night sweats, enlarged lymph nodes, and diarrhea on an HIV symptom checklist as compared with nondepressed men. However, men classified as depressed solely on the basis of affective–cognitive depression items also reported greater frequencies of some physical symptoms than non-affectively–cognitively depressed men. Thus, as

---

[1]Depression in this sense does not necessarily equal clinical depression as defined by psychiatric diagnostic schemes. For simplicity, depressive mood and psychological distress determined by clinical rating scales and psychological tests are used interchangeably with depression.

noted by Perry and Fishman (1993), although physical symptoms of depression overlap with disease processes, illness symptoms are also independently related to affective distress, suggesting that HIV symptom onset leads to depression. Similarly, Lyketsos, Hoover, et al. (1993) found that members of the MACS cohort classified as depressed on the CESD reported significantly more diarrhea, fatigue, fever, skin rashes, and weight loss than did nondepressed cohort members. Overall, depressed individuals report more HIV-related illness symptoms and have lower T-helper cell counts, again pointing to the comorbidity of distress and disease and suggesting a reciprocal process between them.

Assessment instruments of anxiety also overlap with symptoms of HIV infection. Autonomic nervous system reactivity that causes agitation, nausea, dizziness, tremors, perspiration, skin rashes, and gastrointestinal disturbance may be mistaken for signs of advancing HIV disease or medication side effects (Sherr, Davey, & Strong, 1991). Conversely, medical illness and medication side effects may be misattributed to anxiety. Misattribution of physical symptoms of HIV infection to anxiety may be a part of the patient's denial that can interfere with seeking medical treatment (Ostrow, 1990). The mirroring of symptoms between distress and physical illness can become a vicious cycle between increased anxiety and perceptions of progressing illness.

Several methodological procedures can correct for the overlap between disease and distress symptoms. For the most part, researchers have considered behavioral and physical symptoms of depression and anxiety conceptually important and retained these items on assessment instruments. Other studies, however, have controlled for symptom overlap by altering instruments. For example, Kertzner et al. (1993) removed overlapping indicators of anxiety and HIV infection from the Hamilton Rating Scale for Anxiety, resulting in a measure that mostly reflected cognitive and affective dimensions. Similarly, J. L. Martin and Dean (1993b) included only somatic complaints that are not associated with HIV infection in their measures of psychological distress. Burrack et al. (1993) altered the CESD, omitting items related to anorexia, fatigue, restless sleep, and poor concentration to formulate a measure of "affective depression" with a clinical cutoff score defined as one standard deviation above the mean for the subset of items. Other studies have used previously derived subscales of the CESD to examine independent effects of somatic symptomatology, negative emotions, positive emotions, and interpersonal dimensions (Lyketsos, Hoover, et al., 1993; Ostrow et al., 1991). Yet another approach has been to use statistical techniques to control for symptom overlap. For example, Kelly, Murphy, Bahr, Koob, et al. (1993) partialed both length of time since testing HIV positive and number of HIV-related symptoms out of the depression measure in multiple regression analyses. This methodology allowed investigation of predictors of depression while controlling for the potential confounds of overlapping symptoms. Through each of these methods, researchers have attempted to minimize the influence of illness-related symptoms on elevations of measures of psychological distress.

A final measurement problem in this literature has been an overreliance on single items to assess complex constructs. For example, Joseph et al. (1990) used a single item from the Hopkins Symptom Checklist to measure suicidal intention. Similarly, Perry, Jacobsberg, and Fishman (1990) relied on a single item from the Beck Depression Inventory to detect suicidal ideation and intention. As an assessment of death anxiety, Catania, Turner, Choi, and Coates (1992) used one item from the Brief Symptom Inventory. The low reliability of single items therefore limits several study findings.

PSYCHOLOGICAL DISTRESS REACTIONS

Multiple factors interact in HIV-related distress, including perceived responsibility for having contracted HIV, the potential for having unknowingly placed others at risk, and changes in physical appearance that may occur in late stages (Frierson & Lippmann, 1987; Nichols, 1985). HIV-related depression is also fostered by a sense of pessimism and hopelessness (Rabkin, Williams, Neugebauer, Remien, & Goetz, 1990). Knowing others infected with HIV and suffering multiple losses also exacerbate psychological distress (J. L. Martin, 1988). Cultural variations occur with respect to behavioral and physical manifestations of psychological distress, because some cultures promote expressing anxiety and depression through somatic symptomatology that may mimic symptoms of HIV infection (Karasu et al., 1993; Maj, 1990; Ostrow, 1990).

Psychological distress among people with HIV infection is as diverse as the epidemic itself (Moore et al., 1994; Wolf, Balson, Dralle, et al., 1991). Reactions to HIV infection may include feelings of sadness, worry, despair, and confusion, as well as other affective, cognitive, and behavioral responses. Several medical events occur over the course of HIV infection that serve as markers for vulnerability to psychological distress. People who receive HIV-positive antibody test results undergo multiple medical examinations, must make important treatment decisions, and are bombarded with information about illness-related milestones. Distress occurs in response to the initiation of treatment, the development of symptoms, the onset of opportunistic illnesses, the occurrence of the first AIDS-defining conditions, and declines in immunologic markers. Figure 4.1 presents HIV-infection-related events and their potential meaning. Early in

AIDS-Related Event	Psychological Meaning
HIV+ test result	Certainty of HIV infection
Decision to initiate treatment	Information seeking & sorting
Declining T-Helper cells	Monitoring of HIV activity
Development of early HIV symptoms	Recognition of advancing HIV disease
Development of opportunistic illnesses - AIDS diagnosis	Entering final phases of HIV disease
First Hospitalization	Physical debility & increased dependence

Figure 4.1

HIV-related life events and their psychological meaning.

HIV infection, routine T-helper lymphocyte counts can become the focus for self-monitoring disease progression (Clement & Hollander, 1992; MacDonell et al., 1990). At later times, hospitalizations have strong emotional impact, shattering denial and other coping strategies that may have been effective during asymptomatic periods. Because many events, including fluctuations in T-helper cell counts and hospitalizations, are of limited prognostic value, the evaluation of irrational reactions to events is clinically essential.

The result of simultaneous HIV-related events can be emotionally devastating. Individuals with high-risk behavior histories often seek HIV testing after developing symptoms. Thus, immediately upon learning that one is HIV-positive, it is also necessary to make treatment decisions. Advanced immune suppression can mean that a newly diagnosed patient will simultaneously suffer opportunistic illnesses, exacerbating an already catastrophic event. In contrast, when events of HIV infection occur sequentially over a longer period of time, distress reactions may not be of clinical significance (J. B. W. Williams et al., 1991).

The most frequently diagnosed clinical syndrome associated with HIV infection is adjustment disorder with features of anxious, depressed, or mixed mood (O'Dowd, Natali, Orr, & McKegney, 1991). O'Dowd et al. (1993) identified two thirds of 183 persons with HIV infection in New York City as having adjustment disorder. Rundell, Paolucci, Beatty, and Boswell (1988) diagnosed adjustment disorder in 64% of admissions to an Air Force HIV clinic. Chuang, Jason, Pajurkova, and Gill (1992) also found that the most prevalent psychiatric diagnosis in HIV infection is adjustment disorder, and this diagnosis best differentiated HIV-positive from HIV-negative patients. O'Dowd and McKegney (1990) found that 42% of HIV-positive injection drug users, most of whom were women of color, were diagnosed with adjustment disorder. However, this rate was only slightly higher than that of a non-HIV-infected medical patient comparison group. McKegney and O'Dowd (1992) reported that one third of patients with AIDS and other HIV-positive patients referred for psychiatric evaluations were diagnosed with adjustment disorder, a rate comparable to non-HIV-infected medical patients. Interestingly, a similar situation exists for cancer patients, where 68% of patients with a *DSM-III-R* diagnosis have an adjustment disorder (Derogatis et al., 1983). It is the necessary presence of an identified stressor, such as a medical illness, for the diagnosis of adjustment disorder that is apparent in these findings.

Adjustment disorder can be chronic and recurrent. Maladjustment is greatest when the source of distress is unresolvable, as is the case with HIV infection (D. Miller & Riccio, 1990). Persistent maladjustment is also more likely among people with a history of psychological disturbances (American Psychiatric Association, 1987), as is the case for a large number of people with HIV infection. Depression, anxiety, somatization, and other emotional distress reactions, although not mutually exclusive of each other, are addressed individually in the following sections.

Depression

Depression has been the most frequently studied psychiatric condition among HIV-positive patients. In addition to the enormous challenges posed by confronting a life-threatening illness, several characteristics of HIV infection have led investigators to hypothesize that patients will experience clinical depression. Studies of cancer patients show strong relationships between past histories of emotional disturbance and depression after cancer diagnosis (Engel, 1980; S. E. Taylor & Aspinwall, 1990). Similar relationships are observed in HIV infection. For example, Perry, Jacobsberg, Fishman, Frances, et al. (1990) reported that 43% of men and 49% of women at risk for HIV infection who elected to undergo HIV antibody testing had a history of mood disorders, a rate nearly seven times that of age-matched community samples. Similarly, more than one third of injection drug users have depressive disorders unrelated to HIV infection (Tross & Hirsch, 1988), 34% of HIV-negative African American gay men exceed the depression cutoff on the CESD (Cochran & Mays, 1994), 33% of people with HIV infection report a lifetime occurrence of depression (J. B. W. Williams et al., 1991), and HIV-positive military benefit recipients exhibit high lifetime rates of depression (Carey, Jenkins, Brown, Temoshok, & Pace, 1991).

Characteristics of HIV infection may also increase risk for depression. Knowing that treatments are limited and that HIV infection is incurable leads to pessimism. Negativistic thinking is fueled by the knowledge that HIV infection will eventually lead to physical deterioration, social disruptions, and occupational limitations (Maj, 1990). Despite these and other characteristics of HIV infection, it is not possible to conclude that depressive symptoms are entirely situational. Although depression may be a response to HIV-related stressors (Ostrow, 1990), depression may also result from HIV infection of the central nervous system, or may co-occur with an underlying substance abuse disorder (Maj, 1990). Like depression in general, it is estimated that 50% of individuals with HIV infection who are depressed will eventually have recurrent depression during the course of their illness (Karasu et al., 1993).

Depression has been reported, to varying degrees, in several studies of HIV-positive patients. Although less common than once believed, depressed mood is among the most frequent psychological reactions to HIV infection (Rabkin, 1994). Studies of HIV-positive gay men (e.g., Cochran & Mays, 1994; Mulder et al., 1992), injection drug users (Lipsitz et al., 1994), and army personnel (e.g., Ritchie & Radke, 1992), hemophiliacs (e.g., D. Miller & Riccio, 1990), as well as heterogeneous samples (e.g., Perry, Jacobsberg, Fishman, Weiler, et al., 1990, 1993), have all found that people with HIV infection are more likely depressed than non-HIV-infected populations. Dew, Ragni, and Nimorwicz (1990) reported that 42% of HIV-positive hemophiliacs met *DSM-III-R* criteria for depression, and Bornstein et al. (1993) found that 29% of asymptomatic gay men exceeded the clinical cutoff on the Beck Depression Inventory. Using the CESD, Kelly, Murphy, Bahr, Koob, et al. (1993) found that their sample of mostly gay men, all of whom were HIV positive, obtained a mean score of 25.09 ($SD = 12.7$), with the clinical cutoff for depression being 16. Also using the CESD, Cochran and Mays (1994) found that 32% of asymptomatic and 47% of symptomatic HIV-positive gay men met the cutoff. Similarly, Cleary, Van Devanter, et al. (1993) found that 31% of HIV-positive blood donors exceeded the cutoff for depression on the CESD at the time of HIV test result notification, as well as at follow-up assessments. Using the Profile of Mood States (POMS), Wolcott, Namir, Fawzy, Gottlieb, and Mitsuyasu (1986) reported that 28% of people living with AIDS evidenced symptoms of mood disturbances.

Studies using clinical and diagnostic interviews to evaluate depression have obtained similar results. Atkinson et al. (1988) reported that 65% of people living with AIDS met diagnostic criteria for recurrent major depression. It is noteworthy that most of the depressed patients in the Atkinson et al. study had a previous diagnosis of depression that preceded their

HIV infection. Also using psychiatric diagnoses, Bornstein et al. (1993) reported that 19% of HIV-positive gay and bisexual men had a *DSM-III-R* affective disorder. Similar results have been reported in other studies (e.g., Frierson & Lippmann, 1987). Interpretation of these findings must, however, include the fact that high rates of pre-HIV histories of depression occur in several study samples. For example, Lipsitz et al. (1994) found that 30% of HIV-positive injection drug users were diagnosed with a depressive disorder, a rate considerably higher than community samples but not different from HIV-negative injectors.

As noted earlier, depression among HIV-positive persons, measured by both self-report and interview assessments, may be inflated because of symptom overlap between depression and HIV infection. To control for this potential confound, Belkin et al. (1992) used a depression screening instrument that was void of behavioral and physical symptoms of depression. Belkin et al. found that 41% of men and 54% of women with HIV infection showed substantial evidence of depression, relative to 22% of non-HIV-infected primary care medical outpatients screened on the same instrument. Thus, studies using clinical diagnostic interviews as well as self-report assessments have found depression to be common among HIV-positive individuals.

Although depressed mood is associated with HIV infection, some studies have found that relatively few HIV-positive patients are clinically depressed. For example, R. C. Kessler et al. (1988) reported that only 12% of people with HIV infection scored beyond the psychiatric outpatient mean on the Hopkins Symptoms Checklist Depression Scale, with most scores falling between psychiatric outpatients and the general population. Likewise, O'Dowd and McKegney (1990) found that although 33% of injection drug users with AIDS were depressed, the rate of depression was similar to the 35% depression among HIV-negative medical patients. A study of gay men found similar rates of depression for HIV-positive and HIV-negative men; previous history of an affective disorder was the best predictor of depression regardless of HIV serostatus (Perkins et al., 1994). In two large cohorts of gay men, approximately 20% of the HIV-positive men exceeded clinical cut-offs on the CESD (Burrack et al., 1993; Lyketsos, Hoover, et al., 1993). Finally, J. B. W. Williams et al. (1991) found that HIV-positive gay men scored relatively low on the Hamilton Rating Scale for Depression. Williams et al. also found that depression among HIV-positive men was not significantly different from depression observed in their HIV-negative counterparts. Therefore, although depression is common to HIV infection, affective disturbances are not universal or even usual in this population and do not necessarily reach clinical proportions.

The symptoms of depression for HIV-infected persons are not substantially different from those seen in people who suffer other catastrophic life events. Depression consists of four interactive dimensions: emotional–affective symptoms (e.g., sadness, crying), cognitive symptoms (e.g., pessimism, negativistic beliefs), behavioral symptoms (e.g., lethargy, diminished motivation), and vegetative symptoms (e.g., anorexia, sleep disturbances; Golden, Gersh, & Robbins, 1992). People who are HIV positive and depressed likely experience all four dimensions of depression, with protracted sadness, demoralization, diminished self-esteem, sense of worthlessness, disturbances in eating and sleeping, psychomotor retardation, and social withdrawal (J. C. Holland & Tross, 1985; Treisman, Lyketsos, Fishman, & McHugh, 1993). Some features of depression, however, have been discussed as particularly prominent among clinically and subclinically depressed people with HIV infection. For example, one study reported depressed affect as the most frequently endorsed indicator of depression on the CESD in the Chicago MACS cohort (Ostrow et al., 1986). Bornstein et al. (1993) noted that psychomotor slowing in depression has a significant effect on concentration, attention, and memory and could lead to mistaken concerns about early HIV encephalopathy. However, depression has not been reliably associated with neuropsychological test performance decrements in people with HIV infection.

Social dimensions of depression appear particularly relevant to HIV infection. It is well recognized that social supports insulate people from depression. Because HIV infection has thus far been concentrated in groups that are on the fringe of the dominant middle class, individuals with HIV infection appear particularly vulnerable to depression. Varying degrees of stability in social relationships may influence depressive mood in important ways. For example, men who identify themselves as exclusively homosexual reported lower levels of depression than did bisexual men (Ostrow, Joseph, et al., 1989). Men who are exclusively homosexual may have stronger bonds to supportive networks in gay communities and may therefore have greater opportunities to establish high-quality, secure relationships. Relationships and social integration may therefore affect the prevalence and course of depression in people with HIV infection (Dew et al., 1990; Kiecolt-Glaser, Fisher, et al., 1987). Even when social networks are well established, however, depression itself alters the nature of close personal relationships and disrupts social interactions (D. Miller, 1990).

Depression can result in occupational problems, including absenteeism and declining productivity (Karasu et al., 1993). Here again, HIV disease interacts with depression, because similar social and occupational dysfunctions ensue as a result of HIV-related stigmatization, discrimination, and physical limitations. Social disruptions related to HIV infection, such as denied access to public services and delayed health care, can exacerbate depressive reactions (Tross & Hirsch, 1988). HIV-related depression includes demoralization stemming from multiple intrapersonal and interpersonal losses, disabilities, and prejudices (Treisman et al., 1993).

Another feature of depression particularly relevant to HIV infection is the hopelessness of having an incurable, degenerative, and stigmatizing disease. Rabkin et al. (1990) have provided the most extensive study of hope in HIV-AIDS. Rabkin et al. found expected correlations between hopelessness and depression in a sample of HIV-positive gay men in New York City. In this study, 24% of the sample obtained elevated scores on the Beck Hopelessness Scale, classifying them with moderate to severe hopelessness. Rabkin et al. also found that hopelessness was closely related to depression, over and above HIV status and number of HIV symptoms. This is an important finding because unlike most measures of depression, including the Beck Depression Inventory, hopelessness is primarily a cognitive and affective response and is not contaminated by overlapping physical symptoms of HIV infection. Similar findings were reported by D. Miller and Riccio (1990) in a study of hopelessness among HIV-positive hemophiliacs. Thus, hopelessness is a primary component of depression for many HIV-positive people. It should be noted that the role of hope in depression among HIV-positive women has not yet been studied and that the degree to which these findings generalize to women is not known.

Similar to hopelessness, lack of perceived control over the course of HIV infection is related to the onset and course of depression. Knowledge that treatments have limited success is associated with depression among HIV-positive blood donors (Cleary, Van Devanter, et al., 1993). Female blood donors with HIV infection have low levels of perceived control over the course of HIV infection as well as high levels of depression (Cleary,

Van Devanter, et al., 1993). Kelly, Murphy, Bahr, Koob, et al. (1993) showed that viewing chance as the locus of control for HIV–AIDS significantly predicted CESD depression scores, over and above number of HIV symptoms and length of time since testing HIV positive. Thus, a sense of having little control, albeit mostly consistent with reality, potentially contributes to hopelessness and depression in HIV infection.

Several other factors covary with depression in HIV infection. With respect to age, for example, more severe depression occurs among younger persons with HIV infection in samples of homosexually active men (Ostrow, Monjan, et al., 1989) and blood donors (Cleary, Van Devanter, et al., 1993). Low self-esteem, diminished social functioning, low socioeconomic status, and limited participation in health-promoting behaviors are also associated with depression in HIV infection, although the direction of these relationships is not clear (Cleary, Fowler, et al., 1993; Ostrow, Monjan, et al., 1989). Finally, bereavement, as would be expected, is often reflected in the depression of people with HIV–AIDS.

Grief and Bereavement

Although grief is a normal response to loss, deaths of loved ones have potential detrimental psychological and physical effects (Calabrese et al., 1987; Karasu et al., 1993). Two factors appear important in determining responses to AIDS-related losses: the number of losses incurred over a period of time and the HIV serostatus of the bereaved person. Multiple losses to AIDS close in time result in severe emotional disturbance (J. L. Martin, 1988; J. L. Martin & Dean, 1993a). Nearly one third of bereaved gay men in a New York City cohort experienced two or more losses in the past year, and nearly half of those men had three or more losses in that time (J. L. Martin & Dean, 1993b). Such rates of death among young adults have been virtually unknown outside of war (Capitanio, 1994).

Bereavement over AIDS-related deaths appears most pronounced among people who are themselves HIV positive. Given that HIV is principally spread through sexual behavior and needle sharing, people with HIV infection experience multiple losses because of the prevalence of HIV in their social networks (J. L. Martin & Dean, 1993b). Witnessing the degenerative effects of HIV infection, the onset of AIDS, and the eventual death of a friend or relationship partner provides vivid images that prompt thoughts of one's own impending illness. Observing someone with HIV infection become ill may lead to the belief that one is nearing final stages of HIV infection (J. L. Martin & Dean, 1993a). People bereaved over an AIDS-related death may seek mental health services to adjust to their own AIDS-related concerns rather than to work through bereavement and grief (J. L. Martin, 1988). In a 7-year prospective study of gay men in New York City, J. L. Martin and Dean (1993b) found that men who were both HIV positive themselves and bereaved over the loss of someone to AIDS consistently reported greater distress on every measure administered over the course of the entire study. Thus, multiple losses to AIDS substantially contributes to the psychological distress of HIV infection.

Trends in psychological reactions to AIDS-related deaths, however, have changed over the course of the epidemic. Neugebauer et al. (1992) observed a pattern of decreasing adverse effects of loss over the second decade of AIDS among gay men in New York City. Neugebauer et al. concluded that the expanding scope of the epidemic has led to a gradual normalization and expectation for death at young ages. Neugebauer et al. suggested that social and political mobilization against AIDS in gay communities may buffer against severe psychological distress. J. L. Martin and Dean (1993b) observed similar diminishing trends in bereavement intensity in New York City gay communities during their longitudinal study. Although bereavement was closely tied to psychological distress among gay men in 1985, this association was not observed in 1990. Martin and Dean noted that one's own health and physical functioning seemed to replace AIDS-related loss as the focus of concern among gay men.

There are several personal losses associated with having HIV infection. Loss of activity, mobility, and social functioning lead to grief that mirrors bereavement due to death (Kubler-Ross, 1969). In addition, people with HIV infection, like those with other terminal illnesses, experience anticipatory grief related to impending declines in quality of life. Unfortunately, grief and bereavement stemming from self-reflective processes in HIV infection have not yet been empirically investigated.

Suicidal Risk

Depression and hopelessness in response to HIV infection has led to the recognition that HIV-positive persons may be at increased risk for suicide.

People with HIV infection have higher levels of suicidal ideation and more frequent suicide attempts when compared with their non-HIV-infected counterparts (e.g., Zamperetti et al., 1990). Perry, Jacobsberg, and Fishman (1990) reported that suicidal thoughts, but not attempts, occurred after receiving HIV test results in over 15% of individuals who tested HIV positive. Pergami et al. (1993) found high rates of attempted suicide among people seeking HIV testing; a history of self-inflicted harm was found for 14% of people who were getting tested and who subsequently tested HIV positive, and for 22% of those who were to test HIV negative. However, after receiving HIV test results, 21% of HIV-positive individuals attempted suicide, compared with none of those who tested HIV negative. Similarly, Belkin et al. (1992) reported that 17% of HIV-positive men and women considered attempting suicide at least once in the previous week. In a study of HIV-positive U.S. Air Force personnel, Brown and Rundell (1989) found that 21% of men and 7% of women had thought about suicide. O'Dowd and McKegney (1990) also reported that 15% of injection drug users with AIDS had inclinations to attempt suicide. However, O'Dowd and McKegney found a comparable rate of suicidal ideation among non-HIV-infected medical patients.

In a prospective study, Perry, Jacobsberg, and Fishman (1990) used the suicidal ideation item on the Beck Depression Inventory as an index of suicidal tendency. This study found that 30% of people undergoing HIV antibody testing reported suicidal ideation before being tested, whereas 27% of HIV-positive and 17% of HIV-negative individuals continued to consider suicide 1 week after receiving their HIV test results. Perry et al. found that suicidal ideation occurred in 16% of both HIV-positive and HIV-negative people two months following test result notification. Thus, thoughts of suicide in relation to HIV testing may be greatest before result notification and within the first weeks of receiving results.

Studies have reported that suicides attempted by people with HIV infection occur relatively early in HIV disease (Marzuk et al., 1988), with risk for suicide most elevated among people with early symptoms of infection (McKegney & O'Dowd, 1992; O'Dowd et al., 1993). In a large study of medical patients referred for psychiatric evaluation, McKegney and O'Dowd found that 39% of HIV-positive people who had not been diagnosed with AIDS had thoughts of suicide, with rates that exceeded both HIV-negatives and people living with AIDS. AIDS patients were comparable in suicide risk to non-HIV-infected medical patients facing other life-threatening illnesses. A study of male HIV-positive asymptomatic Army personnel found that 55% had considered suicide since their initial diagnosis (Ritchie & Radke, 1992). O'Dowd et al. (1993) reported that having HIV infection and symptoms of illness were as strong predictors of suicidal ideation as was a prior history of suicide attempts. O'Dowd et al. also found that individuals with AIDS experienced fewer suicidal ideations than both those with early HIV symptoms and those who were asymptomatic. The onset of symptoms may therefore be an important factor in suicidal ideation. Individuals diagnosed with AIDS who are not currently ill, either because their diagnosis was based on T-helper cell counts or because an AIDS-defining condition was successfully treated, may also be at increased risk for suicide because of increased energy to commit the act (Frierson & Lippmann, 1988).

Belkin et al. (1992) and Donlou et al. (1985) both reported close associations between suicidal ideation and HIV symptom intensity and chronicity. In both studies, physical symptoms mediated relationships between depression and suicidal tendencies, with people most likely to think about suicide when simultaneously having physical symptoms of HIV infection and clinical depression. Along with the physical decline of a progressive illness, the threat of long-term dependency leads to increased risk for suicide (Marzuk et al., 1988). Rabkin, Wilson, and Kimpton (1993) found that individuals who expressed a wish to die, although not necessarily to commit suicide, almost always did so under the threat of serious debilitating illness, particularly when faced with an impending hospital admission. Similarly, Belkin et al. (1992) reported that the association between physical symptoms of HIV disease and suicidal ideation was mediated by the number of days that a person had been bed-bound. In this study, physical symptoms and immobility predicted thoughts about suicide.

For some, thoughts of suicide may also intensify at later points in HIV infection. Rather than being in response to the knowledge of being HIV positive, later considerations of suicide may reflect despair and hopelessness in the face of debilitating illnesses. For example, Rabkin, Remien, Katoff, and Williams (1993) found that one third of those who experienced multiple HIV symptoms and survived at least 3 years with an AIDS diagnosis reported a desire to die at some point during the course of their disease. The risk for suicide in symptomatic HIV infection and AIDS is between 17 (Kizer, Green, Perkins, Doebbert, & Hughes, 1988) and 66 times higher than for non-HIV-infected comparison groups (Marzuk et al., 1988). A lack of more recent studies, however, limits generalizing these findings to the current state of the epidemic.

Common predictors of suicidal tendencies in HIV infection parallel well-established predictors of suicide risk in general. Risk for suicide is greatest among people with HIV infection who have preexisting or coexisting cognitive and affective disturbances (Marzuk et al., 1988), substance use disorders (Perry, Jacobsberg, & Fishman, 1990), and poor social supports (Frierson & Lippmann, 1988). Consistent with non-HIV-infected populations (R. L. Martin, Cloninger, Guze, & Clayton, 1985a, 1985b; Mayou & Hawton, 1986), O'Dowd et al. (1993) reported that an inpatient psychiatric history was significantly associated with suicidal tendencies across stages of HIV infection and that risk was greatest among those with a prior history of attempting suicide. O'Dowd et al. also found that 90% of HIV-positive people who attempted suicide indicated that their first attempt was unrelated to their HIV infection status. Furthermore, similar to non-HIV-infected samples, methods of attempting suicide are highly diverse in HIV infection (Marzuk et al., 1988). Drug overdose is common, particularly with drugs used to treat HIV infection. For example, antiretroviral drugs such as zidovudine have been used in several attempted suicides (e.g., Terragna, Mazzarello, Anselmo, Canessa, & Rossi, 1990). These drugs are likely implemented in suicide attempts because of their widespread use and availability to most HIV–AIDS patients and because of their well-known toxicities.

Outside of documenting its prevalence, few studies have investigated the dimensions underlying suicidal risk in HIV infection. Schneider, Taylor, Hammen, Kemeny, and Dudley (1991) investigated predictors of suicidal ideations among 100 HIV-positive and 112 HIV-negative men in the Los Angeles MACS cohort. Notification of positive HIV test results, onset of symptoms, number of close friends diagnosed with HIV, knowing someone who died from AIDS, and perceived risk of developing AIDS significantly predicted intentions to attempt suicide. Not having a close friend or confidant, and feelings of loneliness, also predicted suicidal ideations. In contrast, suicide risk for HIV-negative men was predicted, as expected, only by depression and loneliness. Path analysis showed that AIDS-related events and perceived risk of developing AIDS were significantly stronger predictors of suicide intent among HIV-positive men than these factors were for HIV-negative men. Further analyses showed that AIDS-related events specifically predicted suicidal ideations independent of current dysphoria.

Although suicide risk in HIV infection is related to pessimism, depression, hopelessness, and grief, suicide risk may also emerge from decisions to "rationally" end one's life to avoid the protracted pain, dependence, and economic decline associated with advanced HIV disease (Frierson & Lippmann, 1988; Glass, 1988; Zich & Temoshok, 1990). Planning to avoid suffering by hastening death is common among the terminally ill and elderly, who often seek information about the lethality of suicide methods (Humphry, 1991; McIntosh, Santos, Hubbard, & Overholser, 1994). Rabkin, Remien, et al. (1993) found that 25% of long-term survivors with AIDS made arrangements to end their lives should their condition advance to where their quality of life would deteriorate. Because there are motivational distinctions between decisions to end one's life because of physical suffering rather than because of hopelessness and despair, psychological interventions are likely to differ. Also, with advancing disease, people may refuse treatment and seek to control the course of their life and death. Psychological despair of advancing disease may therefore inhibit accepting medical interventions and life-sustaining supports (Fogel & Mor, 1993). Caregivers may also be asked to help hasten death. One study found that 12% of caregivers of gay men who died of AIDS in San Francisco acknowledged increasing medication doses to hasten death for the person they were caring for (Folkman, 1994). Issues surrounding rational and assisted suicide in HIV infection are important but have not yet received research attention.

Anxiety

Anxiety disorders and nonclinical anxiety reactions are among the most frequent responses to HIV infection. As noted earlier, people with high-risk behavior histories have pervasive worries of being HIV positive. More than 48% of individuals who decline to receive their HIV antibody test results indicate that they would rather not know their HIV serostatus because if they were HIV positive they would worry excessively and be unable to cope (Lyter et al., 1987). Among HIV-positive gay men, R. C. Kessler et al. (1988) reported that 12% of their cohort scored above normal levels on a measure of obsessive–compulsiveness. Among HIV-infected hemophiliacs, Dew et al. (1990) found that 45% of their sample showed greater anxiety than an HIV-negative comparison group. Similarly, Pace et al. (1990) reported that 23% of HIV-positive Air Force personnel had generalized anxiety disorder and that 19% had a simple phobia. A clinic chart review of depressed patients with HIV infection showed significantly more use of antianxiety medications than among a non-HIV-infected depression comparison group matched on sociodemographic characteristics, suggesting frequent comorbidity of depression and anxiety in HIV infection (Hintz, Kuck, Peterkin, Volk, & Zisook, 1990).

Anxiety, like depression, is composed of cognitive, affective, behavioral, and somatic symptoms. Physical symptoms of anxiety stem from autonomic nervous system reactivity, including gastrointestinal, psychomotor, visual, and dermatological disturbances (Maj, 1990; D. Miller, 1990). As discussed earlier, physical symptoms of anxiety can be misattributed to HIV disease. Comorbidity of somatic symptoms of anxiety and symptoms of HIV infection therefore makes it difficult to disentangle the etiology of physical symptoms.

People with HIV infection feel vulnerable to disease, body disfigurement, prejudices, and becoming dependent on others (Nichols, 1985). There is often concern about eventually developing physical disabilities (Snyder et al., 1992), social rejection, and isolation (Maj, 1990). Finally, because HIV is transmissible, HIV-positive individuals feel pressure to protect others from infection while simultaneously protecting themselves from rejection and isolation. Loss of friends to AIDS may also serve as a salient reminder that HIV infection leads to early death, further heightening anxiety (J. L. Martin, 1988; J. L. Martin & Dean, 1993a). Cues such as AIDS-related newspaper articles, television news stories, public service announcements, and comments by friends all provoke anxiety.

The uncertainties of HIV infection contribute substantially to anxiety, particularly at the onset of early symptoms (Chuang et al., 1989, 1992; J. C. Holland & Tross, 1985; Maj, 1990). In addition, the lack of curative treatments for HIV infection leads to mistrust of medications. Because most antiretroviral medications are taken several times a day, they too serve to constantly remind asymptomatic persons that they have HIV infection.

The progressive and degenerative nature of HIV infection is expected to result in death anxiety (R. J. D. George, 1992). People with HIV infection indicate that the prospect of dying is a major source of anxiety (Wolcott et al., 1986). Catania, Turner, et al. (1992) found that 85% of HIV-positive gay men reported worries and concerns related to death, relative to 64% of HIV-negative gay men. Death anxiety is greatest among men experiencing symptomatic HIV infection (Catania, Turner, et al., 1992) and increases with the length of time since a person tested HIV positive (Kurdek & Siesky, 1990). Worries about physical decline and fearing dependence on others for basic needs are closely associated with the dying process, and these concerns supersede fears of death itself (Nichols, 1985).

As is the case with depression, it should be noted that anxiety can stem from previous histories of affective disturbance. Anxiety varies over the course of HIV infection, and so results depend on when assessments are conducted and which instruments are used. Although anxiety is a common concomitant of HIV infection, such symptoms rarely develop fully into clinical anxiety disorders (Ostrow, 1990).

Somatization and Hypochondriasis

Somatization provides an example of how HIV infection can be intermeshed with psychological distress. *Somatization* is the tendency to amplify somatic symptoms of psychological distress and attribute them to physical illness in the absence of corroborating organic pathology (Bakal, 1992; Lipowski, 1988). Symptom expectations can produce vague and diffuse physical complaints. In HIV-related somatization, minor physical discomforts associated with distress can heighten concerns about becoming ill. Misperceptions of innocuous sensations may feed and exacerbate distress, intensifying stress responses that are open to further misinterpretation (Warwick, 1989).

Physical health commonly preoccupies people who recently received a positive HIV test result. Repeated body checking and palpating for swellings, discolorations, blemishes, and other physical changes indicative of HIV-related illnesses can take on an obsessive character (Maj, 1990; Frierson & Lippmann, 1987; Ostrow, 1990) and can become maladaptive and disabling (R. C. Kessler et al., 1988). Preoccupations with physical functioning and compulsive symptom checking may develop from premorbid histories of obsessive–compulsive behaviors among both HIV-positive (D. Miller, 1990), and non-HIV-infected medical patients (Burns & Howell, 1969). AIDS-related events, such as declines in immunologic markers, testing anniversaries, or illness among friends, can serve as external cues for disease progression and contribute to somaticizing. For example, J. L. Martin and Dean (1993a) found that bereavement over an AIDS-related death increases preoccupations with signs of physical decline and promotes a sense of developing AIDS. This finding is consistent with descriptions of somatic preoccupations in non-HIV-infected populations, where a death can increase a sense of vulnerability to that illness (Barsky, Wyshak, & Klerman, 1990).

HIV-related somatization can be initiated or aggravated by non-HIV-related illnesses, such as a cold or the flu. Symptoms of relatively innocuous illness can lead to perceptions of progressing to AIDS. Early symptoms of HIV infection, such as persistent fever or diarrhea, can bring about somaticizing reactions. However, physical signs of HIV disease appear less important in somatization than attributional processes. Ostrow, Monjan, et al. (1989) found that gay men with HIV infection who reported swollen lymph nodes experienced significant psychological distress, regardless of whether enlarged lymph nodes were actually detected upon physical examination. R. C. Kessler et al. (1988) demonstrated that physical illness mattered less in HIV-related somatization than perceptions that HIV disease was progressing. Perry, Ryan, Ashman, and Jacobsberg (1992) found that although markers of immune system functioning are not related to concurrent psychological distress, knowledge of T-helper cell counts and intrusive thoughts of somatic functioning did predict distress. In addition, people notified of declines in their immune system functioning become preoccupied with physical illness compared with people with stable immune systems. The use of T-helper cell counts as a benchmark for immune system functioning may also become a means for self-monitoring disease progression. When T-helper cells decline, patients may erroneously expect illness symptoms to quickly follow, and these expectations increase somatic anxiety.

HIV-related somatization appears similar to a condition referred to as *transient hypochondriasis* (Barsky et al., 1990), a subclinical form of hypochondriasis, characterized by multiple and diffuse somatic complaints attributed to undetected medical illnesses. Several aspects of transient hypochondriasis suggest that it may occur in HIV infection. Transient hypochondriasis tends to develop in the context of a life-threatening and terminal medical condition and is related to perceptions that treatments are ineffective (Barsky, Cleary, Sarnie, & Klerman, 1993; Barsky et al., 1990). Distortions of physical symptoms tend to focus on a specific ailment (Jenike & Pato, 1986). Finally, people most susceptible to transient hypochondriasis tend to have fewer coping strategies than those who are free of these symptoms (Barsky et al., 1990).

Somatization and physical preoccupation are not universal to HIV infection. R. C. Kessler et al. (1988) found that HIV-positive gay men often underdetected recognizable symptoms of HIV-related illnesses, where only 9% to 14% of men who had medically diagnosed lymphadenopathy detected enlarged lymph nodes themselves. Similar underdetection occurred for fever and weight loss. Thus, not all patients with HIV infection become preoccupied with physical functioning and symptom checking. Many probably do not recognize actual illness symptoms because they lack awareness of their meaning or are unaware of proper methods of self-detection. Finally, like so many aspects of HIV and AIDS, somatization and hypochondriasis among women with HIV have not yet been examined.

Anger and Guilt

Anger is a common reaction to a life-threatening illness. Guilt, on the other hand, typically accompanies diagnosis of sexually transmitted diseases. It is therefore surprising that anger and guilt are not regularly assessed in studies of psychological responses to HIV infection. In one of only a few studies investigating anger in HIV infection, McCusker et al. (1988) found that HIV-positive gay men were angrier than their HIV-negative counterparts. Anger, frustration, uncertainty, and social rejection contribute to angry reactions to HIV infection (J. C. Holland & Tross, 1985).

As expected in reactions to sexually transmitted diseases, guilty feelings are a part of HIV infection (Christ & Wiener, 1985; Dilley, Ochitill, et al., 1985). Self-blame, shame, and self-devaluation are among the first emotional responses to an HIV-positive test (Chuang et al., 1992). These emotions most often stem from beliefs about having engaged in behaviors that resulted in infection (Nichols, 1985; D. Miller & Riccio, 1990), beliefs that HIV infection is a form of moral retribution or punishment

(Catalan, 1988; Frierson & Lippmann, 1987), and the social disapproval of others (Christ & Wiener, 1985). Guilty feelings also arise after surviving lovers and friends who die of AIDS. Survivor guilt was typical among Nazi holocaust survivors (Niederland, 1968) and occurs in AIDS-devastated communities for similar reasons. HIV-related guilt may become internalized homophobia among men who contracted HIV through homosexual practices. Finally, guilty feelings may arise about having possibly infected others before or after testing HIV positive.

Anger and guilt both come from attributions of blame for HIV infection. Anger can be directed outward toward the person believed to have transmitted the virus to the infected person, medical caretakers unable to cure the disease, or society for failing to respond with urgency and compassion (Chuang et al., 1992). Anger directed inward is similar to guilt and can stem from beliefs about having taken irresponsible risks, failing to recognize risky situations, or falsely trusting what appeared to be safe situations. Guilt is also fostered by social stigmas attached to sexual and drug-use behaviors and may stem from discrepancies among behavior, moral beliefs, and social judgments. Anger and guilt are therefore emotional reactions that warrant careful consideration in clinical evaluations.

Summary of HIV-Related Distress Reactions

The literature on the psychological sequelae of HIV infection suggests that depression, anxiety, and somatization are the most prominent and intensely experienced psychological reactions to HIV infection. However, it is not possible to discern from studies whether these emotions are the most commonly experienced or merely the most frequently studied. Psychological reactions to HIV infection are consistent with those known to occur in response to other life-threatening circumstances (Farrer, 1986; Reich & Kelly, 1976). Like HIV infection itself, psychological reactions are both chronic and phasic. Depression, anxiety, and somatization ebb and flow over the course of HIV infection, subsiding at some points and later surfacing in response to both internal and external events.

The psychological and social demands of HIV infection change over the course of HIV disease (Chuang et al., 1989; Ostrow, 1990). For example, psychological distress commonly occurs with notification of HIV-positive test results and subsides shortly after an adjustment period. Distress often recurs in conjunction with knowledge of drops in T-helper cell counts, the onset of HIV-related illnesses, and the death of a friend or partner to AIDS (Maj, 1990; D. Miller, 1990; Ostrow, 1990). Suicide risk increases, decreases, and changes meaning with repeated episodes of illness (Chuang et al., 1989). An emotional roller coaster therefore best describes the catastrophic life events that occur over the course of HIV disease (e.g., J. L. Martin & Dean, 1993a; Nichols, 1985), with reactions changing unpredictably at each phase.

EMOTIONAL REACTIONS AT EACH PHASE OF HIV INFECTION

It is useful to describe the psychological dimensions of HIV infection in the context of phases of HIV disease progression. Although there are several cohorts of HIV-positive people, only a few studies have reported changes in psychological functioning over the natural history of HIV infection. Psychological reactions are usually reported at one point in time, such as notification of HIV test results, asymptomatic periods, the onset of early symptoms, or during AIDS. An approximate chronological representation of psychological sequelae follows the three major phases of HIV infection: absence of detectable symptoms, onset of early symptoms, and late illness (R. C. Kessler et al., 1988). This layout of psychological sequelae assumes a sequential unfolding of the disease where people learn that they are HIV positive while still asymptomatic. However, people who learn their HIV status after developing symptoms of HIV-related illnesses are likely to have different reactions. In such cases, each phase of disease yields more complex and intensified emotions. Therefore, rather than a linear progression, psychological reactions to HIV infection represent cycles of emotions usually initiated by HIV–AIDS-related events (see Figure 4.2). Although certain reactions are not tied to particular points in HIV infection, the stages of disease provide a useful framework for conceptualizing psychological reactions.

Asymptomatic Phases

Psychological reactions tend to be intense early in HIV infection (Chuang et al., 1989), regardless of whether a person expects beforehand that he or she is HIV positive. Receiving a positive test result sets off a cascade of

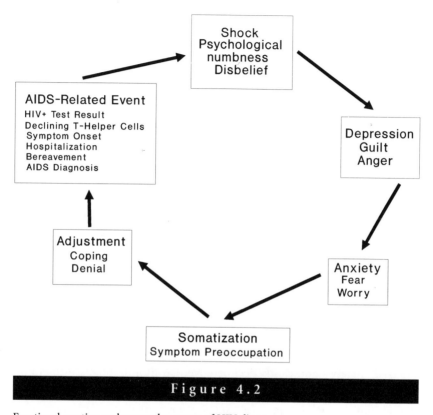

Figure 4.2

Emotional reaction cycles over the course of HIV disease.

psychological responses that are best characterized as an acute distress reaction, including confusion, bewilderment, and emotional turmoil (Maj, 1990). Initial reactions to testing HIV positive include psychological numbness and disbelief (Forstein, 1984). Cognitive dysfunction, psychomotor slowing (Ostrow, 1989), and feelings of fear, sadness, guilt, and anger are also common (Catalan, 1988; Nichols, 1985). Atkinson et al. (1988) reported that most people with HIV infection who develop generalized anxiety disorder report the onset of symptoms at the time of HIV serologic testing. Maj (1990) reported that as many as 90% of recent diagnoses of HIV infection result in acute distress. Initial responses to HIV-positive test results therefore mirror other catastrophic stress reactions (Faulstich, 1987; Nichols, 1985).

Acute distress following diagnosis with HIV infection may include symptoms of depression and somatization (D. Miller & Riccio, 1990). Perry, Fishman, et al. (1992) found that more than one third of people with early HIV infection showed signs of immediate emotional distress, and one third of this group met diagnostic criteria for *DSM-III-R* clinical diagnoses. Similarly, Cleary, Van Devanter, et al. (1993) reported that 31% of HIV-positive blood donors are clinically depressed at the time that they receive their test results and remain depressed for over 2 weeks. Hopelessness, maladaptive behaviors, health-compromising behaviors (Ostrow, 1990) and increased potential for suicide have all been observed early in HIV infection (Glass, 1988).

Initial reactions to testing HIV positive precede long periods of psychological adaptation, eventually progressing toward acceptance. Early in the adaptation process, denial is a short-term compensatory mechanism (Ostrow, 1990). Denial may include repeated HIV testing and numerous calls to physicians and counselors (D. Miller, 1990). Even upon intellectually accepting HIV seropositivity, emotional disbelief often persists (Ostrow, 1990).

Prospective studies show that distress declines over repeated assessments. Rabkin et al. (1991) found that symptoms of depression and generalized anxiety significantly declined over a 6-month interassessment interval. Cleary, Van Devanter, et al. (1993) also reported reduced depression 2 weeks following HIV test result notification, with similar declines in distress following diagnosis reported by other investigators (e.g., R. C. Kessler et al., 1988). Most compelling, however, has been a prospective study in New York City that showed severity of depression in HIV-positive individuals to significantly decline 6 months after notification of HIV test results (Perry et al., 1993). Overall psychological distress 1 year after receiving results for asymptomatic HIV-positive individuals did not significantly differ from their HIV-negative counterparts. In another study, HIV-positive asymptomatic patients responded more favorably to antidepressant medications than did people with early and late symptomatic HIV disease (Hintz et al., 1990), suggesting that HIV-related depression, at least early in the course of infection, responds well to treatment.

Early Symptomatic Phases

The onset of HIV-related symptoms gives new meaning and urgency to being HIV positive (J. L. Martin & Dean, 1993a). The first signs of illness can cause a resurgence of depression, anxiety, somatization, and other mood disturbances (Chuang et al., 1989). Early symptoms tend to prompt generalized anxiety, despair, tension, physical preoccupation, and substance use relative to both asymptomatic and late symptomatic periods (Atkinson et al., 1988; Hinkin et al., 1992; J. L. Martin & Dean, 1993b). The first physical signs of disease can signal the progression of infection, creating thoughts of soon developing AIDS. Symptoms may also fuel beliefs that medications and other treatments have not impeded the progression of the virus (Tross & Hirsch, 1988).

In addition to first onset of symptoms, the frequency of illnesses elicits psychological reactions. Numbers of symptoms significantly correlate with emotional distress and subjective impressions of declining physical health (Wolcott et al., 1986). Depression assessed by self-report instruments correlates with HIV symptoms, even when affective and somatic symptoms of depression are assessed independently (Belkin et al., 1992; Hays, Turner, & Coates, 1992; Kalichman et al., 1995; Kelly, Murphy, Bahr, Koob, et al., 1993; Ostrow, Monjan et al., 1989; Rabkin et al., 1991). One study showed that people with symptomatic HIV infection scored significantly higher on the Beck Depression Inventory and the State–Trait Anxiety Inventory than both HIV-positive asymptomatic and HIV-negative people (E. M. Martin, Robertson, et al., 1992). Ostrow, Monjan, et al. (1989) reported that individuals with HIV-related symptoms were five times more likely to be depressed. Belkin et al. (1992) found that 35% of individuals with between 4 and 8 constitutional symptoms of HIV infection were depressed, compared with 24% of those with 3 or less symptoms. Belkin et al. reported that 64% of people with more than 14 physical symptoms of HIV infection were depressed, suggesting a linear relationship between number of symptoms and levels of depression. In contrast with relationships between symptoms of HIV infection and depression, two studies have failed to identify associations between number of HIV symptoms and feelings of hopelessness (Rabkin et al., 1990; Zich & Temoshok, 1990). This lack of association may be accounted for by the absence of overlap between symptoms of HIV infection and hopelessness.

Detecting one's own HIV-related symptoms is directly related to psychological distress (R. C. Kessler et al., 1988; Ostrow et al., 1986). Although severity of symptoms correlates with distress, immune markers for HIV disease progression have not been consistently related to measures of depression (Perry, Fishman, et al., 1992). Perceptions of symptoms alone do not, however, explain dysphoria with advancing HIV disease, suggesting that multiple factors contribute to the association between illness and distress (R. C. Kessler et al., 1988). Finally, early symptoms of HIV infection rarely cause physical disability and are usually followed by a return to asymptomatic phases and improved psychological functioning.

Later Symptomatic Phases and AIDS

Acute psychological distress typically returns with an AIDS diagnosis (Tross & Hirsch, 1988; Woo, 1992). However, following an initial reaction, people living with AIDS are actually less distressed than people at both asymptomatic and early symptomatic phases of infection (Catalan, 1988; Chuang et al., 1989; O'Dowd et al., 1993). These findings differ from those reported in studies of other chronic illnesses, where severity of depression usually increases with severity of medical illness (e.g., Koenig, Meador, Cohen, & Blazer, 1988; Rodin & Voshart, 1986). With other terminal illnesses, depression increases over time because the course of disease tends to be persistently debilitating. In contrast, HIV infection is characterized by long asymptomatic periods followed by symptom onset and return to asymptomatic phases. With a diagnosis of AIDS may come a sense of relief because a person now knows the extent to which HIV infection has progressed (McKegney & O'Dowd, 1992). People with AIDS usually have had time to adjust to earlier symptoms and illnesses. The distress that accompanied earlier symptoms of HIV disease may serve to prepare a person for AIDS. Because HIV infection has long asymptomatic periods, people are significantly older when they have AIDS than when first testing HIV positive, and older people tend to adjust better to chronic illness (Cassileth et al., 1984).

People with AIDS, however, are not free of psychological distress. Belkin et al. (1992) found significant correlations between functional limitation and both cognitive and affective symptoms of depression. Long-term survivors with AIDS indicate that the most intolerable aspects of HIV disease include the prospects of protracted pain, declining mental abilities, loss of vision, urinary incontinence, and loss of privacy and personal control (Rabkin, Wilson, & Kimpton, 1993). Cognitive disturbances from late-stage involvement of HIV in the central nervous system, potentially resulting in delirium and dementia, further complicate psychological functioning in later phases (Glass, 1988).

CONCLUSION

Depression, anxiety, somatization, anger, and guilt characterize the emotional roller coaster of HIV infection. These emotions change rapidly over the course of HIV infection in conjunction with uncertainty about the course of illness. Distress results from testing for HIV antibodies, receiving HIV test results, making life-style adjustments to an HIV-positive status, searching for symptoms, observing others along the spectrum of disease, and fearing the progression of one's own disease. These events have unique sequences and psychological meaning for each individual.

HIV infection is an underlying degeneration of the immune system that manifests itself as a variety of opportunistic illnesses, with no single pattern of symptoms or illnesses. With immune suppression, some people develop one opportunistic infection, whereas others develop multiple infections and malignancies. Individual patterns of HIV disease are multidetermined by pre-HIV health status, lifetime exposure to microbes, ability to fight diseases, and life-style factors. Likewise, psychological adaptation to HIV-related events is characterized by an underlying emotional reaction of which there is not a single, universal pattern. As HIV infection advances, some people experience depression, others have anxiety or somatization, and still many others do not experience depression or anxiety. Individual expressions are determined by factors stemming from psychological history, previous health-related experiences, and available coping resources.

Educating HIV-positive clients about the comorbidity of physical symptoms of disease and psychological distress may assist them to examine their own HIV-related experiences objectively. It is important that HIV-positive clients not discount or dismiss physical symptoms as emotional responses. Mislabeling physical symptoms as depression, anxiety, or somatization can lead to avoidance of medical examinations, with deleterious outcomes. Conversely, somatization can result in avoidance of mental health care. Understanding the interrelatedness of physical symptomatology and emotional reactions may increase one's sense of control. Neuropsychological symptoms signaling HIV involvement of the central nervous system pose similar problems of comorbidity. Lapses in memory, transient states of confusion, and decreased ability to concentrate may indicate the advance of HIV disease or reflect depression or anxiety. However, the neuropsychological effects of HIV infection are complex in their own right and require careful examination.

5

Neuropsychological Sequelae

Although the human immune system is the principal site of HIV infection, numerous other organ systems become infected by the virus. HIV brain infection and AIDS-related opportunistic illnesses of the central nervous system pose some of the most feared HIV-related health problems. Early in the epidemic, HIV was thought to cause an inflammation of the brain (encephalitis) only associated with late-stage HIV infection (Snider et al., 1983). It was also believed that AIDS-related neuropsychological impairment was caused by cytomegalovirus infection of the brain (Sharer, 1992). However, studies conclusively demonstrated that HIV itself crosses the blood–brain barrier and infects brain tissue (Levy, Shimabukuro, Hollander, Mills, & Kaminsky, 1985; Navia, Cho, Petito, & Price, 1986; Shaw et al., 1985). Early on, a large number of people with AIDS were thought to develop severe cognitive impairment. The diagnostic label *AIDS dementia complex*, introduced in 1987, served to describe the clinical constellation of neuropsychological symptoms in cases of AIDS (R. W. Price & Sidtis, 1992; Worley & Price, 1992). AIDS dementia complex is diagnosed in 3% of adults and 14% of children with AIDS (CDC, 1994b). It is believed that most HIV-positive people will develop HIV infection of the central nervous system (Collier et al., 1992) and that between 30% and 60% of all AIDS patients develop symptoms of central or peripheral nervous system disease. In addition, AIDS patients can have opportunistic infections of the nervous system, including toxoplasmosis, Cryptococcal meningitis, progressive multifocal leukoencephalopathy (PML), and non-Hodgkin's lymphomas. Diseases that can cause neuropsychological impairment are characterized by a wide spectrum of clinical symptoms and functional disabilities.

HIV infection of the brain and opportunistic illnesses of the nervous system must be distinguished. Originally, AIDS dementia complex was defined by cognitive and behavioral deterioration in the absence of an AIDS-defining condition of the central nervous system (Aronow, Brew, & Price, 1988; Egan, 1992). The parameters for a diagnosis of AIDS dementia complex were self-evident: AIDS reflects the morbidity of neuropsychological impairment relative to other complications of HIV infection; *dementia* denotes acquired and persistent declines in cognitive functioning observed over the course of late-stage infection; and *complex* reflects a triad of cognitive, motor, and behavior dysfunctions (see Table 5.1; R. W. Price & Brew, 1991; Worley & Price, 1992). Like other forms of dementia, such as Alzheimer's and Huntington's diseases, AIDS dementia complex involves persistent impairment in multiple spheres of mental activity, including, but not limited to, psychomotor control, attention, concentration, language, memory, visual–spatial skills, emotion, reasoning, and cognitive flexibility. Like organic mental disorders in general, the essential feature of AIDS dementia complex is a loss of intellectual abilities of sufficient severity to interfere with social or occupational functioning (American

Table 5.1

Clinical Manifestations of HIV-Related Dementia

Domain	Early manifestations	Late manifestations
Cognitive	Reduced attention and concentration, increased forgetfulness	Generalized dementia
Motoric	General slowing, clumsiness, disrupted walking	Paraplegia
Behavioral	Apathy, agitation	Mutism

Table 5.2

Clinical Staging of AIDS Dementia Complex

Stage	Symptoms and characteristics
0 (normal)	Normal mental and motor function.
0.5 (subclinical)	Either minimal or equivocal symptoms or motor dysfunction characteristic of HIV-related dementia, or mild signs but without impairment of work or capacity to perform activities of daily living; walking and strength are normal.
1 (mild)	Unequivocal symptoms, neuropsychological test performance, or functional, intellectual, or motor impairment characteristic of HIV-related dementia but able to perform all but the most demanding work or daily living tasks; can walk without assistance.
2 (moderate)	Cannot work or maintain demanding aspects of daily life, but able to perform basic activities of self-care; may require assistance in walking.
3 (severe)	Major intellectual incapacity or motor disability, including carrying on conversations, performing daily living tasks; requires walker or personal support in walking, usually motor slowing and clumsiness of arms.
4 (end stage)	Nearly vegetative; intellectual and social comprehension and responses are at very low levels; nearly or absolutely mute; paraplegic with incontinence.

Psychiatric Association, 1987). Although it occurs at all ages, AIDS dementia complex has a greater likelihood of afflicting children (Egan, 1992). In addition to loss of functions from dementia, children with AIDS experience several developmental delays, motor disturbances, and structural abnormalities of the brain (Janssen et al., 1991). Table 5.2 presents the diagnostic staging scheme used for AIDS dementia complex.

DIAGNOSIS AND CLASSIFICATION

Classifications of central nervous involvement of HIV infection have undergone several revisions. Because AIDS dementia complex had a specific and identifiable etiological agent, the *DSM-III-R* criteria for organic mental disorder and the ninth edition of the *International Classification of Diseases* (World Health Organization, 1979) criteria for dementia associated with other illnesses appeared to provide an appropriate diagnosis. The manifestations of AIDS dementia complex are also included among conditions deemed sufficient for an initial diagnosis of AIDS (Janssen et al., 1991). For a number of reasons, however, AIDS dementia complex is now viewed as an incomplete description of the neurocognitive effects of HIV infection. First, although AIDS dementia complex describes a loss of cognitive and motor functioning not attributable to opportunistic infections, malignancies, or systemic HIV disease, dementia does not correctly characterize HIV-related central nervous system disturbances because the cognitive, motor, and behavioral triad does not invariably exist (Markowitz & Perry, 1992; Vitkovic & Koslow, 1994). Second, HIV infection of the brain occurs early in the course of HIV disease, inconsistent with the notion that central nervous system involvement is only associated with AIDS. Finally, earlier and less severe neurological symptoms associated with HIV infection do not approach levels of dysfunction that characterize dementias.

Several new diagnostic labels are now replacing AIDS dementia complex, including HIV-associated neurobehavioral deficit (Bornstein et al., 1992), and *HIV-related* or *HIV-induced organic mental disorder* (Markowitz & Perry, 1992; Perry & Marotta, 1987). The most widely used nomenclature was introduced by the Working Group of the American Academy of Neurology AIDS Task Force (Janssen et al., 1991). The system distinguishes two subclasses of HIV-related disorders: *HIV associated minor cognitive/motor disorder* and *HIV associated dementia complex.* HIV associated minor cognitive/motor disorder is diagnosed in patients with mild functional impairment, including minimal disruption of their social relationships, occupation, or everyday living (Worley & Price, 1992). Severe neuropsychological impairment is diagnosed as HIV associated dementia complex, denoting progressive HIV encephalopathy. The major distinction between the minor and severe subclasses is the degree of functional impairment. The diagnostic classification system, therefore, reserves the term *dementia* for cases with cognitive impairment consistent with other forms of dementia (Worley & Price, 1992). Thus, although HIV associated dementia complex still constitutes an AIDS case-defining condition, manifestations of HIV associated minor cognitive/motor disorder are insufficient for an AIDS diagnosis (Janssen et al., 1991).

HIV associated dementia complex constitutes a combination of clinical symptoms consistent with disturbances of both subcortical and frontal lobe functioning, including cognitive slowing, memory impairment, and behavioral disinhibition (Egan, 1992; R. W. Price & Sidtis, 1992). Available evidence strongly suggests that HIV infection of the brain predominantly affects subcortical brain structures, with attention deficits and cognitive slowing the most predominant features of HIV-related impairment (Krikorian & Worbel, 1991; Martin, Sorensen, Edelstein, & Robertson, 1992; Perdices & Cooper, 1990; Sharer, 1992), and impaired functions of the cerebral cortex, such as language, the least common (Ho, Bredesen, Vinters, & Daar, 1989). Damage to the basal ganglia, three large subcortical structures that play critical roles in the functioning of motor systems, results in involuntary movements such as tremors and reduced motor speed without paralysis (Kandel, Schwartz, & Jessell, 1991).

HIV ENCEPHALOPATHY

Structural damage to the brain because of HIV disease is well established, but clinical signs of higher-order cortical dysfunction, such as verbal responsiveness, aphasia, or emotional reactions, rarely occur (Bornstein et al., 1992; Janssen et al., 1991). HIV-related encephalopathy involves nonspecific disturbances including clouding of consciousness, dysfunctions in short-term memory, and psychomotor slowing (Ostrow, 1990). HIV infection can involve myelopathy, diseases of the spinal cord where dysfunction of the lower extremities is greater than cognitive impairment. Other conditions include peripheral neuropathy, diseases of the peripheral nerves causing both sensory numbness and pain in up to 35% of people with AIDS; and myopathy, slow and progressive weaknesses of the arms and legs (Koppel, 1992). Although neurological symptoms overlap with other AIDS-related conditions, particularly in later HIV disease, HIV associated minor cognitive/motor disorder and HIV associated dementia complex occur independently of other manifestations of HIV infection.

Unfortunately, many of the mechanisms of HIV-related nervous system dysfunction remain poorly understood. HIV-related neuropsychological disturbances do not appear invariably progressive. Symptoms can be static or somewhat reversible, but the determinants of any particular course of disease are unknown. We also do not know whether minor and severe forms of impairment are the same disease entity expressed in different degrees or whether people with minor forms of cognitive decline inevitably progress in severity (Janssen et al., 1991).

HIV-RELATED DISEASE OF THE NERVOUS SYSTEM

HIV was isolated from the brain tissue of people with AIDS very early in the U.S. HIV epidemic (e.g., Ho et al., 1989; Shaw et al., 1985). Autopsies of people who died from AIDS consistently found that 70% to 90% of cases showed significant central nervous system disease (Anders, Guerra, Tomiyasu, Verity, & Vinters, 1986; Bornstein, 1993; Koppel, 1992), with structures most affected by HIV involving information transfer across brain regions including central white matter, the thalamus, areas of the brain stem, and basal ganglia (Markowitz & Perry, 1992).

In addition to postmortem studies, brain imaging research has identified structural damage. Both computed tomography (CT) and magnetic resonance imaging (MRI) have shown that a substantial number of AIDS patients have cerebral cortical atrophy (widening of cortical sulci), scattered brain lesions, and ventricular dilation (Markowitz & Perry, 1992). Electrocephalograhy (EEG) has also identified abnormalities in both slowed Alpha rhythms, associated with states of relaxed wakefulness, and diffuse Theta waves, normally associated with sleep in adults (Kandel et al., 1991; Koppel, 1992). However, structural damage and electrical disturbances in AIDS are not directly linked to functional impairment; some people show clinical signs of dementia without apparent HIV encephalitis, whereas others show gross abnormalities on CT and MRI scans but do not indicate problems in functioning (Sharer, 1992).

AIDS may also involve spinal cord disease, including vacuolar myelopathy, potentially resulting in spasms of the extremities and significant leg weakness (Koppel, 1992; Sharer, 1992). The peripheral nervous system can become involved with polyneuropathy, which causes painful burning or numbness in the feet and lower legs, or inflammatory demyelinating polyneuropathy, resulting in slowed nerve conduction (Janssen et al., 1991).

HIV appears to enter the central nervous system shortly after viral transmission. HIV antigens are found in the cerebrospinal fluid soon after infection (Brew et al., 1989), and some longitudinal studies have detected HIV in the cerebrospinal fluid of asymptomatic cases within 6 to 24 months following HIV seroconversion (Bornstein, 1993; McArthur et al., 1988; Resnick et al., 1985). HIV infection of the central nervous system principally occurs in monocyte-derived cells, including macrophages and microglia, cells sharing the same origin as T-helper lymphocytes and carrying out immunological functions in the brain (Giulian, Vaca, & Noonan, 1990; Sharer, 1992; Worley & Price, 1992). HIV does not, however, directly infect neurons or oligodendrocytes (cells that form insulating myelin sheaths that wrap around axons; Bornstein, 1993; Markowitz & Perry, 1992). HIV infection of macrophages in the brain does, however, both cause the loss of neurons and damage cell dendrites, effectively disabling neurons (Sharer, 1992). Table 5.3 summarizes the areas of the brain most commonly affected by HIV and associated symptoms.

HIV-related neurological damage may have several mechanisms, including autoimmune responses, where cell destruction is caused by immune system attacks on HIV-infected immunological cells. Synergy of HIV with other pathogens may cause additional damage (Markowitz & Perry, 1992). However, most neuronal damage seems to be caused by toxins, either created by viral components of HIV or released from HIV-infected

Table 5.3

Areas of the Brain Most Commonly Affected by HIV

Structures	Symptoms
Frontal lobes	Apathy, depression, trouble concentrating, loss of organizational skills
Limbic system & temporal lobes	Memory loss and language impairment
Basal ganglia	Impaired eye movements, involuntary movements, tremor
Brain stem	Disturbed gait, eye-movement dysfunctions, visual disturbances
Demyelination	Delayed information processing, slowed responses, impaired fine motor skills, incontinence

neighboring cells (Perry & Marotta, 1987). Neurotoxic products of HIV include the viral envelope glucoprotein *gp*120, which disrupts neurons by causing imbalances in intracellular chemistry (Bornstein, 1993; Sharer, 1992). Uninfected macrophages respond to HIV envelope proteins by releasing cytokines, a cascade of which interferes with interneuron communication. Brain cells infected by HIV, particularly the macrophages and microglia, release additional neurotoxins that compromise metabolic activities of neurons (Deicken et al., 1991; Giulian et al., 1990; Sharer, 1992). Diffuse encephalopathies caused by metabolic and toxic disturbances are also identified by MRI scanning conducted with AIDS patients (Bottomley, Hardy, Cousins, Armstrong, & Wagle, 1990).

Concurrent with primary HIV infection of the brain, damage often results from systemic diseases, opportunistic infections, and malignancies within and outside of the nervous system. For example, systemic disease, such as pneumonia, can result in hypoxia that compromises brain functioning (Janssen et al., 1991; Levenson, 1989; R. W. Price & Brew, 1991; Worley & Price, 1992). In addition, reduced cerebral blood flow early in HIV infection can cause encephalopathy (Schielke et al., 1990). Co-infection with other viruses, including HTLV-I, HTLV-II, and cytomegalovirus, may also contribute to brain damage (I. Grant & Heaton, 1990). Finally, neurologic symptoms may stem from iatrogenic factors, such as direct effects and side effects of treatments for HIV infection and associated ailments (Markowitz & Perry, 1992). For example, most antiretroviral medications, including zidovudine, ddC, and ddI, can cause neuropathy and even seizures in extreme cases (Koppel, 1992). Like other aspects of HIV disease, multiple sources of damage co-occur and become superimposed because of underlying immune suppression (Markowitz & Perry, 1992). Multiple etiologies and interrelated symptoms cause complex neuropsychological impairments in AIDS cases, as well as a variety of neuropsychological disturbances across the HIV disease spectrum. Before reviewing specific neuropsychological impairments related to HIV associated minor cognitive/motor disorder and HIV associated dementia complex, it is important to note several methodological constraints in this literature.

METHODOLOGICAL ISSUES

Research on neuropsychological impairment resulting from HIV disease began in response to a crisis and without the benefit of previous studies.

HIV-related neuropsychological impairment research shares many of the problems encountered by early research on other forms of neurological disease and dementias (I. Grant & Heaton, 1990). Studies commonly use diverse assessment batteries, ranging from brief mental status screening examinations to full neuropsychological batteries. Research has often failed to include external behavioral indices of daily functioning to corroborate neuropsychological testing data (Markowitz & Perry, 1992). Finally, non-neurological factors may cause direct and indirect effects on test results. Issues of sample selection, sample sizes, and criteria used to define degrees of impairment also limit study findings.

Confounding Factors

Studies of HIV-related neuropsychological impairment have generally failed to control simultaneous causes of disrupted test performance. For example, depression potentially confounds neuropsychological studies by compromising cognitive processing speed, attention, concentration, and motor functioning (Hinkin et al., 1992; Van Gorp, Satz, Hinkin, Evans, & Miller, 1989). Decreases in motivation that occur with depression may also adversely affect neuropsychological test performance. For example, depression scales correlate with neuropsychological test scores, and depression scores have accounted for some observed neuropsychological deficits in HIV disease (E. N. Miller et al., 1990). In contrast with earlier findings, however, there is substantial evidence that depression does not seriously threaten the interpretation of neuropsychological test findings from most people with HIV infection (Markowitz & Perry, 1992). Many studies fail to identify meaningful associations between measures of depression and functional impairment (I. Grant et al., 1993), performance on standardized neuropsychological batteries (Bornstein, 1993; Hinkin et al., 1992), screening measures of cognitive functioning and attention (Belkin et al., 1992), and tests of memory (Egan, Chiswick, Brettle, & Goodwin, 1993). Relationships between depression and neuropsychological testing may be attenuated because of the restricted range of minimal neuropsychological impairment during asymptomatic HIV infection and the severe impairment of later phases of HIV associated dementia complex.

Other potential confounds in this literature threaten internal validity. Concomitant HIV-related opportunistic illnesses, past and current prescription and illicit drug use, sleep deprivation, and nutritional status may potentially confound neuropsychological studies. In addition, education and socioeconomic status may influence neuropsychological test performance, particularly in studies of gay men with higher education and of injection drug users, whose education and socioeconomic status are typically low (Krikorian & Worbel, 1991; Selnes & Miller, 1992). Antiretroviral medications may confound studies because they disrupt neuropsychological performance through fatigue and reduced concentration (Koppel, 1992; Markowitz & Perry, 1992). On the other hand, zidovudine, particularly at higher doses, may reduce cognitive symptoms of HIV associated dementia complex and therefore improve neuropsychological test performance (Bornstein, 1993; Catalan & Burgess, 1991; Koppel, 1992; Schmitt et al., 1988; Worley & Price, 1992). In either case, studies of neurological functioning of people taking zidovudine and perhaps other antiretroviral medications could be confounded by effects and side effects of these drugs (Clifford, Jacoby, Miller, Seyfried, & Glicksman, 1990). However, the degree of confound in specific studies is often not known, because evidence is inconclusive that antiretrovirals affect cognitive performance, and in fact, some studies fail to document such effects (e.g., Egan et al., 1992).

Sample Selection and Sample Sizes

The majority of studies on neuropsychological sequelae of HIV infection have investigated predominantly White gay men who have high levels of education, are from higher socioeconomic statuses, and are members of cohorts followed in U.S. epidemic centers. Although some studies have targeted injection drug users (e.g., Egan et al., 1992; Maxwell et al., 1991), few have represented heterogeneous samples of people with HIV infection, and few have included women (Van Gorp, Lamb, & Schmitt, 1993). Also limiting most studies outside of longitudinal cohorts is ignorance of when participants seroconverted, making it impossible to track effects of HIV on the central nervous system over time (I. Grant & Heaton, 1990). Additional sampling problems result from methods used for defining symptomatic and asymptomatic comparison groups. For example, Janssen et al. (1991) included men with constitutional symptoms of HIV infection in a group classified as asymptomatic, even though constitutional symptoms would have defined these same men as symptomatic in studies using the CDC staging system.

This literature also tends to draw conclusions from small samples, often with less than 30 participants (e.g., I. Grant et al., 1987; Van Gorp et al., 1989). A literature review of 56 studies of AIDS-related dementia included only 7 reports with more than 50 participants and 17 with more than 20 (Perry & Marotta, 1987). Studies with small sample sizes have also tended to use large batteries of neuropsychological tests, conducting multiple statistical comparisons without correcting for chance associations. For example, Krikorian and Worbel (1991) used eight measures of neuropsychological functioning and two measures of psychological distress in a study of 48 participants divided into three groups that were compared using multivariate stepwise statistical techniques—all factors that seriously limit the reliability of results. Most early studies found evidence for neuropsychological impairment in asymptomatic HIV infection that has failed to replicate in subsequent studies with larger sample sizes.

Criteria for Defining Impairment

The prevalence of neuropsychological deficits in a given sample is a function of the criteria used to define impaired neuropsychological test performance (Bornstein et al., 1992). Studies using lenient criteria to define impairment, such as scores falling within one standard deviation of the mean of a control group, will necessarily differ in prevalence rates from studies using more stringent criteria, such as greater than two standard deviations above a control group mean. More extensive test batteries also yield higher rates of impairment because of the greater likelihood of identifying performance deficits. Stringent criteria and less extensive test batteries are therefore less sensitive to subtle neuropsychological changes. To address these problems, some studies have used multiple performance criteria for defining impairment, internally controlling for differences among criteria (e.g., E. N. Miller et al., 1990). Thus, rates of neuropsychological impairment at various points along the HIV disease spectrum are directly affected by definitions of test performance.

Other Methodological Issues

The literature on neuropsychological sequelae of HIV infection is limited by the characteristics of comparison and control groups. For example, groups of HIV-positive and -negative people are often confounded by history of substance abuse. Furthermore, tests selected for study inclusion necessarily limit the scope of neuropsychological functions investigated. Finally, studies usually lack non-psychometric data to corroborate neuropsychological test findings (Bornstein, 1993; Markowitz & Perry, 1992). Such external data are essential because neuropsychological test performance does not necessarily translate to impaired occupational, social, and everyday functioning.

NEUROPSYCHOLOGICAL MANIFESTATIONS

Although HIV enters the central nervous system shortly after infection (R. W. Price et al., 1988) and many individuals with AIDS suffer cognitive decline, little is known about the mechanisms and course of HIV-related neuropsychological disorders. Available research can, however, describe neuropsychological decrements at early, asymptomatic, and later phases of HIV disease. Figure 5.1 shows the typical time line of neurological disorders in relation to the course of HIV disease, with most central nervous system manifestations occurring at later stages of AIDS. Unfortunately, most studies of neuropsychological sequelae of HIV infection have relied on cross-sectional research designs. Only a few studies have used longitu-

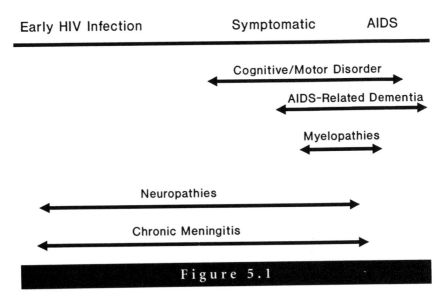

Figure 5.1

Manifestations of nervous system disease over the course of HIV infection.

dinal prospective designs to provide data on the progression of neuropsychological impairment. Because study participants are usually grouped on the basis of early, asymptomatic, and later infection, each phase can be described by characteristic types and degrees of neurological impairment.

Early HIV Infection

Although most people do not experience cognitive or motor symptoms early in the course of infection, a small number of newly infected persons have some signs of neurological impairment. Acute meningitis and meningoencephalitis occur soon after HIV crosses the blood–brain barrier (Bornstein et al., 1992; Markowitz & Perry, 1992; R. W. Price et al., 1988). When they occur, early neurological symptoms usually overlap with other acute symptoms. Early nervous system infection has symptoms common to non-HIV-related meningitis, including fatigue, headache, sensitivity to light (photophobia), pain around the eyes and facial areas, and leg weakness (Tindall et al., 1992; Worley & Price, 1992).

The prevalence of early neurological symptoms differs across HIV subgroups, particularly age groups. Infants and young children demonstrate early nervous system involvement more often than adolescents and adults, with progressive encephalopathy in children beginning as early as 2 months (Janssen et al., 1991). Young children with HIV infection usually fail to reach developmental milestones, such as sitting up and walking, or lose abilities they once had achieved (Ho et al., 1989; Janssen et al., 1991). Children with HIV infection otherwise show the same features of neuropsychological impairment observed in adults. The course of central nervous system involvement varies in children and, as in adults, can be either progressive or stable (Aronow et al., 1988; Worley & Price, 1992). Unfortunately, little is known about possible differences in neuropsychological symptoms between men and women with early infection.

Asymptomatic HIV Infection

Much research, discussion, and controversy has been devoted to possible central nervous system dysfunction before significant immune suppression and opportunistic illnesses (I. Grant & Heaton, 1990). Several studies with small sample sizes and extensive testing batteries have demonstrated HIV-related neuropsychological impairment prior to other HIV-related illnesses (e.g., I. Grant et al., 1987). Early neuropsychological dysfunction would suggest that HIV can cause insidious damage to the central nervous system prior to symptomatic HIV disease (Markowitz & Perry, 1992). Using a one-standard-deviation difference from a control group mean as a criterion for neuropsychological impairment, Bornstein et al. (1992) classified 26% of HIV-positive men as neurocognitively impaired, relative to 15% of HIV-negative men. Bornstein et al. showed that degrees of neurocognitive impairment for the HIV-positive sample were twice the magnitude of those observed among HIV negatives. The study also found that neuropsychological impairment was not accounted for by clinical depression and that neuropsychological test performance agreed with self-reported ratings of functional limitations. In another study, Saykin et al. (1989) found that asymptomatic HIV-positives met study criteria defining neuropsychological impairment significantly more often than did a control group, but HIV-positive people on average performed within normal limits. Thus, studies that find neuropsychological deficits in asymptomatic HIV infection suggest that only a subgroup, and probably a small group at that, evidences such decline.

The MACS cohort provided data from 727 HIV-positive asymptomatic gay men, 84 men with symptoms of HIV disease, and 769 HIV-negative men (E. N. Miller et al., 1990). Using an extensive neuropsychological battery, including the Trail Making Test, Digit Span, a verbal fluency test, the Grooved Pegboard Test, the Symbol Digit Modalities Test, and the Rey Auditory Verbal Learning Test, the study did not identify any significant differences between HIV-positive asymptomatic and HIV-negative men. Using a two-standard-deviation difference from the HIV-negative group mean as a criterion for impairment, Miller et al. classified 6% of HIV-positive men as impaired relative to 4% of HIV-negative men. When the criterion for impairment was relaxed to one standard deviation from the control group mean, Miller et al. classified 37% of HIV-positive and 34% of HIV-negative men as neurocognitively impaired. Miller et al. also failed to find relationships between immunologic markers and neuropsychological functioning. Subdividing men on the basis of duration of HIV infection also did not show any associations with impairment. These findings strongly suggest that neuropsychological deficits in asymptomatic individuals are rare and that changes that do occur are usually modest.

The degree to which these results are generalizable to women, however, is not known.

Additional research has failed to find neuropsychological impairment in otherwise asymptomatic HIV-positive people. Selnes et al. (1990), also from the MACS, administered a battery of neuropsychological tests to 238 HIV-positive and 170 HIV-negative men over a period of one and a half years. The study did not find significant differences between the two groups in neuropsychological changes over time. Furthermore, HIV-positive men did not decline in neuropsychological functioning over time. Consistent with these findings, Egan et al. (1992) found no significant cognitive impairment prior to the onset of other HIV-related symptoms in a large cohort of HIV-positive injection drug users. Other studies using more extensive neuropsychological batteries (e.g., E. M. Martin et al., 1993) and experimental memory tasks (e.g., Clifford et al., 1990) have failed to distinguish asymptomatic HIV-positive from HIV-negative persons, and studies that have identified central nervous system electrophysiological and structural changes in HIV-positive individuals, such as EEG abnormalities and cerebral atrophy, have not consistently related such abnormalities to clinical impairment.

Little evidence, therefore, supports the notion that HIV associated dementia complex is a progressive disorder that has an early onset and evolves during asymptomatic periods (Bornstein et al., 1992; Catalan & Thornton, 1993). An absence of detectable cognitive decline over asymptomatic HIV infection further suggests that HIV-related neuropsychological impairment follows the development of substantial immune suppression and usually coincides with opportunistic illnesses, although not necessarily opportunistic illnesses of the central nervous system (Selnes et al., 1990). When the immune system functions relatively healthily, viral expression of HIV remains generally suppressed in the central nervous system. Therefore, a competent immune system may delay the onset of HIV-related cognitive disruptions, encephalitis, and opportunistic illness (Sharer, 1992). In summary, although some people may have acute meningitis near the time of seroconversion, asymptomatic phases of HIV infection are rarely associated with impaired occupational, social, or everyday functioning (Worley & Price, 1992). However, these conclusions remain tentative because some studies, mostly with small sample sizes and extensive batteries, have identified a small subgroup of asymptomatic HIV-positive individuals with cognitive deficits. In contrast with the controversy over cognitive and motor impairment in asymptomatic phases of HIV infection, there is greater acceptance of the more frequent neuropsychological deficits in later phases of HIV disease.

Later HIV Infection and AIDS

Neuropsychological dysfunctions of HIV infection are most likely to occur at times of severe immune suppression (Mapou & Law, 1994). Studies have found neurocognitive deficits in 40% to 50% of people with symptoms of HIV infection and 33% to 87% of people with AIDS (I. Grant et al., 1993; R. W. Price & Brew, 1991; R. W. Price et al., 1988). As many as 15% of AIDS cases demonstrate abnormal brain structures on CT and MRI scans (Ostrow, 1990). Studies of the clinical symptomatology of HIV-associated neurological impairment suggest that one third of cases eventually develop severe impairment, one third show mild disturbances, and one third experience few or no neurocognitive symptoms (Bornstein, 1993). Even when neuropsychological impairment does occur, only a minority of HIV-positive people progress to dementia (Egan et al., 1992). Thus, although many individuals with later HIV infection do not demonstrate serious cognitive decline, a sizable proportion of AIDS cases do have some degree of neurological impairment.

A broad range of neurocognitive disturbances occur in later-stage HIV infection. The earliest symptoms include diffuse and nonspecific symptoms such as lethargy; social withdrawal; psychomotor slowing; attention, concentration, and retrieval deficits; derailed train of thought; increased difficulty with complex tasks; forgetfulness; clumsiness; and complaints of slowed thinking (Janssen et al., 1991; R. W. Price & Brew, 1991; Sharer, 1992; Worley & Price, 1992). These symptoms reflect HIV associated minor cognitive/motor disorder. Severe cognitive disturbances of HIV associated dementia complex most often occur late in HIV infection and include declines in social, occupational, and daily functioning; confusion; disorientation; motor losses; and eventual degeneration into a vegetative state.

HIV-related neurocognitive impairment reflects the subcortical brain structures that are known to be most damaged by HIV (Koppel, 1992). Most commonly, declines occur in information-processing speed and efficiency; impaired memory and learning; and motor disabilities. Cognitive slowing is, however, the most widely observed feature of HIV-associated neurocognitive impairment (Derix, de Gans, Stam, & Portegies, 1990; I. Grant et al., 1993; Navia, Jordan, & Price, 1986). Reaction-time tasks index cognitive-processing speeds because these measures are sensitive to cognitive dysfunctions without ceiling effects. Simple reaction-time tasks, where a key is pressed as quickly as possible in response to the onset of a stimulus, consistently show that people with HIV infection have slower response times than do HIV-negative control groups (e.g., E. M. Martin, Sorensen, Edelstein, & Robertson, 1992). In addition, choice reaction-time tasks, where a key is pressed as quickly as possible with one hand in response to a target stimulus and another key is pressed with the other hand in response to a different stimulus, have demonstrated cognitive slowing in HIV infection. E. M. Martin, Sorensen, Edelstein et al. (1992) found that both asymptomatic and symptomatic HIV-positive gay men have slower decision-making speed in choice reaction time relative to their HIV-negative counterparts. Similar results have been found on choice reaction-time tasks with injection drug users (Egan et al., 1993). In a study of hemophiliacs with known dates of HIV seroconversion, duration of time since contracting HIV infection correlated with declines in decision speed as indexed by choice reaction time (Kokkevi et al., 1991). It should be noted, however, that most reaction-time differences occur between symptomatic HIV-positive and HIV-negative groups rather than among gradations of performance within HIV positives.

In addition to slowed cognitive processing speed, attention and concentration deficits also occur among some individuals with HIV infection. E. M. Martin, Sorensen, Robertson, Edelstein, and Chirurgi (1992) found that HIV-positive men performed less accurately on a subtle visual attention task relative to HIV-negative men. Another study using the same sample reported by E. M. Martin, Sorensen, Robertson, et al. (1992) showed further evidence for disrupted attention processes using the Stroop color–word naming task (E. M. Martin, Robertson, Edelstein, et al., 1992). HIV-positive men had more difficulty than HIV-negative men with controlled cognitive functions on a Stroop task that relies on effortful, voluntary actions that place greater demands on attention. Additional evidence from divergent neuropsychological measures has also suggested that cognitive and perceptual information-processing disturbances occur at later stages of HIV infection (e.g., Egan et al., 1993).

HIV infection, particularly during later symptomatic phases, also involves deficits in learning and memory. People with HIV infection perform less accurately than HIV-negative control groups on tests of long-term and short-term memory and on verbal learning tasks (Bornstein et al., 1992; Egan et al., 1993; Krikorian & Worbel, 1991; Wilkie, Eisdorfer, Morgan, Loewenstein, & Szapocznik, 1990). In one study using a neuropsychological battery, HIV-positive gay men differed in short-term and long-term verbal memory when compared with a medical patient control group matched for education and socioeconomic status (Sinforiani et al., 1991). HIV-positive injection drug users have also demonstrated short-term memory deficits relative to control groups (McKegney et al., 1990).

Cognitive deficits in HIV infection are also related to psychomotor functioning. E. N. Miller et al. (1990) found that symptomatic men in the MACS cohort showed the greatest degree of neurocognitive deficits on measures of manual dexterity and psychomotor speed, including the Grooved Pegboard Test, Symbol Digit Modalities, and the Trail Making Test. HIV-positive injection drug users also have difficulty with the Finger Tapping Test, an index of fine motor speed (McKegney et al., 1990). Motor slowing, leg weakness, and loss of mobility can occur in the absence of other cognitive and intellectual dysfunctions (Markowitz & Perry, 1992; Worley & Price, 1992). In summary, information-processing speed, attentional processes, learning, memory, and motor abilities are affected by HIV infection. Deficits are most apparent when measured by sensitive cognitive tasks at later infection stages.

The risk for neuropsychological impairment increases as HIV disease progresses. Twenty-five percent of people with AIDS develop clinically significant cognitive impairment within 9 months of their first AIDS-defining condition, and another 25% show impaired functioning within 1 year of diagnosis (Markowitz & Perry, 1992). Rather than starting out slowly and gradually progressing during asymptomatic phases, HIV-associated neuropsychological impairment seems to follow the onset of systemic HIV manifestations, and its progression usually occurs rapidly (I. Grant & Heaton, 1990; Selnes et al., 1990). Although both longer duration of infection and accelerated rates of T-helper cell declines are associated with neuropsychological impairment (Bornstein, 1993), deteriorated immune functioning does not reliably predict neurocognitive dysfunction (Markowitz & Perry, 1992). Because progression of central nervous system disease does not necessarily follow immune suppression, both immune and neurological declines are correlated but not causally linked (I. Grant & Heaton, 1990). Cognitive disturbances coincide with immune suppression, making it likely that neuropsychological impairment will occur with illnesses (Egan et al., 1992; E. N. Miller et al., 1990). Later HIV infection therefore involves simultaneous vulnerability to HIV-related symptoms, HIV-related neurological disorders, and opportunistic illness (Selnes et al., 1990). Immune system decline in later HIV infection results in the nervous system itself becoming vulnerable to opportunistic infections and malignancies that have entirely different neurocognitive consequences.

OPPORTUNISTIC ILLNESSES OF THE CENTRAL NERVOUS SYSTEM

Advanced immune suppression leads to increased susceptibility to infections and malignancies of multiple organ systems, including the nervous system (see Table 5.4). Diagnoses of AIDS-related central nervous system

Table 5.4

AIDS-Related Diseases of the Central Nervous System

Manifestation	Causal agent
Opportunistic viral infections	Cytomegalovirus
	Herpes simplex I & II
	Herpes zoster
	Papovavirus (PML)
Fungal and protozoan infections	Toxoplasmosis
	Cryptococcus
	Candida
	Mycobacterium
Malignancies	Primary lymphoma
	Metastatic lymphoma
	Metastatic Kaposi's sarcoma
Cerebrovascular conditions	Hemorrhage
	Infarction

opportunistic illnesses are made through CT and MRI scanning, attempts to medically treat neurological symptoms, and brain biopsy. Among the less frequent initial AIDS diagnoses, nervous system disorders often develop during late stages of AIDS.

Cytomegalovirus

This infection is highly prevalent, with 95% of HIV-positive gay men carrying antibodies for cytomegalovirus (Markowitz & Perry, 1992). Although an infrequent manifestation, cytomegalovirus can cause meningoencephalitis, resulting in clouding of consciousness and other disabling symptoms (Worley & Price, 1992). Cytomegalovirus infection causes several other neuropsychological disturbances (McArthur, 1987). More commonly, cytomegalovirus infects the retinas (CMV retinitis), a serious threat of partial and complete blindness. Cytomegalovirus can also cause demyelination of brain white matter and a subacute encephalitis (Koppel, 1992). Cytomegalovirus may synergistically interact with HIV and other viruses to cause an array of nervous system disorders.

Progressive Multifocal Leukoencephalopathy (PML)

This demyelinating disease is caused by activation of a latent papovavirus infection (McArthur, 1987). Progressive deterioration of white matter occurs because the papovavirus attacks oligodendrocytes, resulting in loss of nerve fiber insulation (Krupp et al., 1992). Changes in mental status, memory loss, motor weaknesses, loss of vision and other sensory functions, and decreased mobility are common consequences of PML (Koppel, 1992; Krupp et al., 1992). Symptoms of PML develop gradually and significantly reduce AIDS survival time.

Toxoplasmosis

The protozoan Toxoplasma *gondii* principally affects the central nervous system as a generalized encephalopathy as well as by causing massive brain lesions (Koppel, 1992; Mariuz & Luft, 1992). Toxoplasmosis is the most common central nervous system infection in adults with AIDS (Koppel, 1992). Toxoplasmosis encephalopathy includes headache, fever, confusion, lethargy, changes in personality, and delirium (Bredesen, Levy, & Rosenblum, 1988). Focal neurologic damage resulting from brain lesions can cause seizures and specific functional deficits (Levy, Kaminsky, & Bredesen, 1988; R. W. Price & Brew, 1991; Worley & Price, 1992). In general, cerebral toxoplasmosis progresses rapidly and seriously threatens permanent brain damage. However, once diagnosed, there are several available medications that effectively treat toxoplasmosis and provide relatively fast symptom relief (Aronow et al., 1988).

Cryptococcal Meningitis

Caused by the fungus cryptococcus, an encapsulated yeast, Cryptococcal meningitis is the most common central nervous system fungal infection in AIDS, affecting up to 25% of cases (Koppel, 1992; Masci et al., 1992). The symptoms of Cryptococcal meningitis are similar to those of other meningitides, including neck stiffness, headache, photophobia, lethargy, changes in mental functioning, confusion, and sometimes nausea and vomiting. Symptoms can range from mild to severe (Aronow et al., 1988; Worley & Price, 1992) and can result in encephalitis, causing symptoms that mimic depression (Markowitz & Perry, 1992).

Lymphoma

Central nervous system lymphomas occur in 5% of AIDS cases (Worley & Price, 1992). Although the brain is rarely the site of primary lymphoma, people with AIDS are nearly 100 times more likely to develop primary central nervous system lymphoma than the general population (Koppel, 1992). In addition, B-cell lymphomas that originate as systemic disease can spread secondarily, resulting in metastatic lymphoma to the central nervous system, causing single or multiple lesions (Levy et al., 1988). Symptoms include headache, lethargy, and damage to cranial nerves, as well as focal damage caused by specific sites of tumor growth.

Other Nervous System Complications

HIV-related conditions may become disseminated to the central and peripheral nervous systems, although most of these occurrences are relatively rare. Herpes simplex viruses I and II can cause encephalitis and meningitis, with acute symptoms of headache, fever, seizures, and abrupt behavioral changes (Koppel, 1992). In addition to its characteristic painful outbreaks of rash, herpes zoster virus can also cause encephalitis (Koppel,

1992). Candidiasis, a common fungal infection in HIV, can cause brain abscesses in people with AIDS (Koppel, 1992). Coccidioidomycosis and histoplasmosis, also fungi, can cause chronic meningitis (Koppel, 1992). Mycobacterium infection can cause meningitis and brain abscesses (Aronow et al., 1988). Neurosyphilis may develop or recur with suppressed immunity and is more difficult to treat than primary syphilis (Aronow et al., 1988). Spread of Kaposi's sarcoma to the central nervous system is also possible, although rare (Levy & Bredesen, 1988). In addition to infections and malignancies, people with AIDS can suffer strokes because of changes in cerebral vascular walls and blood flow, as well as cerebral hemorrhage resulting from HIV-related changes in blood clotting factors (Koppel, 1992). Finally, it should be noted that many causal mechanisms of HIV-related diseases of the nervous system are still unknown, particularly diseases affecting the peripheral nervous system.

NEUROPSYCHOLOGICAL ASSESSMENT

Neuropsychological testing in HIV infection is most useful for evaluating subjective reports of decline in cognitive functions, including but not limited to attention, concentration, abstraction, reasoning, visual–perceptual skills, problem solving, mental and motor processing speed, and language (Egan, 1992). Neuropsychological evaluations inform clinicians of cognitive deficits and can disconfirm mistaken beliefs about losses in cognitive abilities (Greenwood, 1991). Factors such as expectancies, anxiety, depression, and systemic illness can contribute to reports of the presence or absence of early neuropsychological symptoms (Markowitz & Perry, 1992). Because most cognitive changes in HIV infection are subtle, clinical mental status exams lack adequate sensitivity for reliable assessment (I. Grant & Heaton, 1990; Markowitz & Perry, 1992). Therefore, comprehensive neuropsychological evaluations that assess multiple mental faculties, although time consuming, labor intensive, and expensive, remain the most effective method for evaluating cognitive capacities.

Several authorities have suggested comprehensive neuropsychological assessment batteries that provide optimal sensitivity to neurocognitive deficits associated with HIV infection. For example, Janssen et al. (1991) suggested assessing attention and concentration (Trail Making Test A; Continuous Performance Test), information processing speed (Trail Making Test A and B; Digit Symbol Modalities; choice reaction time task), motor functioning (Finger Tapping Test; Grooved Pegboard Test; Thumb–Finger Sequential Test), abstract reasoning (Wisconsin Card Sorting Test; Halstead Category Test), visual–spatial skills (Weschler Adult Intelligence Scale–Revised Block Design), concentration (Serial Sevens; Digit Span), memory and learning (Rey Auditory Verbal Learning Test; California Verbal Learning Test; Weschler Memory Scale Verbal Reproduction and Logical Prose Tests), and speech–language abilities (Verbal Fluency Test, Vocabulary, Boston Naming Test). Although Janssen et al. recommended these areas of assessment and suggested tests for measuring them, they did not propose a standardized testing battery.

To address the need for a standardized neuropsychological battery for use with HIV infection, a workshop sponsored by the National Institute of Mental Health assembled a 7- to 9-hour battery for assessing HIV-related cognitive impairment (N. Butters et al., 1990). Tests were compiled with the intention of maximizing sensitivity to cognitive functions most affected by HIV infection. Both widely used standardized clinical tests and tasks taken from experimental cognitive psychology were included to broaden the battery's complexity and increase its sensitivity. The battery included 10 neurocognitive domains assessed by 26 tests (see Table 5.5). Administration of the full battery was intended to cast a broad net across a wide range of cognitive and motor functions.

Unfortunately, administration of the battery recommended by N. Butters et al. (1990) posed several limitations. Including experimental cognitive psychology tasks limits the use of the battery in many clinical settings. Furthermore, experimental psychology procedures do not provide normative testing data and cannot define clinical diagnostic criteria (N. Butters et al., 1990). The battery is also long and taxing for both the test taker and administrator. For these reasons, Butters et al. suggested an abbreviated form of the battery that requires only 1 to 2 hours to administer.

Clinical findings from a neuropsychological battery usually lack sufficient sensitivity and specificity to diagnose HIV-related neuropsychological impairment (Janssen et al., 1991; Markowitz & Perry, 1992). Neuropsychological testing is most limited early in the course of HIV-related central nervous system disease. When present, early symptoms are usually subclinical and cannot be reliably detected by standard clinical instruments (Martin, Sorensen, Robertson, et al., 1992). In addition, although neu-

Table 5.5

Neuropsychological Test Battery Recommended by a Workshop Sponsored by the National Institute of Mental Health

Cognitive function	Assessment instrument
Premorbid intelligence	*WAIS-R Vocabulary
	National Adult Reading Test
Attention	WMS-R Digit Span
	*WMS-R Visual Span
Processing speed	Sternberg Search Task
	Simple and Choice Reaction Time
	*Paced Auditory Serial
	Addition Test
Memory	*California Verbal Learning Test
	Working Memory Test
	Modified Visual Reproduction Test
Abstraction	Category Test
	Trails Making Test A and B
Language	Boston Naming Test
	Letter and Category Fluency Test
Visual–spatial ability	Embedded Figures Test
	Money's Standardized Road-Map Test of Direction Sense
	Digit Symbol Substitution
Construction ability	Block Design Test
	Tactile Performance Test
Motor abilities	Grooved Pegboard
	Finger Tapping Test
	Grip Strength
Psychological distress	Diagnostic Interview Schedule
	*Hamilton Depression Rating Scale
	*State–Trait Anxiety Inventory
	Mini-Mental Status Examination

NOTE: Source: Butters et al., 1990. WMS-R = Weschler Memory Scale—Revised; WAIS-R = Weschler Adult Intelligence Scale—Revised
*Tests included in the abbreviated battery recommended by Butters et al. (1990).

ropsychological tests can suggest focal lesions, underlying disease processes cannot be determined. The interpretation of neuropsychological tests therefore requires consultation with neurologists and infectious disease specialists (Ostrow, Grant, & Atkinson, 1988; Tross & Hirsch, 1988).

Differential diagnosis of cognitive dysfunction and affective disorders can pose another obstacle to neuropsychological assessment, particularly in earlier phases of infection (J. C. Holland & Tross, 1985). Even when symptoms of depression and anxiety are somewhat distinct from those of mild neurocognitive impairment, negative emotions can disrupt neuropsychological test performance. Neurological conditions are often accompanied by overlapping symptoms with psychological distress, including indifference, apathy, social withdrawal, emotional blunting, and lethargy (Navia et al., 1986). Reduced motivation, attention, and concentration can impede neuropsychological assessment, so most batteries include evaluations of negative affective states.

People with asymptomatic HIV infection may report neuropsychological impairment when test results fail to identify even subtle cognitive deficits. Thus, subjective complaints, neurological signs, and brain imaging often do not correspond with laboratory findings (I. Grant et al., 1987; Janssen et al., 1991; Markowitz & Perry, 1992). Neuropsychological evaluations in HIV infection require substantial expertise, including familiarity with HIV disease of the central nervous system, AIDS-related opportunistic illnesses, and corroborating information of occupational, social, and everyday functioning. Interdisciplinary approaches help to fully evaluate cognitive functions in HIV infection and to assure careful medical follow-up.

HIV-ASSOCIATED FUNCTIONAL INCAPACITIES

Physical disabilities that may result from neurological complications of HIV infection range from complete absence of impairment to severe disability. People with central nervous system HIV infection, determined through either examinations of cerebral spinal fluid or radiological imaging, are often completely asymptomatic of neuropsychological impairment. In HIV associated minor cognitive/motor disorder, most complex daily living skills are usually minimally disrupted (Janssen et al., 1991).

Asymptomatic HIV infection usually does not involve cognitive and motor dysfunctions (Selnes et al., 1990). Early symptoms of HIV infection may include slowed information-processing speed and deficits in verbal memory, but neither of these cognitive domains is affected to the degree of impairment seen in everyday functioning (Sinforiani et al., 1991). Apathy, mental slowing, social withdrawal, and avoidance of complex tasks may occur and pose problems in differential diagnosis with clinical depression, especially as HIV-related illnesses emerge (Markowitz & Perry, 1992). Although decrements in cognitive functioning may mark the onset of progressive cognitive losses (I. Grant & Heaton, 1990), mild forms of impairment do not provide prognostic indicators of HIV associated dementia complex.

HIV associated dementia complex and most opportunistic infections and malignancies of the central nervous system pose serious threats to daily functioning in later phases of HIV infection. Impairment can be progressive and affect multiple cognitive and motor abilities. Opportunistic illnesses may cause diffuse damage or focal lesions. Cognitive and motor disorders related to HIV infection most likely co-occur with systemic manifestations of HIV disease and opportunistic illnesses outside of the nervous system (Markowitz & Perry, 1992). Concerns may eventually arise about home safety, wandering, confusion, severe memory loss, and basic motor disturbances. Cognitive and motor impairments also limit coping and adaptation, further complicating efforts to adjust psychologically to HIV disease (Krikorian & Worbel, 1991).

CONCLUSION

The prospect of losing mental and sensory abilities is one of the most frightening aspects of HIV disease. People who expect to develop cognitive dysfunctions often become hypervigilant and monitor their day-to-day activities and performance of even simple tasks. Typical forgetfulness or lack of concentration under stress can be misinterpreted as the beginnings of dementia. Although neuropsychological testing helps to evaluate subjective complaints of cognitive decline, most tests do not detect subtle symptoms. In addition, individuals with HIV infection are usually aware of the potential for neuropsychological impairment and may have known others who have developed neurocognitive dysfunctions. Thus, expectations for HIV-related neuropsychological symptoms create anxieties that amplify normal lapses in cognitive functioning.

HIV-positive individuals, their families, and others in their support networks often benefit from education and counseling about the risks of cognitive decline (Markowitz & Perry, 1992). HIV patients should be aware that significant deterioration in mental abilities rarely occurs before systemic illness and that many people with HIV infection do not ever decline in neurocognitive functioning. Counseling may educate about how symptoms of depression, anxiety, and medication side effects can mimic HIV-related neuropsychological symptoms. HIV-positive individuals should be informed of the distinctions between HIV-related encephalopathy and opportunistic illnesses of the central nervous system, as well as the different treatment options available for each. Finally, counseling may emphasize that if neuropsychological disorders should develop, they are most often treatable, and clients should be encouraged to seek evaluation and treatment.

Perhaps as much as any other dimension of HIV disease, central nervous system involvement demands the integration of services from a multidisciplinary intervention team. Neurologists, infectious disease specialists, and radiologists definitively diagnose HIV-related nervous system conditions. Functional evaluations offered by neuropsychological assessment help to determine the degree of impairment suffered. Behavioral interventions may help ameliorate functional impairments, including altering environmental obstacles to facilitate occupational and daily functioning, as well as learning and memory aides. Functional adaptation improves through interventions already widely used by neuropsychologists and rehabilitation specialists to treat neurocognitive disorders, regardless of their cause.

6

Social Sequelae

Epidemics have far-reaching social consequences. Public knowledge that an invisible microbe is causing illness and death can bring irrational fears and widespread panic. The history of world epidemics shows that fears ultimately cause the persecution of those associated with the disease. For example, the 14th-century plague was viewed as divine punishment for sinful behavior; the uninfected often became so terrified they blamed the epidemic on already socially ostracized groups (Kishlansky et al., 1991). Many towns in Germany where plague ran rampant sought out Jews as scapegoats, putting many innocent people to death. Similarly, the cholera epidemic of the 1930s was viewed as a moral punishment for unclean and sinful behavior (Herek, 1990). Not until the early to middle 1900s did various forms of prejudice against cancer patients begin to give way to care and compassion, although many discriminatory practices against cancer patients still exist (Stahly, 1988).

The social sanctions suffered by victims of disease fit well under the broader rubric of *social stigmatization*. The term *stigma* refers to a visible mark, such as a brand or tattoo, used to disgrace, shame, condemn, or socially ostracize (Herek, 1990). Stigmas are therefore socially ascribed to discredit those who bear a mark of social disapproval (Goffman, 1963).

Discrediting occurs when a stigma is openly known and visible to others and stigmatization occurs to the extent that a person loses social stature and becomes socially ostracized (Goffman, 1963).

The social construction of HIV–AIDS in the United States has made it among the most stigmatizing medical conditions in modern history. AIDS is viewed as much more than a transmissible and lethal disease (Herek, 1990). HIV-related stigmatization is a second branch of the HIV epidemic, an epidemic of fear, prejudice, and discrimination against people with HIV infection and AIDS (Kegeles, Coates, Christopher, & Lazarus, 1989). Although the contributing factors may differ in different cultures, stigmatization of HIV infection occurs across societies (Woo, 1992). In the United States, several factors contribute to the stigmatization of HIV infection, including the following: misinformation about risks of HIV transmission, prejudicial attitudes against groups most affected by the epidemic, the sexual and drug-using behaviors that transmit HIV, and fears more generally associated with sickness and death (Herek & Glunt, 1988; see Figure 6.1).

HIV- and AIDS-related stigma includes all of the adverse attitudes, beliefs, and behaviors directed at individuals perceived as HIV infected (Herek & Glunt, 1988). Herek (1990) identified six general dimensions of social stigmas: (a) *concealability*, the extent to which a condition is hidden or apparent to others; (b) *disruptiveness*, the extent to which it interferes with social interactions and relationships; (c) *aesthetics*, the degree to which others react to the condition with dislike or disgust; (d) *origin*, the amount of responsibility attributed for causing or maintaining the stigmatized condition; (e) *course*, the degree to which the condition is alterable or progressively degenerative; (f) and *peril*, the degree to which the condition will physically, socially, or morally contaminate others. Using these dimensions, Herek illustrated the stigmatization associated with HIV–AIDS as follows: Although concealable early in its course, later stages of HIV infection and AIDS are rarely hidden from others; HIV infection interferes with social relationships; the disease physically disables and disfigures and is therefore aesthetically repellent; its origin is often, although not always, blamed on behaviors and life-style; the course of HIV infection is degenerative and not alterable; and HIV is a high-peril condition in that it poses risks to others. Thus, HIV infection represents the negative aspects of all six stigmatization dimensions (see Figure 6.2).

Whether related to medical illness or other culturally constructed con-

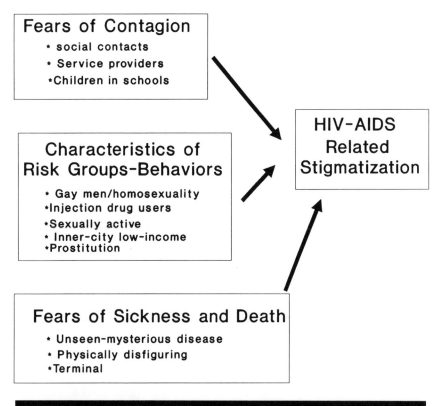

Figure 6.1

Factors contributing to HIV-related social stigmatization.

ditions, social stigmas serve instrumental functions (Pryor, Reeder, Vinacco, & Kott, 1989). Stigmas provide a means for retaining social distance and allow a sense of personal security (Kegeles, Coates, Christopher, & Lazarus, 1989; Mondragon, Kirkman-Liff, & Schneller, 1991). Moralistic judgments that hold people responsible for contracting HIV infection serve the purpose of distinguishing between "people like them" and "those like us" (McDonell, 1993). However, stigmas play out in subtle and unexpected ways. For example, what may appear as supportive attitudes toward people with HIV infection, treating individuals as "special" or with "holiness," patronizes and results in a form of paradoxical stigmatization (Herek, 1990).

People suffer countless social repercussions related to HIV and AIDS. Family, friends, employers, co-workers, and health care providers can all

Dimension of Stigmatization	Characteristics of HIV-AIDS
Concealability	AIDS is apparent at later Stages of disease
Disruption	AIDS is disabling and degenerative
Aesthetics	Body disfigurement in later stages of AIDS
Origin	Persons blamed for contracting HIV infection
Course	Degenerative and irreversible
Peril	Poses actual and fictive risks to others

Figure 6.2

Characteristics of AIDS along six dimensions of social stigmatization.

contribute to social prejudice, discrimination, and isolation. To varying degrees, most people conceal their HIV status from others, often at the cost of their personal welfare. The following sections review the attitudes and fears that contribute to stigmatization toward people with HIV infection. Specific attention is paid to how social stigmas are expressed among human service professionals. The chapter concludes with a discussion of education as a means of combating HIV-related stigmas.

BASES FOR HIV-RELATED STIGMATIZATION

Prejudice against people with HIV infection and AIDS primarily stems from three distinct, although not mutually exclusive, sources (Crandall,

1991; V. Price & Hsu, 1992; Taerk, Gallop, Lancee, Coates, & Fanning, 1993). First, social stigmas result from realistic and unrealistic fears of contracting HIV. Although fears can relate to a lack of knowledge about HIV and its transmission, misinformation alone does not completely account for avoidance of people with HIV infection. Second, the groups most affected by HIV infection have been socially ostracized prior to the HIV epidemic. Social stigmas that extend beyond HIV itself therefore serve as a foundation for AIDS stigmatization. Finally, the negative course of HIV infection corresponds to cultural attitudes and fears about death and dying, and the tendency to avoid the terminally ill. Each source of stigmatization is discussed in detail below.

Fears of Contracting HIV Infection

Fears of contracting the virus are a major contributing factor to HIV-related stigmas. These fears, for the most part, are grounded in misinformation and misperceptions (Bartlett, 1993a). Many negative attitudes toward HIV infection surfaced early in the epidemic when little was known about AIDS and its cause. Attitudes toward people with HIV infection have not, however, improved despite new information and understanding of the disease.

Studies continue to show that the public lacks accurate information about HIV infection and AIDS. For example, Herek and Capitanio (1993) conducted a random phone survey of over 1,100 men and women across the United States and found a high degree of misinformation about HIV and AIDS, and inaccurate information was associated with negative attitudes toward HIV-infected individuals. Nearly half of the respondents believed that HIV infection could result from casual activities such as drinking from the same glass as a person with HIV infection, using the same toilet seat, being near a person with HIV infection when he or she coughs or sneezes, and insect bites. Another random-digit-dial survey of more than 1,500 people in 44 states and the District of Columbia showed that 16% believed that insects could transmit HIV (CDC, 1991c). In yet another random-digit-dial phone survey of 1,204 people, Mondragon et al. (1991) found associations between misperceptions of HIV transmission from low-risk activities and hostile feelings toward people with AIDS. Similarly, Kegeles, Coates, Christopher, and Lazarus (1989) found that one third of survey respondents believed that they could contract HIV from a physician carrying the virus. Similar fears of casual HIV transmission, including sharing kitchen utensils and bathroom facilities, create a major source of concern among caregivers of people with AIDS (Frierson, Lippmann, & Johnson, 1987). Much of the public therefore fears contracting HIV infection through casual social contacts despite the fact that no cases of HIV transmission have occurred through these means. Misperceptions of HIV transmission potentially lead to hostility and avoidance of people with HIV infection (Kegeles, Coates, Christopher, & Lazarus, 1989; Mondragon et al., 1991).

Several other factors contribute to fears of contracting HIV through casual contacts. Concern about even the most remote possibilities of contracting HIV stem from its high mortality rate (Schneiderman & Kaplan, 1992). The paradox, of course, is that a great deal of concern is exerted over contacts with very low probabilities of HIV transmission while people continue to freely engage in sexual behaviors that carry high risk for HIV transmission (Gelman, 1993). People are well known to inaccurately judge risks, with risks of low-probability events overestimated (Slovic et al., 1982). Frequencies and salience of media images of a particular transmission route are a major source of risk misperceptions. For example, media coverage of six cases of HIV transmission that apparently occurred in one dental practice contributed to near social hysteria over contracting HIV from dentists, which in turn brought about guidelines from the CDC and the American Dental Association. Policy initiatives for mandatory HIV antibody testing for dentists and to limit the practices of dentists with HIV infection resulted from this one unusual case.

Fears of contracting HIV motivate avoidance and ultimately lead to the isolation of people with HIV infection. Herek and Capitanio (1993) found that 12% of people surveyed would intentionally avoid a close friend if he or she learned that they were HIV positive, 16% would prohibit HIV-infected children from attending schools, 20% would avoid an infected co-worker, and 50% would avoid a neighborhood grocer if they knew he or she was HIV positive. Isolating individuals with HIV infection in medical hospitals is also a common practice that stems from early policies that were based on incomplete information. Isolation of patients with HIV infection is supported by noninfected patients. A survey of hospitalized patients found that 55% would object to sharing a room with an HIV-positive patient because of unfounded fears of contracting HIV (Seltzer, Schulman, Brennan, & Lynn, 1993).

Public misperceptions about HIV transmission may translate to broad-based health policies that reflect prejudicial attitudes (Kegeles, Coates, Christopher, et al., 1989). Fears of HIV transmission have justified prohibiting people with HIV infection from entering the United States despite widely held views by public health experts that such policies only serve discriminatory functions (Gilmore, Orkin, Duckett, & Grover, 1989). Fears of contracting HIV infection can form the basis for discriminatory practices in the workplace (Leonard, 1985). At their worst, fears of HIV have led to recommendations to isolate people with HIV–AIDS. Kegeles, Coates, Chistopher, et al. (1989) found that 29% of survey respondents favored tattooing or otherwise visibly marking individuals who are HIV positive. The study also found that 21% to 40% of respondents supported isolating people with AIDS from neighborhoods and public places. Some have even called for quarantines of people with HIV infection, even though such actions may have a public health backlash and result in increased HIV infections (D. A. Smith & Smith, 1989). Although nowhere in the United States has there been a serious policy to isolate individuals with HIV infection, several states have enacted legislation to restrict the liberties of people with HIV who are known to engage in high-risk behaviors (Gostin, 1989). For example, restrictive measures have been taken against people with HIV infection in Colorado who exposed others to the virus through negligent, reckless, or criminal behavior (Woodhouse, Muth, Potterat, & Riffe, 1993). Related policy initiatives involve mandated reporting of HIV infection to public health authorities, a practice that will likely inhibit seeking HIV antibody testing (Kegeles, Coates, Lo, & Catania, 1989). Still, the public supports isolating people with HIV and AIDS, and some countries have instituted quarantine sanitariums (Kirby, 1988).

Risk Group Characteristics

HIV-related social stigmas are overlaid upon negative attitudes associated with behaviors and life-styles that existed before the HIV epidemic (Herek, 1990; Herek & Glunt, 1988). Prejudice and fears are related to behavior long viewed as deviant, such as homosexuality and drug abuse (Mondragon et al., 1991). Public perceptions of AIDS combine with sociocultural perceptions of the subgroups most visibly affected by the epidemic (Herek & Glunt, 1988). Discrimination against people with HIV infection has therefore arisen out of prejudice against gay and bisexual men, the sexually promiscuous, and injection drug users (Kegeles, Coates, Christopher et al., 1989; Treiber, Shawn, & Malcolm, 1987; Tross & Hirsch, 1988).

Before designated AIDS, the syndrome was originally classified as *Gay-Related Immune Deficiency* (GRID) and commonly referred to as the *Gay Plague* (Herek & Glunt, 1988). Media images of gay activists protesting political silence about the syndrome, coupled with the first widely recognized celebrities afflicted with HIV being gay men, served to strengthen perceptions of AIDS as a gay disease (Triplet, 1992). Antigay hostility, prejudice, and intolerance became closely associated with HIV (Herek, 1990). Shortly later in the U.S. epidemic, injection drug use was associated with HIV infection. This new dimension did not reduce stigmas because drug use supports perceptions of AIDS as a disease of moral retribution.

Socially condemned behaviors that afford efficient transmission of HIV create perceptions of personal responsibility for contracting the virus (McDonell, 1993). Blame leads to anger and to a lack of compassion. The greatest degree of blame for the epidemic is attributed to those HIV-positive individuals believed to have known about the risks they were taking but still chose to do so (McDonell, 1993). Thus, people with HIV infection compose two socially defined groups: innocent victims who had no knowledge of their risk and are not held accountable (e.g., infected infants, hemophiliacs, and transfusion recipients), and those perceived as guilty and held accountable (e.g., gay men, injection drug users, prostitutes, and the unmarried sexually active; McDonell, 1993). Thus, blame attributed to people with HIV infection corresponds to views of a just world. Unfortunately, like other aspects of HIV infection, research in HIV-related stigmatization has underrepresented non-injection-drug-using women, heterosexuals, and ethnic minorities. Because these groups have life experiences that differ from those of gay men, there are considerable gaps in our understanding of HIV-related social stigmas (Rabkin, Remien, Katoff, & Williams, 1993).

Associations between HIV–AIDS and previously stigmatized groups have had a number of adverse effects. Individuals who already suffer social discrimination confront further injustices related to their illness. Homophobia, prejudice against injection drug users, and dismay for people perceived as sexually promiscuous inhibit the potential power of public education efforts. Misinformation that feeds prejudice is not easily corrected (Gallop et al., 1991; Mondragon et al., 1991). Beliefs about HIV–AIDS, homophobia, and prejudices against addicts hinder policymakers from taking positive action (Herek, 1990). The links among negative attitudes, misperceptions, and misinformation further propagate HIV-related stigmas by exacerbating fears of terminal illness.

Negative Attitudes Toward Death and Dying

Western cultures have highly negative views of death and dying. Death is associated with darkness, despair, and the unknown (Kalish, 1985). Fears of death influence the social and medical treatment of the terminally ill. People with HIV–AIDS are socially ostracized and experience prejudices typically expressed against the terminally ill. HIV infection reminds healthy people of their own mortality and ultimate finality. Thinking of individuals with HIV infection as inherently different has the protective function of distancing oneself from the disease (Herek & Glunt, 1988) and therefore enables one to escape thinking about one's own vulnerability and mortality (Taerk et al., 1993).

Negative attitudes toward HIV infection reflect fears of social loss from death. Health care professionals commonly avoid working with the terminally ill because they fear becoming attached to patients who they know will die (Kalish, 1985). Nurses who lose multiple patients with HIV infection report extreme distress (Gordon, Ulrich, Feeley, & Pollack, 1993). Further concerns among health care providers include working through reactions of families and friends during periods of bereavement and grief (Weinberger, Conover, Samsa, & Greenberg, 1992). Thus, negative attitudes toward death, dying, and the terminally ill contribute to social stigmas of HIV infection and AIDS.

EFFECTS OF HIV-RELATED STIGMATIZATION

Psychological Effects

Social stigmas become a source of chronic stress for people living with HIV infection (Lyter et al., 1987). Victims of social stigmatization can become bitter, hostile, suspicious, and alienated (Crandall & Coleman, 1992).

HIV-related stigmas contribute to anxiety, depression, and interpersonal distrust (Crandall & Coleman, 1992). Social stigmatization occurs across all phases of HIV disease and interferes with coping and adjustment (Crandall & Coleman, 1992).

During asymptomatic HIV infection, when people do not suffer physical debilitation, people with HIV remain potentially discreditable (Goffman, 1963). Threats of stigmatization may inhibit disclosure of HIV infection, therefore cutting off potential social support and creating another source of psychological vulnerability. For example, individuals who do not disclose their HIV infection to others may still overhear derogatory remarks about people with AIDS (Grossman, 1991). Individuals who conceal asymptomatic infection and later become ill can suffer serious distress from unwanted disclosures (Grossman, 1991). Crandall and Coleman (1992) found that stigma, depression, and anxiety were highest among those whose risk behavior histories either were not disclosed to anyone or had become completely public. Selective disclosure of HIV seropositivity to close and trusted confidants correlated with adjustment.

Internalized stigmas are another contributing factor to psychological distress. People with HIV infection commonly view the disease as punishment and believe that HIV infection has contaminated all aspects of their life (Schwartzberg, 1993). Moulton et al. (1987) found that the degree to which people attributed the cause of HIV infection to themselves positively correlated with psychological distress and dysphoria. In contrast, attributing HIV infection to chance or another person corresponds with lower distress. Moulton et al. found that people with AIDS frequently feel guilty about contracting HIV as well as the possibility that they might have infected others. Similarly, many HIV-positive gay men develop internalized homophobia, where hatred and fear regarding homosexuality turn inward (Siegel, 1986). Wolcott et al. (1986) found that gay men with AIDS held negative attitudes toward their own homosexuality and toward disclosure of their sexual orientation. People who contract HIV through heterosexual contact or injection drug use may also internalize responsibility and blame that translates into self-reprehension and distress.

Effects on Interpersonal Relationships

Loss of social support, feelings of isolation, and fear of abandonment commonly occur with life-threatening illnesses (Dilley, Ochitill, et al., 1985).

Although seeking social support is an important coping strategy (Leserman, Perkins, & Evans, 1992), and social relationships critically effect psychological adjustment and emotional well-being (Crandall & Coleman, 1992), many people with HIV infection socially isolate themselves (McDonell, 1993). Like other stigmatized groups (Kleck, 1968), people with HIV infection withdraw from social situations and leave themselves vulnerable to psychological distress (Crandall & Coleman, 1992). People with HIV infection often stop working, as well as limit their participation in social activities, cutting themselves off further from potential sources of support (Crandall & Coleman, 1992).

HIV-related stigmas influence the amount of social support that others willingly offer (Turner, Hays, & Coates, 1993). Stigmas and fears make it less likely that individuals with HIV infection will receive support (Bor, Prior, & Miller, 1990; Kelly, Murphy, Bahr, Koob, et al., 1993). In a study of over 100 HIV-positive gay men, Crystal and Jackson (1989) found that 31% had been rejected by at least one family member and that 38% had been abandoned by friends. Pergami et al. (1993) found that 27% of HIV-positive women experienced changes in their social networks following notification of HIV infection and that nearly two thirds suffered severe disruptions to their sexual relationships. Turner et al. (1993) found similar relationship problems in the lives of gay men with HIV infection, particularly among family members who were previously unaware of their sexual orientation. Acceptance of one's own homosexual orientation opens up opportunities to discuss HIV-positive serostatus and, therefore, positively influences availability of support.

As much as stigmas may affect available social supports, they also affect perceptions of received social support. A perceived lack of opportunities for support leaves people vulnerable to distress and maladaptive coping (Green, 1993). Even within what at one time may have been a socially supportive network, people with HIV infection may find themselves removed from friends. It is therefore common for people with HIV infection to develop bonds among themselves, as a group with similar experiences (Crandall & Coleman, 1992).

Associations between HIV-related stigmatization and the quality of interpersonal relationships are reciprocally determined (Crandall & Coleman, 1992). Stigmas set up expectations for social rejection among people with HIV infection and can cause withdrawal from social relationships. Rejection by family members, friends, and co-workers further reinforces beliefs about being abandoned. Broken social bonds and disrupted supportive networks are therefore the product of social stigmas, through both intrapersonal and interpersonal processes.

Health Effects

Stigmas present several potential adverse health outcomes. Concerns over discrimination and stigmatization often translate into avoiding HIV testing (Kegeles, Coates, Lo, et al., 1989; O'Dowd, 1988). Fear of harassment and job discrimination therefore precludes opportunities for early medical interventions (Herek, 1990; Kegeles, Coates, Lo, et al., 1989). HIV infection can result in loss of health insurance because of the infection being deemed a preexisting condition, lost employment, or other technicalities (Herek, 1990). Although not entirely due to social perceptions of HIV disease, discontinued health insurance benefits occur in the context of social stigmatization and therefore becomes incorporated into a broader framework of experiences. Stigmatization also originates from within the health care system, directly affecting the delivery of medical and mental health services. People with HIV often compare themselves to lepers in the health care system, with impersonal attitudes among hospital staff and isolation within health care facilities (Frierson & Lippmann, 1987).

SOCIAL DISCRIMINATION

Discrimination against people with HIV infection originates from the same fears and prejudices that give rise to other forms of stigmatization (Triplet & Sugarman, 1987; Weiss & Hardy, 1990). For example, foster parents of children with HIV infection fear contracting HIV and express concerns over suffering stigma and discrimination themselves for raising the child (F. L. Cohen & Nehring, 1994). Ridicule, interpersonal violence, housing eviction, loss of insurance, denial of health and dental care, loss of supportive services, and loss of employment are also common (Herek, 1990; Lyter et al., 1987; Siegel, 1986; Tross & Hirsch, 1988). Discrimination occurs for most HIV-positive gay men, injection drug users, school-age children, and prostitutes (Triplet & Sugarman, 1987). Crystal and Jackson (1989) found that 11% of the HIV-positive gay men in their study had lost their housing because of fears and discrimination. A number of gay men in the Chicago MACS cohort reported discrimination specifically attributed to their HIV seropositive status. For example, 6% of men in the cohort were denied services by rental agents or bankers, 6% had been harassed by the police, another 6% experienced physical violence or attempted violence, and 3% experienced work-related discrimination. Family members and caregivers of HIV-positive people also often suffer similar forms of social discrimination (Frierson et al., 1987). For many, the most destructive forms of discrimination involve employment, health care, and mental health services.

Employment Discrimination

HIV infection is frequently concealed from employers (Siegel, 1986). Workplace discrimination can include reduced responsibilities, isolation from co-workers or the public, lay-off, or termination (Leonard, 1985). Isolation or termination causes loss of social relationships and a diminished sense of self-worth. Although job termination on the basis of illness is legal when physical limitations prohibit the performance of required duties, there is protection against discrimination for disabled individuals (Leonard, 1985; Terl, 1992). HIV–AIDS falls under the Federal Rehabilitation Act of 1973, which prohibits discrimination against "otherwise qualified" disabled individuals (Gostin, 1989). However, laws and employment practices vary across states, and those who suffer illegal termination outside of high-AIDS-incidence areas will likely lack adequate legal support and advocacy.

HIV-positive people in service-providing occupations are especially vulnerable to discrimination. Employers, like many people, hold irrational beliefs that HIV-positive employees will threaten the health of customers or clients. HIV-positive teachers, hair stylists, cooks, food servers, sales clerks, receptionists, and other service providers often become victims of employment discrimination. Even employers who know that HIV is not transmitted on the job may realistically fear that the public will not understand and that their business could be adversely affected if an HIV-positive employee became known. Like family members and friends, employers may fear displacement of HIV- related social stigmas on them. To an even greater extent, HIV-positive dentists, physicians, and other medical professionals must limit their practice to noninvasive procedures, and for some, like dentists, this is the equivalent of not practicing. Despite universal precautions against HIV transmission and the fact that only a few providers have ever infected patients, the public does fear dental and medical services from HIV-positive practitioners. However, stigmatization runs in the opposite direction as well, with health care providers expressing discomfort about working with HIV-positive patients.

Social Stigmatization by Medical Professionals

Stigmas and prejudices from health service providers are particularly troublesome. Studies consistently show that many medical professionals hold attitudes toward people with HIV mirroring those of society in general (Silverman, 1993). Medical staff report anxiety-like reactions to HIV-positive patients and feel reluctant to offer them treatment (Rosse, 1985). Wallack (1989) found that 87% of physicians and nurses experience more anxiety about caring for AIDS patients than other patient groups. An AIDS-related phobia identified among physicians is characterized by fear, night terrors, and avoidance (Horstman & McKusick, 1986). A similar HIV-caregivers syndrome consists of trauma-like symptoms (Silverman, 1993). Nurses who care for hemophilia patients are troubled by fears of contracting the virus (Gordon et al., 1993). Caring for people with HIV infection can be more stressful than working with other equally serious medical disorders (P. Reed, Wise, & Mann, 1984; Silverman, 1993).

Several factors contribute to reluctance to provide health services to people with HIV infection. In one study, Kegeles, Coates, Christopher et al. (1989) found similar perceptions among health care workers as those held by the general public. Willingness to provide services was predicted by fears of contracting HIV from patients, worries about contact with hazardous materials such as injection needles or surgical instruments, negative attitudes toward homosexuals and injection drug users, and death anxiety raised by terminally ill patients. Knox and Dow (1989) found that fears of contracting HIV infection and death anxiety interrupted the delivery of health services to patients with HIV infection.

Because HIV is transmitted through blood, medical professionals who perform invasive procedures most commonly fear HIV infection (O'Donnell, O'Donnell, Pleck, Snarey, & Rose, 1987). In one study, 60% of medical personnel expressed concern over risks of HIV infection, with the greatest fear occurring among surgeons and emergency room physicians (Weinberger et al., 1992). Wallack (1989) found that 65% of hospital staff physicians and 63% of nurses felt at risk for contracting HIV infection even when following infection control guidelines. Thus, fears of HIV transmission persist despite practicing well-established occupational precautionary guidelines (Blumenfield, Smith, Milazzo, Seropian, & Wormser, 1987). Concern over occupational HIV transmission among health care workers is explained by distrust of technology, instrumentation, information, and authorities (Gallop, Lancee, Taerk, Coates, & Fanning, 1992; Wallack, 1989). Health care workers are aware that standard precautionary procedures reduce risk but do not guarantee protection against accidental HIV transmission (Taerk et al., 1993).

Inaccurate estimates of the relative risks of various medical procedures fuel fears of occupational transmission (Gallop et al., 1991). Professionals may believe that HIV transmission occurs from ways in which no one has ever become infected. Even highly knowledgeable medical professionals exaggerate odds of contracting HIV infection (Gallop, Taerk, Lancee, Coates, & Fanning, 1992). Fears of HIV transmission by medical procedures exceed actual risks (Gallop, Lancee, et al., 1992). Risks related to medical accidents, such as needlestick injuries, are the product of three probabilities: the probability of the injury × the probability that the patient involved is HIV positive × the probability of risk of HIV transmission associated with that type of accident. Using needlestick injuries as an example: the odds of a piercing needlestick among health care professionals is less than 1 in 100 blood draws (McGuff & Popovsky, 1989); the probability of a patient having HIV infection varies with geographical location and medical specialty, but for example, the odds of a cardiac care patient in Seattle being HIV infected is less than 1% (CDC, 1992f); and the chance of HIV transmission occurring from a needlestick injury with an HIV-infected needle is also less than 1% (Marcus & CDC Cooperative Needlestick Surveillance Group, 1988). Thus, the estimated probability of contracting HIV from an occupational needlestick accident is a small fraction of 1%. Under most conditions, therefore, risks through medical accidents, even relatively common accidents like needlesticks, are exceedingly low. The same factors that foster exaggerated risk perceptions in the general public cause medical professionals to overestimate their risk.

Factors unrelated to fear of HIV transmission, however, influence avoidance of patients with HIV infection. Homophobia and negative attitudes toward injection drug users contribute to professional resistance to work with HIV-positive patients (Bliwise, Grade, Irish, & Ficarrotto, 1991). In a survey of over 1,100 physicians, Gerbert, Maguire, Bleecker, Coates, and McPhee (1991) found over one third uncomfortable caring for patients with injection drug addictions, reflecting sentiments toward drug users even without HIV infection. Like the general public, medical professionals often view HIV infection as a disease of choice because of the behaviors associated with HIV transmission (Taerk et al., 1993). For example, nurses prefer to care for patients infected through blood transfusions as opposed to those infected through homosexual activity (Gallop, Lancee, et al., 1992). Kegeles, Coates, Christopher et al. (1989) also found that between 25% and 33% of health care providers preferred to treat individuals infected with HIV through blood transfusion compared with HIV-positive gay men and injection drug users. Many medical professionals also experience greater personal discomfort with HIV–AIDS patients than with other medical patients because of the association between HIV infection and socially disapproved behaviors (Treiber et al., 1987).

In two early and widely replicated studies, Kelly, St. Lawrence, Smith, Hood, and Cook (1987a, 1987b) found that medical professionals exhibited negative attitudes toward patients with HIV infection. Kelly et al. studied medical students (1987a) and physicians (1987b) using an experimentally controlled case vignette to independently manipulate characteristics of a patient, including the type of disease (AIDS or leukemia) and the sexual orientation of the patient (heterosexual or homosexual). The case vignette used by Kelly et al. read as follows:

> Following graduation from college, Mark accepted a management trainee position with a large computer manufacturing firm. His solid work performance won him the respect of his supervisors and he has advanced rapidly on the corporate ladder. At 32, he is the youngest division manager in the firm and has 55 employees working for him. Mark has always been active in his leisure time. In the summer he spends many weekends sailing on a small sloop he bought several years ago and often plays a game of tennis in the evening after work. He usually takes his vacation during the winter months so he can enjoy his favorite winter sport, skiing.

Within the last year Mark's life has changed in unexpected ways. For some time, he just didn't feel his usual self. He was frequently tired, felt run down and unenergetic, and had constant bouts of colds, flu, and infections which took longer than usual to heal. He had always been in excellent health. He finally decided to see a physician. After several visits and a number of tests, Mark learned that he has AIDS. The diagnosis came as a searing shock to Mark and has dramatically changed his life. Physically, he fights a constant battle against fatigue and recurrent illnesses which seem to last unceasingly. Although he continues to exercise, he can barely walk a mile each morning instead of the four miles he used to run in the morning before he left for work. He has lost weight and looks sallow. Friends who haven't seen him for a while comment on his changed appearance when they meet. Mark doesn't know whether or not to tell them he has AIDS. Mark has done quite a bit of reading recently about AIDS and knows that he will probably die in the next year or two, but hopes by taking care of himself that he may live a little longer.

Loneliness has become a major problem for the first time in Mark's life. Mark has always had a constant circle of friends and an active social life. Yet, the first few friends he turned to for emotional support after learning he had AIDS seemed uncomfortable with him. Recently, when he returned to the doctor's office for a checkup, the staff seemed unsupportive and distant. As his illness progresses, he realizes his job performance is not up to its old standards. He has not told anyone at work that he has AIDS, but people are beginning to ask questions and comment on his changed appearance. He's becoming very anxious about losing his job and feels that it's just a matter of time before either he isn't able to work any longer or is fired. He's doing the best he can on the job, but the constant illnesses and fatigue have taken their toll and he just doesn't have as much energy anymore.

Life has become a strain at home, too. After telling his partner, Robert, that he has AIDS, Mark has felt very alone. For a week or two, Robert was sympathetic and supportive. When Mark first told him he had AIDS, Robert held him as they both cried and Robert said he'd be there faithful until the end to help care for Mark. But now Robert is increasingly distant and reserved. Robert seems more preoccupied with himself these days and has become very uncaring. Although they have been together for nine years and had a stable, affectionate relationship, Robert now stays away from the apartment almost all of his waking hours, comes in late, and then sleeps on the sofa in the living room instead of in their bedroom. Two nights ago Robert told Mark he is planning to move out as soon as he finds another place to live. They've meant a lot to one another and both cried some during that conversation, but Robert explained that he is feeling very confused right now and needs a chance to get off by himself and think things through.

When Mark told his parents about his illness, although they had always had a good relationship with one another, they became very emotional. They haven't offered him much emotional support or understanding and just don't seem to want to talk about it.

There are several noteworthy aspects of the Kelly et al. (1987a, 1987b) case vignette. The early sections of the vignette describe the patient in positive and personal terms. The patient is a responsible and productive 32-year-old on an ambitious and successful career path. His leisure activities reflect middle- to upper-middle-class interests, including skiing, sailing, and tennis. The vignette therefore sets a context with which many of the medical professional participants could identify. The onset of illness and the patient's declining health presented a tragic tone, but with the patient remaining courageous through difficult times. Thus, the patient's plight likely evoked sympathy. Following the positive description of the patient and his tragic illness, the patient's sexual orientation was introduced in the vignette. The context of the vignette probably minimized attributions of blame to the patient and levels of discomfort treating the patient. The study results therefore represent conservative estimates of stigmatizing attributions ascribed by health care professionals.

Using this same case vignette with physicians, Kelly et al. (1987b) identified several negative attitudes held toward HIV-infected patients. Physicians believed AIDS patients to be more responsible for their illness and less deserving of sympathy than leukemia patients. Physicians were also less willing to interpersonally interact with AIDS patients than with leukemia patients, even in situations as innocuous as casual conversations.

Among medical students, Kelly et al. (1987a) found that negative attitudes corresponded with homophobia; however, this association did not repli- cate in the sample of practicing physicians. Kelly et al. concluded that dis- comforts of medical service providers ultimately limit interactions with HIV-positive patients, interfering with service delivery and quality of care, conclusions that have since been empirically supported (McDonell, 1993).

Stigmatization of HIV-positive patients by health care providers may also develop out of concerns over their own repercussions for treating HIV-infected patients (Bliwise et al., 1991). Providers may feel helpless and ineffective when dealing with HIV–AIDS patients, particularly when pro- fessionals have had minimal training and limited experiences with HIV infection (Weinberger et al., 1992). Few resources, limited support, and increased workloads associated with these difficult cases lead medical pro- fessionals to fear excessive stress and burnout (Silverman, 1993). Because most HIV-infected patients are uninsured, they may pose a financial lia- bility to health care professionals (Weinberger et al., 1992). Finally, health care providers have expressed concern over the possibility of spreading HIV infection to their friends and family should they become infected while on the job (Treiber et al., 1987). As many as two thirds of profes- sionals report that friends or family members express similar concerns about contact with them should their practice include HIV-positive pa- tients (Blumenfield et al., 1987).

Stigma in HIV infection often interferes with professional service de- livery (McDonell, 1993). For example, medical professionals frequently fail to discuss HIV disease processes with their HIV-positive patients (Ger- bert, Maguire, & Coates, 1990; R. O. Valdiserri, Tama, & Ho, 1988). In the Netherlands, the majority of physicians and nurses surveyed avoided in- vasive medical procedures with HIV-positive patients (Storosum et al., 1991). Medical students in the United States have preferred not to per- form invasive procedures with HIV-positive patients, including routine blood draws (Imperato, Feldman, Nayeri, & DeHovitz, 1988). Medical stu- dents have also reported that concerns about AIDS have influenced their choice of specialty areas and that they believe they should have the right to refuse treatment to AIDS patients (Strunin, Culbert, & Crane, 1989). Another study found that 53% of hospital staff admitted that they had avoided performing procedures on patients with HIV infection (Wallack, 1989). Gerbert, Maguire, et al. (1991) showed that although physicians feel a sense of responsibility for providing care, 50% would prefer not to work with AIDS patients if given a choice. Van Servellan, Lewis, and Leake (1988) reported that 23% of nurses surveyed indicated that they would not accept AIDS case assignments. Blumenfield et al. (1987) found that nearly half of nurses surveyed indicated that they would transfer out of their current position if required to treat HIV-positive patients on a regular basis. Thus, negative attitudes have the potential to interfere with quality medical care. Although studied to a lesser extent, similar types of fears and prejudice occur among mental health professionals.

Social Stigmatization by Mental Health Professionals

Unlike many other health services, mental health professionals working in nonmedical settings do not have any occupational risk for HIV infection. Nevertheless, fears and negative attitudes are common among mental health professionals. Social stigmatization of HIV-positive individuals here again stems from homophobia, prejudice against injection drug users, and death anxiety. In a study of hospital-based social workers, Dhooper, Royse, and Tran (1987–1988) found 80% unwilling to accept clients with AIDS into their caseloads. Social workers feared contracting HIV infection from HIV-positive clients, suggesting widespread misinformation and prejudice. Dhooper et al. also found that social workers lacked empathy for HIV-positive clients and attempted to maintain distance from them. Fear of AIDS among social workers in the Dhooper et al. study correlated with homophobia; homophobic respondents were most afraid of contact with HIV-positive clients. Kegeles, Coates, Christopher et al. (1989) surveyed a more heterogeneous sample of mental health professionals and found that they also avoided treating individuals with HIV–AIDS in their counseling practices.

Clinical psychologists express generally negative attitudes toward people with AIDS relative to other medical patients (St. Lawrence et al., 1990). Using the same experimentally controlled case vignette used by Kelly et al. (1987a, 1987b), St. Lawrence et al. found that psychologists held AIDS patients more responsible for their illness and less willing to see them in their practice relative to identical cases of leukemia patients.

Crawford, Humfleet, Ribordy, Ho, and Vickers (1991) surveyed clinical psychologists, counseling psychologists, and social workers in 13 U.S.

cities using a case vignette modeled after the one used by Kelly et al. (1987a, 1987b). Mental health professionals were again hesitant to see clients they believed to have HIV infection, and avoided contact with HIV-positive people. Crawford et al. replicated Kelly et al.'s findings, demonstrating that mental health professionals perceived people with AIDS as more responsible for their medical condition than other medical patients. Crawford et al. showed that negative attitudes toward AIDS were associated with homophobia, again replicating the Kelly et al. (1987a) medical student findings. Importantly, however, Crawford et al. (1991), St. Lawrence et al. (1990), and Kelly et al. (1987a, 1987b) used practically the same experimental case vignette in their respective studies. Thus, findings replicated but may not generalize to situations that differ from the case description.

In summary, stigmatization of HIV infection by mental health professionals appears to mirror that of medical professionals and the general public. Professionals, like the general public, distrust authoritative sources of information about HIV transmission and commit cognitive errors that result in overestimation of risk for infection. Thus, widely held social and cultural values fuel most negative attitudes toward people with HIV infection. Prejudices cause many to conceal personal aspects of themselves. Sexual orientation and drug abuse are both concealed to avoid social stigmas. For similar reasons, people with HIV infection do not always disclose their HIV-positive status.

DISCLOSURE OF HIV SEROSTATUS

People who suffer from stigmatized medical conditions, especially when symptoms are not visible, often hide their diagnoses from others (Kleck, 1968). The social and personal costs associated with HIV infection cause many with HIV–AIDS to keep their condition to themselves (Crandall & Coleman, 1992). Individuals may hide their status from others for fear of straining friendships and potentially damaging already stressed family relationships (Herek, 1990). Siegel and Krauss (1991) identified four considerations among HIV-positive gay men that influenced disclosure of their HIV status: fears of rejection, the wish to avoid pity, the wish to spare loved ones emotional pain, and concerns about discrimination. People may want to maintain as much normalcy in their lives as possible and protect others from worrying about them (Herek, 1990). For example, HIV-positive parents often do not disclose their health status to their children out of fear that they too will suffer psychological harm from stigmatization (Pliskin, Farrell, Crandles, & DeHovitz, 1993). Families have expressed concerns about word getting out about an HIV-positive family member, particularly because of associations between HIV and stigmatized behaviors (Frierson et al., 1987).

Concealment of HIV infection decreases the availability of social support (Herek, 1990). Stress from the effort of concealing a positive HIV status partially stems from the necessity of structuring interactions to minimize risks of disclosure (Herek, 1990). Selective disclosure of HIV status tends to divide one's world into those who know and those who do not know. Living a "double life" can involve lying about absences from work, concealing medications, and covering up illnesses (Siegel & Krauss, 1991). In a study of Hispanic men with HIV infection, Marks, Richardson, Ruiz, and Maldonado (1992) found disclosure of HIV status to be a highly selective process and that disclosures increased as HIV disease advanced. In this study, men disclosed to their sexual partners and close friends more often than to their families. Disclosure of HIV serostatus and communication about HIV infection with friends and family result in satisfaction with social supports (Turner et al., 1993). Thus, disclosure of HIV infection helps gain social support but also risks loss of support.

A particularly important example of self-disclosure of HIV status involves telling sexual partners. To the degree sexual partners are placed at risk, HIV-positive individuals are obligated to inform their sexual partners of their HIV status. However, many people with HIV hesitate telling sexual partners that they have tested HIV positive, and most people do not know their partner's HIV status (Dawson et al., 1994). HIV-negative or unknown-HIV-status sexual partners are least often informed because of fears of rejection and abandonment (Marks, Richardson, et al., 1992).

Social barriers inhibit disclosure of HIV status to sexual partners. Perry et al. (1994) found that nearly one third of HIV-positive men and women had not disclosed their HIV status to past or present sexual partners. In a study of HIV-positive gay men, Marks, Richardson, and Maldonado (1991) found that 52% kept their HIV-positive status a secret from at least one sexual partner. Although 69% of men with one sex partner had disclosed their HIV status to their partner, only 18% of men with five or more sexual partners had disclosed to at least one. Thus, the likelihood of self-disclosure of HIV infection decreased in proportion to the number of reported sexual partners. In addition, men who disclosed their HIV-positive status to HIV-negative sexual partners tended to engage in safer sexual practices, whereas those who disclosed to HIV-positive partners were more likely to practice unprotected intercourse. Thus, the nature of the relationship and beliefs about the effects of disclosure on the relationship affect willingness to disclose.

Some studies show that fears that disclosure inevitably leads to abandonment may be unfounded. For example, Schnell et al. (1992) showed that 82% of HIV-positive men had disclosed their HIV status to sexual partners and that most men who did disclose reported stronger relationship bonds after disclosure. It is unfortunately not known which relationship characteristics best predict positive outcomes and how long support by partners is maintained. It is also not known what factors influence women's decisions to self-disclose their HIV status. Fears of abandonment and other harsh reactions likely interfere with women's disclosing to their partners.

As people approach late HIV infection, hiding their HIV status becomes increasingly difficult. Increased frequencies of medical visits, a mass of medications, deteriorating health, changes in appearance, and occupational disability can cause an awareness of infection. The onset of AIDS can precipitate a crisis of forcing disclosure (Crandall & Coleman, 1992). Forced disclosure threatens to uncover a life-style that carries added stigma and prejudice.

CONCLUSION

As the HIV epidemic expands, threats of infection will create new fears and increase perceptions of personal vulnerability. As the number of people needing medical services increases, HIV infection will place even greater demands on an already burdened health care system, again exacerbating negative attitudes toward HIV–AIDS (Herek, 1990). Education is the first line of defense against the parallel epidemic of HIV-related stigma. Even brief education programs can successfully reduce negative attitudes toward HIV–AIDS and remove unfounded fears of contracting HIV infection (Bliwise et al., 1991; Gallop, Taerk, et al., 1992; Riley & Greene, 1993). Crawford et al. (1991) found that mental health professionals who received AIDS education held less negative attitudes and more often accepted people with HIV infection. Education efforts are bolstered by including discussions with HIV-positive public speakers or by the use of videotaped patient interviews (Gallop, Taerk, et al., 1992).

Although necessary, education is insufficient to eliminate HIV-related stigmas. Education efforts with medical students, for example, have shown little effect on misperceptions of risk and negative attitudes (Imperato et al., 1988). Education does not stop people from blaming HIV-positive individuals for having been infected (Herek, 1990). Homophobia and prejudice against injection drug users persist despite education. As the United States epidemic spreads among inner-city ethnic minorities, new dimensions of social stigma based on racial and socioeconomic discrimination will likely emerge. Public and professional distrust in information about the "truth" of HIV transmission will ultimately thwart education efforts (Herek, 1990). Providing factual information about routes of HIV transmission to families with an HIV-positive member has had little effect on dispelling anxieties about casually contracting HIV infection (Frierson et al., 1987). Thus, removing social stigmas attached to HIV infection will require greater change than offered by unidimensional education programs. Removing stigmas increases opportunities for social support and eliminates distress stemming from blame and condemnation. Efforts to dismantle HIV-related stigmas will therefore psychologically benefit people with HIV infection.

PART THREE

Psychological and Social Adjustment

I told my comrades that human life, under any circumstances never ceases to have a meaning, and that this infinite meaning of life includes suffering and dying, privation and death. . . . They must not lose hope but should keep their courage in the certainty that the hopelessness of our struggle did not detract from its dignity and its meaning.

(Victor Frankl, 1963, pp. 131–132)

7

Coping and Adjustment

I t is well documented that most people with HIV adjust after first learning they are HIV positive and continue adjusting over the course of infection (Perry et al., 1993). Coping is a process influenced by multiple competing stressors including social discrimination, poverty, and substance abuse, as well as an individual's social and coping resources. Here, HIV-related coping is defined as the thoughts and behaviors used in dealing with HIV infection (Lazarus & Folkman, 1984). Coping constitutes cognitive and behavioral activities that serve to manage external and internal demands related to HIV infection that are seen as personally threatening (Lazarus & Folkman, 1984). Coping responses must apply to the continuous flow of HIV-related stressors over the course of the disease.

On the basis of research with people facing life-threatening illnesses, S. E. Taylor (1983) proposed the Cognitive Adaptational Model, which provides a structure for describing HIV-related adjustment. Adaptation to life-threatening illness is characterized by three general themes: a search for meaning, attempts to regain mastery or control over the illness, and efforts to enhance self-esteem. Adjustment is a pervasive process and often involves distortions of reality in the service of psychological protection. Deriving meaning and holding unrealistic perceptions of control and an inflated sense of self may normalize and establish psychological stability (S. E. Taylor, 1983; S. E. Taylor & Brown, 1988).

Models of cognitive behavioral coping also help explain adjustment to HIV infection. In their widely accepted model, Lazarus and Folkman (1984) identified seven basic types of coping: self-control, cognitive escape–avoidance, behavioral escape–avoidance, distancing, planful problem solving, seeking social support, and positive reappraisal. In general, these coping strategies comprise two broad clusters of coping behaviors: problem-focused coping and emotion-focused coping (Lazarus & Folkman, 1984; S. E. Taylor & Aspinwall, 1990; Wolf, Balson, Morse, et al., 1991). Problem-focused coping includes cognitions and behaviors that actively seek resolution of specific stressors (problem-solving coping). In contrast, emotion-focused coping is geared toward alleviating immediate distress and emotional turmoil without directly confronting sources of stress.

In adjustment to chronic illness, coping falls within problem-focused and emotion-focused domains. Examples of illness-related problem-focused coping include seeking information about the disease (Felton & Revenson, 1984), calling upon others for help (Dunkel-Schetter, Feinstein, Taylor, & Falke, 1992), and seeking medical advice and treatments (Feifel, Strack, & Nagy, 1987). Strategies for problem-focused coping are similar to confrontational coping behaviors (Feifel et al., 1987) and to a "fighting spirit" observed among cancer patients (Greer, Morris, & Pettingale, 1979). Emotion-focused coping is also common in serious medical illness. Selective ignoring, wishful thinking, blaming others (Felton & Revenson, 1984), focusing on the positive, distancing (Dunkel-Schetter et al., 1992), avoidance (Dunkel-Schetter et al., 1992; Feifel et al., 1987), and acceptance (Feifel et al., 1987; Greer et al., 1979) are all examples of emotion-focused coping.

Coping strategies must address a number of adaptational tasks in chronic illness, including harm reduction, tolerance of negative events, maintenance of positive self-image, establishing emotional equilibrium, and maintenance of interpersonal relationships (J. F. Miller, 1983). Coping mechanisms in HIV infection are similar to those used by people facing other life-threatening illnesses (e.g., Folkman, Chesney, Pollack, & Coates, in press; Griffiths & Wilkins, 1993; S. E. Taylor et al., 1992). It is, however, important to note that illness-related experiences and coping processes differ for men and women and various ethnic groups and HIV risk populations. Adjustment to HIV infection can therefore be conceptualized as coping behaviors that occur within themes of searching for meaning, establishing a sense of control, and enhancing self-esteem. Together, these themes and strategies provide a framework for understanding psychological adjustment to HIV infection.

MEANING, CONTROL, AND SELF-ESTEEM

In her classic descriptions of cancer patients coping with their disease, S. E. Taylor (1983) described three themes in cognitive adaptation to chronic and life-threatening illnesses: meaning, control, and restoring self-esteem. These dimensions also play important roles in adjustment to HIV infection.

Meaning

Meaning is derived through an individual's efforts to understand adversity and human suffering. Perceptions of how one contracted HIV and beliefs about its implications can provide a sense of meaning. Searching for meaning may be conceptualized as an attempt to answer the question "Why me?" Causal attributions are one mechanism by which meaning is therefore ascribed. The need to achieve a sense of meaning is observed among holocaust survivors, combat veterans, victims of violence, and survivors of natural disasters (Schwartzberg, 1993). Similarly, cancer patients want to understand why they developed cancer. Because the exact cause of cancer is unknown, there are numerous explanations that may be incorporated in the search for meaning, including internal attributions (e.g., hereditary factors), external and uncontrollable attributions (e.g., accidents or trauma), and external and controllable attributions (e.g., exposure to toxins, stress, smoking, or diet; S. E. Taylor, 1983). Deriving meaning from terminal illness is also influenced by many cultural and personal factors (A. Kleinman, 1988; Moos & Tsu, 1977). A sense of meaning is not universally achieved by the terminally ill (S. E. Taylor, 1983). When obtained, however, a sense of meaning can bring discovery of beneficial, self-affirming attitudes toward life in general and a new sense of self-knowledge or positive self-regard (Moos & Tsu, 1977; S. E. Taylor, 1983).

A sense of meaning for HIV-positive individuals is often gained through conscious efforts to live each day to its fullest (Nichols, 1985).

What may have once seemed to have been a problem of monumental importance may suddenly appear trivial and irrelevant in a new life context that includes HIV infection (O'Dowd et al., 1993). People with HIV infection commonly experience a sense of personal growth. People state that they achieve a sense of self-awareness, inner strength, resiliency, and consolidation of core beliefs and values as a result of learning they are HIV-positive (W. Borden, 1991; Viney, Crooks, Walker, & Henry, 1991). In a study of HIV-positive gay men, Schwartzberg (1993) found that HIV was perceived as a catalyst for personal growth. A greater appreciation for loved ones, reprioritizing of values and time commitments, and becoming more forgiving and less self-centered often occur after learning one is HIV positive. Schaefer and Coleman (1992) also found that gay men with HIV infection gained a sense of meaning, purpose, and value subsequent to testing HIV positive. Relationships, self-discovery, aesthetic appreciation, and contributing to the lives of others are all potential sources of meaning.

Control

Perceptions of control develop out of a sense of mastery that one has over one's illness. Uncertainties of chronic illness and diminishing perceptions of control are linked to psychological maladjustment (Jenkins & Pargament, 1988; S. E. Taylor et al., 1991). A sense of control buffers the effects of stressful life events and can lead to active coping to facilitate health and foster illness recovery (Jenkins & Pargament, 1988; G. M. Reed et al., 1993). A sense of control over stressful events emerges out of cognitions, coping strategies, attitudes, and dispositions (G. M. Reed et al., 1993). Feelings of control over chronic illness can also develop out of a general personality style that leads to viewing events positively (S. E. Taylor et al., 1991). People who adjust to stressful life events therefore often experience a sense of control. There may, however, be a third set of factors causing both a sense of control and psychological adjustment, such as available social supports or access to medical services (S. E. Taylor et al., 1991).

Feelings of control over chronic illness seem necessary for psychological adjustment, even when perceptions of control are illusory (Lazarus & Folkman, 1984; Somerfield & Curbow, 1992). For example, patients often believe that they can control recurrent cancer through strict compliance with a chemotherapy regimen. However, if cancer recurs, perceptions of control over the outcomes of additional chemotherapy, particularly the possibility of arresting recurrent disease, are also likely to recur (S. E. Taylor, 1983).

Perceptions of control occur in multiple life domains, some of which are remotely affected by illness. Perceived sources of control include oneself, powerful others, God, and chance (Jenkins & Pargament, 1988). More generally, a sense of control originates in one of two ways: internally or externally. Internal control, or personal control, stems from beliefs about actions that can change HIV disease progression. In contrast, external control involves beliefs that powerful external agents or forces control the course of HIV infection (G. M. Reed et al., 1993).

Internal Control

A sense of personal control over stressful life events reduces psychological distress (Folkman et al., in press). Research has shown that perceptions of control over the course of disease correspond to psychological adjustment among women with breast cancer (S. E. Taylor, Lichtman, & Wood, 1984), chronic arthritics (Affleck, Tennen, Pfeiffer, & Fifield, 1987), and people with HIV infection (Folkman et al., in press; Remien, Rabkin, Williams, Katoff, 1992). The greater the uncertainty associated with a medical condition, the more important it is that people have a sense of control. Personal control over the course of illness is also associated with hope for longer survival and improved quality of life (Rabkin et al., 1990). S. E. Taylor et al. (1991) showed that perceived personal control plays a causal role in reducing psychological distress in chronic illness.

A sense of control over the course of chronic illness can become maladaptive in some cases when such beliefs create a false sense of hope, particularly when efforts to control the disease are futile (Burish et al., 1984). Still, most evidence suggests that feelings of control reestablish themselves despite the progression of a chronic illness (S. E. Taylor et al., 1991). Perceived control persists even when situations become apparently uncontrollable. Personal control is durable because it joins with coping strategies. For example, perceived personal control and coping behaviors were associated in a study of almost 500 gay men in San Francisco (Folkman et al., in press). Using path analysis, Folkman et al. showed that perceptions of personal control correspond to a constellation of HIV-related coping strategies. A sense of control among HIV-positive men led to treatment involvement, including planful problem solving, advice and information seeking, and positive appraisals. Similar findings were reported in a sample of 53 long-term AIDS survivors (Remien et al., 1992).

Although it can be seen as a belief or perception, personal control itself can take the form of a coping strategy. In this sense, a person may assume personal control over a particular aspect of illness. For example, compliance with medical treatments can be considered a form of control expressed as a coping strategy. Control and coping can therefore appear similar to each other and often overlap. A sense of control and enacting problem-focused coping can also be related in the opposite manner, with coping strategies giving rise to a greater sense of personal control.

In an unusual example of how coping strategies can bring an increased sense of control, Schneider et al. (1991) found that suicidal thoughts linked to AIDS-related events can function as a means of coping. Schneider et al. found that suicidal ideations may alleviate psychological distress, rather than emerging out of despair. Contemplating suicide helped some individuals continue functioning with a greater sense of personal control in relation to their future. One of the Schneider et al. participants illustrated the finding by stating, "I think that thinking about suicide alternatives is a way for me to cope, or deal with the 'what would I do' question if I were to develop AIDS" (p. 785). This is not to suggest that all suicidal ideations occur to achieve a sense of personal control over HIV infection. Rather, this result illustrates that a need for control can be strong and may occur in subtle and unexpected ways.

The need to control one's own health decisions and physical functioning is observed when people first seek HIV antibody testing (Siegel & Krauss, 1991), as they enter early HIV infection (G. M. Reed et al., 1993; Pakenham, Dadds, & Terry, 1994), and during later stages of AIDS (S. E. Taylor et al., 1991). Control can be exerted over symptoms, HIV-related illnesses, the general course of HIV disease, or a combination of disease processes. S. E. Taylor et al. (1991) found that gay men in the Los Angeles MACS cohort sensed control over day-to-day symptoms, health maintenance, and medical treatment. A sense of control over HIV-related symptoms corresponds to improved psychological adjustment (G. M. Reed et al., 1993), particularly among those suffering moderate to severe symptoms (S. E. Taylor et al., 1991). Perceptions of control may motivate actions to suppress HIV-related symptoms, such as increased relaxation and sleep, improved self-care, and stress reduction (G. M. Reed et al., 1993).

Control may be exerted during HIV-related illnesses. For example, gay men with advanced HIV infection subjectively experience at least some degree of control over the course of HIV, and these perceptions positively correspond to adaptation (G. M. Reed et al., 1993). Perceptions of control appear most adaptive when there is actual control available (S. E. Taylor et al., 1991). For example, individuals with HIV infection often engage in activities that have immediate and tangible health outcomes, including changes in diet, initiating an exercise program, and seeking information about available treatments (G. M. Reed et al., 1993). One of the most common types of control exerted over the course of HIV involves taking responsibility for one's medical care. G. M. Reed et al. (1993) found that 79% of gay men with HIV infection viewed themselves as having control over their medical care and control over the course of infection. Thus, a sense of control over illness progression has psychological benefits across phases of the HIV infection (S. E. Taylor et al., 1991).

External Control

External control beliefs involve forces outside the person thought to exert control over the course of illness, including luck, chance, or other people (S. E. Taylor et al., 1984). Individuals often believe that physicians and other medical professionals have a greater degree of control over the course of HIV than they do themselves. For example, one third of people with HIV infection believe that their physician has control over day-to-day symptoms, and over two thirds believe that physicians have some control over the course of infection (G. M. Reed et al., 1993).

Studies of non-HIV chronic illnesses show that perceptions of external control interact with illness-related factors to influence adjustment. Taylor and her colleagues (S. E. Taylor et al., 1984, 1991) have shown that perceived external control over the course of breast cancer relates to psychological adjustment in women with favorable prognoses. In contrast, beliefs that others control the course of illness correlate with maladjustment among women with poor prognoses. Control ascribed to powerful others is therefore related to adjustment only when others are credited with a positive outcome. Affleck et al. (1987) found that arthritis sufferers who believe physicians control their daily symptoms become distressed, whereas beliefs that physicians control the course of illness relate to psychological adjustment. Thus, the positive or negative value of perceived external control depends on illness status and expected outcomes.

Perceptions of medical professionals' control over HIV infection correspond with poor psychological adjustment (e.g., Kelly, Murphy, Bahr, Koob, et al., 1993), particularly when symptoms of HIV are advanced (G. M. Reed et al., 1993; Remien et al., 1992; S. E. Taylor et al., 1991). People with HIV infection who believe others control their health and medical care are less well adjusted when compared with those who ascribe little control to external sources (S. E. Taylor et al., 1991). Medical care settings generally limit personal control, while facilitating the control of powerful others. Thus, perceptions of external control can be difficult to balance with perceived personal control when individuals are receiving medical treatment. Personal distress can especially occur when control is given over to physicians reluctant to take on HIV-related cases and who are perceived as lacking expertise in HIV disease (G. M. Reed et al., 1993). Like recurrent cancer (S. E. Taylor et al., 1991), HIV infection has a poor prognosis and therefore understandably leads to distress when others are believed to be in control of one's fate.

Self-Esteem

Changes in body image, physical limitations, and loss of social roles adversely affect the self-esteem of chronically ill patients. S. E. Taylor (1983) identified enhancing self-esteem as a theme in the adjustment to chronic and life-threatening illnesses. Self-enhancement is achieved by deriving personal benefit from illness experiences either by comparing oneself with others who are less fortunate or by focusing on aspects of the illness to make one feel well-off (S. E. Taylor, 1983). Taylor found that cancer patients tend to compare themselves with others who are doing worse rather than better than themselves to build up their self-esteem. Downward comparisons enhance personal perceptions by focusing on one's positive relative to other's negative experiences. Unfortunately, little research has been done to evaluate self-enhancement processes in HIV infection. Thus, although people with HIV infection appear to have similar issues of self-esteem as those observed among cancer patients, conclusions must be held until more research is available.

COPING STRATEGIES

Achieving a sense of meaning, control, and self-esteem occur in conjunction with coping strategies that either directly address the illness or address emotional responses to the illness. Factor analysis typically identifies two types of coping strategies: problem-focused coping and emotion-focused coping (Fleishman & Fogel, 1994; Folkman, Lazarus, Dunkel-Schetter, De-Longis, & Gruen, 1986; McCrae & Costa, 1986; Pearlin & Schooler, 1978). Problem-focused and emotion-focused coping constitute different means to achieve psychological balance. The particular coping strategies that an individual with HIV infection may use is determined by multiple factors, including stage of illness, personal coping history, and perceived available coping resources. For example, men living in urban gay communities have access to stable resources that facilitate coping with HIV infection (Neugebauer et al., 1992). In contrast, people with HIV infection living in rural areas lack resources that facilitate adjustment (Bozovich et al., 1992). There is evidence that men and women, ethnic groups, and HIV risk groups differ in their use of coping strategies (Billings & Moos, 1981, 1984; Fleishman & Fogel, 1994). Unfortunately, not enough information is available to allow for conclusions about differences among patterns of coping across segments of the HIV epidemic.

Problem-Focused Coping

Problem-focused coping consists of behavioral and cognitive strategies aimed at solving problems and resolving conflicts (Lazarus & Folkman, 1984) and is used most in situations where a person has a sense of personal control; doing something is potentially constructive (Scheier & Carver, 1987). Direct confrontation of symptoms is a common example of problem-focused coping in chronic illness (e.g., Feifel et al., 1987). Mobilization against chronic disease has positive effects on psychological adjustment (Wolf et al., 1991), global psychological well-being (Kurdek & Siesky, 1990), self-esteem, emotional well-being, subjective health (Namir, Wolcott, Fawzy, & Alumbaugh, 1987), and certain aspects of physical functioning (Mulder & Antoni, 1992). People with HIV infection frequently engage in action-oriented coping behaviors and appear to find these strategies psychologically beneficial (S. E. Taylor & Aspinwall, 1990). An active, "fighting spirit" style of coping relates to positive effects on HIV disease progression (Solano et al., 1993) as well as to adjustment to HIV infection (Leserman, Perkins, & Evans, 1992). However, these relationships are correctional, and health outcomes are likely bidirectionally linked to problem-focused coping. That is, with improved health people feel better and have more energy to engage in activities that in turn promote a sense of positive well-being.

Examples of problem-focused coping include trying to learn more about HIV infection, seeking new treatments, focusing on healthy changes in life-style, and making plans to access new therapies (Fleishman & Fogel, 1994; Longo, Spross, & Locke, 1990). An examination of responses to a coping scale completed by HIV-positive men and women showed that active, problem-focused coping strategies were frequently endorsed (Kalichman, 1995). As shown in Table 7.1, problem-focused coping was common, with over half of respondents endorsing five of the seven strategies. Similarly, long-term survivors use a number of active coping strategies without any one dominant pattern of responses emerging (Remien et al., 1992). Broadly defined HIV-related active coping encompasses cognitive coping, involvement in medical treatment, seeking information, life-style changes, and social activism.

Cognitive Coping Strategies

Problem-focused cognitive coping is characterized by attempts to achieve a perspective that protects against the graveness of HIV or creates mean-

Table 7.1

Problem-Focused Coping Strategies Endorsed by People With HIV Infection

Coping strategy	% endorsing item
Analyzed the problem to understand it better	67
Talked with someone to find out more about the situation	62
Got professional help	45
Made a plan of action and followed it	49
Talked with someone who could do something concrete about the problem	51
Changed something so things would turn out all right	62
Came up with a couple of different solutions	55

ing out of being HIV positive. People with HIV infection commonly adopt a life view that promotes a sense of emotional well-being (Namir et al., 1987; Wolf et al., 1991). Typical cognitive techniques used by people with HIV include meditation, self-hypnosis, and mental imagery (Namir et al., 1987). Plans of action and positive thoughts about the future are also common cognitive coping strategies. Fleishman and Fogel (1994) found that thoughts such as concentrating on how things could be worse and looking toward the brighter side of things were related to lower levels of depressive mood. Kalichman (1995) found that 62% of HIV-positive men and women had rediscovered what was important in their lives after learning they were HIV positive, and 67% indicated that they rehearsed particular actions as a means of coping.

Involvement in Medical Treatment

Becoming active in one's medical care can facilitate adjustment to HIV infection (Namir et al., 1987; Storosum, Van den Boom, Van Beauzekom, & Sno, 1990). Seeking medical treatments, becoming informed about possible treatment side effects, identifying opportunities to enroll in clinical trials and experimental treatments, exploring complementary therapies, and developing alliances with medical professionals are examples of increased involvement (Remien et al., 1992; Siegel & Krauss, 1991). Participation in AIDS clinical trials offers additional psychological benefits, such as an increased sense of control and increased hope (Robiner et al., 1993).

Information Seeking

Identifying and consuming pertinent information are among the greatest needs expressed by the chronic medically ill (Felton & Revenson, 1984), and by people with HIV infection in particular (D. Miller & Pinching, 1989). Namir, Wolcott, Fawzy, and Alumbaugh (1990) found that 85% of HIV-positive gay men had tried to find out more information about their illness. Information seeking is common in HIV infection, with over 62% of HIV-positive men and women indicating that they have discussed with others ways to find out more about HIV and AIDS (Kalichman, 1995).

Sources of information vary, and most people seek materials from multiple resources. Thus, a large number of information services have been established to meet these needs. Federal, state, and local health departments, as well as activist and grass-roots organizations, have produced brochures, booklets, and newsletters for people with HIV infection. Rapid changes in the development, testing, and clinical trials of treatments for HIV infection and HIV-related opportunistic illnesses overwhelm people with information, particularly immediately after they test HIV positive.

Life-Style Changes

People with HIV infection often make changes in their life-style and everyday habits to promote their physical health. Namir et al. (1990) found that 81% of HIV-positive patients began eating more healthily and taking vitamins in response to testing HIV positive. Individuals with HIV infection also report resting more and reducing their use of alcohol and drugs as a means of coping (Siegel & Krauss, 1991). Aerobic exercise is another common change in life-style that buffers stress for people with HIV infection (LaPerriere, Schneiderman, Antoni, & Fletcher, 1990). Changes in life-style bolster a sense of personal control in a similar fashion as do other problem-focused coping strategies. Although such changes improve both psychological and physical well-being, it should be noted that there is no evidence that healthy life-style changes significantly impede HIV infection or clinically alter its course.

Social Activism

Although only 7% of HIV-positive people become involved in political activism as a means of coping (Namir et al., 1990), those who are social activists experience benefits in terms of their psychological adjustment. Those who are not themselves activists may vicariously benefit from knowing others who are.

In summary, action against HIV infection by way of problem-focused coping strategies occurs most frequently in response to aspects of disease that appear controllable, such as medical care, health behavior changes, and social relationships. The realities of HIV infection indicate that most benefits come from attempts to prevent opportunistic illnesses and control symptoms. Forestalling the onset of or curing opportunistic illnesses increases involvement in treatment, information seeking, and life-style changes. However, when problem-focused coping strategies are unsuccessful, or are at least perceived as unsuccessful, or when people respond to aspects of HIV that they feel they have little control over, a shift occurs from problem-focused to emotion-focused coping (Somerfield & Curbow, 1992).

Emotion-Focused Coping

Emotion-focused coping consists of cognitive and behavioral adjustment strategies that do not directly intervene with problem situations (Lazarus & Folkman, 1984). These coping strategies include denial, acceptance, avoidance, escape, distancing, use of distractions, and positive reappraisal (Lazarus & Folkman, 1984). Chronic medical patients can benefit from certain emotion-focused coping strategies (e.g., Derogatis, Abeloff, & Melisaratos, 1979). One model of coping with terminal illness almost exclusively relies on emotion-focused coping. Kubler-Ross (1969, 1975, 1981) described five stages of adjustment to terminal illness and loss: *denial*, experience and expression of *anger*, *bargaining* with external forces perceived as controlling the course of illness, *depression* in the face of continued deterioration, and *acceptance*. Given that emotion-focused coping is effective when a person can have little actual control over the course of illness (S. E. Taylor & Aspinwall, 1990), it is not surprising the Kubler-Ross's model revolves around emotion-focused coping. Consistent with Kubler-Ross's model, Kalichman (1995) found that people with HIV engage in denial, acceptance, avoidance, and distractions as coping strategies. Table 7.2 presents the percentages of HIV-positive people in Kalichman's study who endorsed eight emotion-focused coping strategies.

Table 7.2

Emotion-Focused Coping Strategies Endorsed by People with HIV Infection

Coping strategy	% endorsing item
Turned to work or substitute activity to take my mind off things	44
Looked for the silver lining; tried to look on the bright side of things	64
Told myself things that helped me to feel better	54
Didn't let it get to me; refused to think too much about it	45
Wished that I could change what happened or how I felt	54
Daydreamed or imagined a better time or place than the one I was in	61
Wished the situation would go away or somehow be over with	54
Reminded myself how much worse things could be	63

Denial

Denial may occur at several points in HIV infection. For example, people may avoid getting tested for HIV antibodies despite high-risk histories or even illness symptoms (Lyter et al., 1987; Siegel et al., 1989). Following receipt of an HIV-positive test result, some people engage in denial by believing that HIV infection is not the cause of AIDS (Chuang et al., 1989). Still others do not believe that their test results are accurate and may either get retested or just go on as if they were not tested in the first place (Siegel et al., 1989). HIV infection may also be denied by misattributing symptoms to non-HIV-related causes (Weitz, 1989). Although denial may recur over the course of HIV infection, few long-term survivors with AIDS use denial as a coping strategy (Rabkin, Remien, et al., 1993). Leserman et al. (1992) found that denial among gay men with AIDS was associated with negative moods, particularly anger. Thus, denial can be an effective shelter against emotional distress, but precludes problem-focused coping (Adelman, 1989).

Acceptance and Resignation

Realistic acceptance was proclaimed by Kubler-Ross (1969) as a natural final stage of coping with terminal illness. Kubler-Ross described acceptance as a state of calm that is relatively void of negative and positive emotions. According to Kubler-Ross, however, acceptance does not necessarily represent a constant state, with a sense of acceptance fading in and out over the course of illness. Studies of patients with life-threatening illnesses show that acceptance and resignation are most common among those who have diseases with little chance of cure or long-term remission (Feifel et al., 1987). These same descriptions seem valid in AIDS. Griffiths and Wilkins (1993) found that individuals diagnosed with HIV infection for five years or longer accepted their condition. Long asymptomatic periods of HIV infection may facilitate acceptance of impending illness (Nichols, 1985). Over 54% of people in one study had accepted being HIV positive and believed that nothing could be done to help them (Kalichman, 1995).

Accepting HIV infection is not, however, necessarily associated with psychological adjustment. G. M. Reed, Kemeny, Taylor, Wang, and Visscher (1994) found that realistic acceptance of HIV infection was unrelated to a global index of psychological adjustment. Reed et al. also found that individuals who were resigned to dying of AIDS demonstrated shorter lengths of survival. These findings suggest that personal acceptance of future debilitation, loss of functioning, and death may be related to poorer psychological adjustment in HIV infection. A possible reason for these findings is that acceptance and resignation are inconsistent with confrontational styles of coping and a fighting spirit, both of which are associated with problem-focused coping. Perhaps because AIDS represents multiple opportunistic illnesses, each of which may be successfully treated, AIDS patients believe, and with good reason, that they can live longer if they just get past an AIDS-related condition.

Avoidance

For the most part, avoidance coping corresponds to psychological distress and poor long-term adjustment (Lazarus & Folkman, 1984). Cognitive and behavioral avoidance occurs relatively frequently early in asymptomatic HIV infection as compared with later symptomatic phases (Kurdek & Siesky, 1990). HIV symptomatics rarely use cognitive and behavioral avoidance strategies (Namir et al., 1987). Concern over health and existential issues correlate with use of avoidance coping (Namir et al., 1990). Like other medical conditions, avoidance coping in HIV infection leads to increased psychological distress and dysphoria (Fleishman & Fogel, 1994; Namir et al., 1987; Nicholson & Long, 1990). Women, ethnic minorities, and injection drug users with HIV infection are more likely to use avoidance coping strategies relative to their White gay male counterparts (Fleishman & Fogel, 1994; Leserman et al., 1992). Avoidance coping includes simply trying to forget about being HIV positive, canceling medical appointments, and refusing to discuss HIV infection.

Distraction

Cognitive and behavioral distraction strategies seem to occur with greater frequency than avoidance techniques and, in contrast with avoidance, may facilitate psychological adjustment (Namir et al., 1987, 1990). In one study, 38% of HIV-positive people stated that they had gone on a vacation to cope, and 44% turned to work or some other activity to distract themselves from thoughts of being HIV positive (Kalichman, 1995). People with HIV infection report going out with friends, treating themselves to something special, and thinking about things unrelated to their condition as means of distracting themselves from thinking about being HIV positive (Namir et al., 1987). Movies, theater, and music are also common means of distraction (Remien et al., 1992). Opportunities to divert attention away from being HIV positive diminish in advanced stages of HIV infection. Loss of employment and a dwindling social life limit opportunities for distraction. People with HIV–AIDS must often give up their pets and even hobbies that could serve as distractions, because of risks of contact with disease-causing microbes.

Other Emotion-Focused Strategies

Substance use may provide a temporary escape from the everyday distress that can be associated with HIV infection, as well as an escape from symptoms and illness (Cleary, Fowler, et al., 1993). Alcohol and drug use is common in gay communities and particularly frequent among men at risk for HIV infection (Ostrow, 1994). Unfortunately, little is known about baseline coping among individuals who later become HIV infected, particularly with reference to maladaptive coping. Wishful thinking and intellectualization may also be used to feel better for the moment without directly addressing HIV infection.

OPTIMISM AND SPIRITUALITY

Beyond specific coping strategies, attitudes and personal styles are closely related to adjustment. A positive outlook toward the future and an importance placed on faith and spiritual beliefs may motivate coping responses. Optimism and spirituality are related to meaning, control, and self-esteem: Optimism and hope parallel a sense of personal control and help foster a sense of self-esteem, whereas spirituality is more closely connected to a search for meaning.

Optimism and Hope

For people facing adversity, positive beliefs about the future can promote a sense of self-worth and inner-strength (C. Peterson, Seligman, & Vaillant, 1988; S. E. Taylor & Brown, 1988; S. E. Taylor et al., 1992). For example, coronary heart disease patients who are optimistic about their health and the course of their illness have fewer symptoms than do pessimistic patients (Scheier et al., 1989). Optimism in relation to HIV disease corresponds to a greater sense of control and increased use of problem-focused coping (S. E. Taylor et al., 1992). Knowledge of being

HIV positive evokes a sense of optimism about not developing AIDS that is only seen in individuals who are HIV positive (S. E. Taylor et al., 1992). Perceived control over HIV infection can be characterized as unrealistically optimistic, and serve psychologically self-protective functions (S. E. Taylor et al., 1992). Like personal control, optimism gives rise to problem-focused coping and leads to improved adjustment (Rabkin et al., 1990; S. E. Taylor et al., 1992). Optimism and hope both consist of expectations that something positive lies ahead, imply confidence about the future, and result in positive appraisals about potential illness outcomes (Rabkin et al., 1990). In a study of HIV-positive gay and bisexual men, Pakenham et al. (1994) found that a sense of optimisim was related to psychological adjustment.

In addition to HIV-specific optimism and hope, a more global style of positive thinking, or *dispositional optimism*, may reduce fears and promote problem-focused coping (S. E. Taylor et al., 1992). Dispositional optimism is associated with reductions in psychological distress, alleviation of worries and concerns about AIDS, decreased perceptions of risk of developing AIDS, and the use of problem-focused coping (S. E. Taylor et al., 1992). Long-term survivors with AIDS demonstrate a psychological resiliency that reflects dispositional optimism (Hardy, 1991). Rabkin, Remien, et al. (1993) found that long-term survivors were able to articulate goals and saw the future in a positive light. Thus, positive attitudes, optimistic outlooks, and hope compose a constellation of attitudes that contribute to psychological adjustment in HIV, particularly among people at later stages of infection.

Spirituality

HIV-positive individuals possess a broad range of religious beliefs and diverse spiritual practices, including identification with long-held faith and inquiries into new spiritual expressions (Winiarski, 1991). Once again like other chronic illnesses, existential and spiritual issues emerge out of questioning how the personal tragedy of HIV infection could happen to anyone (D. Grant & Anns, 1988). Thus, spiritual experiences and expression are concerned with a search for meaning and value from illness.

Unlike other life-threatening illnesses, HIV infection is associated with behaviors opposed by many traditional religious institutions (Warner-

na, 1989; Weitz, 1989; Winiarski, 1991; Yates, 1991).
ifection may encounter reprehension rather than sup-
; guidance from spiritual leaders. Thus, it is not un-
viduals with HIV infection to seek new and alternative
moue   l expression. For example, Carson (1990) found that gay
men with AIDS do not achieve spiritual well-being as a result of participating in formal religions, but rather through an individual's ability to respond to existential challenges. In another study of gay men with HIV infection, Somlai and Kalichman (1994) found that men who were
ambivalent toward formal religious doctrines developed new and alternative modes of spiritual expression. Spiritual practices with immediate and
tangible benefits were frequently reported in this sample of HIV-positive
men and women. Figure 7.1 shows the relative frequencies of spiritual
practices, both formal and nontraditional, reported by Somlai and Kalichman.

For many people, facing a life-threatening illness involves reliance on
religious beliefs, particularly if they tended to be religious before becoming ill (J. Holland, 1982). HIV infection can serve as a catalyst for spiritual growth, including a return to religious beliefs, deepening of an existing spirituality, and developing new dimensions to one's spiritual self
(Schwartzberg, 1993). Spiritual needs and practices are common among
HIV-positive people, with more than half of participants in one study indicating that they frequently prayed, 40% reporting they had found new
faith, and 62% often hoping that a miracle would happen in relation to
their being HIV positive (Kalichman, 1995).

Spiritual practices potentially provide multiple sources of comfort, including support from beliefs in connection with a higher power and social support from a spiritual community. Religiosity and spirituality can
reduce the burdens of caregiving for partners of HIV-positive patients who
are themselves HIV positive. Social support, whether through participation in spiritual practices or otherwise, constitutes an important dimension of adjustment in its own right.

CONCLUSION

On the basis of the literature and information gained from interviews with
HIV-positive men and women (Kalichman, 1995), the following ideas are

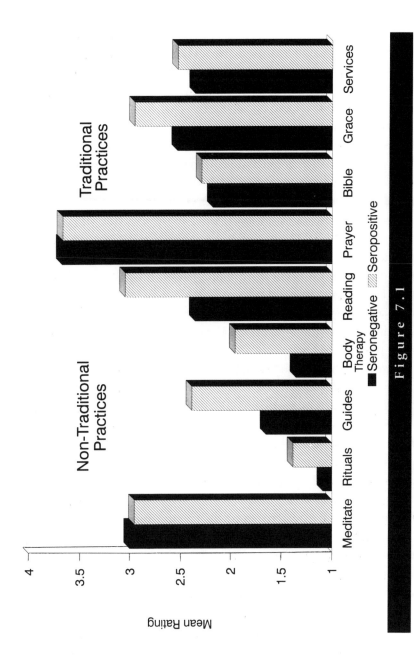

Figure 7.1

Traditional and nontraditional spiritual practices among people with HIV infection. Mean ratings for frequency of practice: 1 = never, 4 = daily.

offered to aid practitioners in promoting adaptive coping with HIV-positive clients.

People with HIV infection may be empowered to chart their own course of health care and medical treatment. Being HIV positive can lead to a sense of demoralization and can halt most plans for the future. People with HIV infection may therefore require encouragement to exert control over their responses to HIV disease and become active participants in their medical treatment. Asking questions and developing a treatment alliance with health care providers should be encouraged. Clinical trials and complementary therapies offer opportunities to become engaged in one's own treatment. Such actions may have positive effects on psychological adjustment as well as health status (Robiner et al., 1993).

Coping can be facilitated by anticipating physical declines. It is important for people with HIV infection to recognize that coping and support needs change over the course of infection. Fatigue, weakness, illness symptoms, and treatment side effects may interfere with psychological adjustment. A lack of initiative and physical disability interfere with coping at later phases of HIV infection. Recognizing these changes before their onset affords the opportunity to build a safety-net of coping supports in advance of physical decline.

The availability and use of multiple coping strategies facilitates adjustment processes. Thus, individuals with a broader range of coping behaviors will have more coping options. Cancer patients who use multiple coping strategies adjust better than those with narrow coping repertoires (Dunkel-Schetter et al., 1992; S. E. Taylor & Aspinwall, 1990). Diversity and flexibility in coping allows ineffective coping responses to be replaced with new strategies, increasing the chances that coping will meet the needs of a given situation.

Distractions from HIV–AIDS decrease psychological distress. HIV infection can consume a person's entire being. Over the course of HIV disease, relationships are often lost and the ability to actively participate in life diminishes. HIV infection usually leads to physical limitations that result in unemployment and restricted social activities. At the same time, regular medical visits increase, medications become routine, and people are surrounded by others with HIV infection and AIDS. Opportunities for distractions become more constricted as infection progresses. Social interactions and keeping busy become valued breaks from intrusive thoughts of being HIV positive.

Clients with HIV infection appear to benefit from actions and practices that provide immediate and tangible coping outcomes. Being HIV positive leads to the realization that life is finite. Recognizing an ultimate end to one's life may create pressure to adjust. Changes in diet, exercise, relationships, and spiritual practices are geared toward meeting immediate needs. Creative writing, painting, gardening, and other forms of personal productivity help to provide a sense of self-worth and purpose (Schaefer & Coleman, 1992).

As the HIV epidemic progresses and more people die of AIDS, psychological numbing, complacency, and hopelessness may replace a fighting spirit. People with HIV infection should be encouraged to look toward future developments in treatment. Advances in antiretroviral (Lundgren et al., 1994), and prophylactic treatments against opportunistic illnesses (Osmond et al., 1994) have increased survival times for people with HIV infection. Although a cure for HIV infection that clears the virus from the body is not in sight, advances in preventing, treating, and curing HIV-related illnesses are occurring at an astounding pace. Hope that people will live longer with a higher quality of life requires active encouragement, support, and opportunities to access medical treatments.

Denial is maladaptive when it interferes with medical treatment decisions and deters proactive health decisions. There are numerous ways that denial is used to cope with HIV infection. For example, some believe that HIV is not the cause of AIDS or that the HIV-antibody test has a high false-positive rate. Such beliefs inhibit seeking medical treatments that can extend and enhance the quality of life. Realistic optimism, as opposed to denial, can increase treatment seeking and promote proactive health decisions, as well as other problem-focused coping strategies.

Substance use as a means of avoidance is common, where alcohol and other drugs are used as an escape from daily life stressors including HIV infection. Substance use can provide a temporary escape from emotional distress of HIV infection. Prolonged substance abuse, however, interferes with problem-focused coping, disrupts social relationships and work attendance, and can become psychologically maladaptive. Eliminating substance use as a means of coping requires adopting optional coping behaviors that meet immediate and tangible needs. Individuals who become substance dependant may require specialized treatment as well as a means of replacing substance use with adaptive coping behaviors.

8

Social Adjustment and Social Support

Interpersonal relationships can help to alleviate psychological distress associated with chronic and life-threatening illness (Cobb, 1976). Social support promotes cognitive and behavioral coping, facilitates a sense of meaning, enhances self-esteem, fosters a sense of belonging, and increases available coping resources (Linn, Lewis, Cain, & Kimbrough, 1993; Wolf, Balson, Morse, et al., 1991). Unfortunately, the chronically ill often lack adequate social support at a time when it is most needed. Depression and anxiety associated with chronic illness can further disrupt relationships and distance people from potential social support (Shinn, Lehmann, & Wong, 1984; Turner et al., 1993).

Social support is related to stress–health relationships, mortality, and other health-related outcomes (Antonucci, 1989; Broadhead et al., 1983; House, Landis, & Umberson, 1988; Ostrow et al., 1991). Although some studies have suggested that social support impedes disease progression (e.g., Jensen, 1983; Shearn & Fireman, 1985), most research has focused on the role of social support in emotional adjustment. Social support is inversely related to depression in diabetes (Littlefield, Rodin, Murray, & Craven, 1990) and is positively related to adjustment to breast cancer (Meyerowitz, 1980; Watson, 1983), hemodialysis (Dimond, 1979), disabilities resulting from stroke (Evans & Northwood, 1983; Schulz, Tompkins, & Rau, 1988), and rheumatoid arthritis (Goodenow, Reisine, & Grady, 1990). Thus, there is compelling evidence that supportive relationships facilitate adjustment to the stressors of chronic illness.

As a construct, social support lacks generally accepted operational definitions (Green, 1993). Social support is defined here as a multidimensional construct that includes support needs, available resources, and satisfaction. In addition, social support refers to multiple aspects of interpersonal relationships, including the number and types of contacts a person has, the functional content of relationships, and the perceived quality or adequacy of support (Green, 1993). In relation to chronic illness, each dimension of social support tends to vary at different stages of disease (Broadhead et al., 1983). Under this conceptualization, perceptions of adequate social support will, by definition, enhance a sense of feeling cared for, loved, informed, and affiliated (Cobb, 1976).

Two conceptual models of health-related social support are described in the literature: models that emphasize the main effects (or direct effects) of support and models that view social support as an immediate buffer of stress. Main-effects models posit that social support directly increases health by information, enhanced self-esteem, or perceived control (S. Cohen, 1988). Stress-buffering models, on the other hand, state that when a person is under duress, social support increases information, emotional well-being, or tangible resources that in turn affect health outcomes (S. Cohen, 1988). Both models of support incorporate information, compassion, and the assistance of others that are either directly or indirectly linked to health and illness.

In addition to the functional aspects of support, the structure of support networks has health implications (Shinn, Lehmann, & Wong, 1984). Structural aspects of support include the frequency of social contacts, the relationships that serve as sources of support, the opportunity to reciprocate support, and the integration of the individual into a supportive network (House et al., 1988; Israel & Antonucci, 1987; Stowe, Ross, Wodak, Thomas, & Larson, 1993). Individual differences in perceived social support, personality dispositions, and the match between support and needs interact to determine the ultimate effects of social support (Lakey & Cassady, 1990). Figure 8.1 summarizes the structural and functional components of social support. Independent of or in conjunction with coping

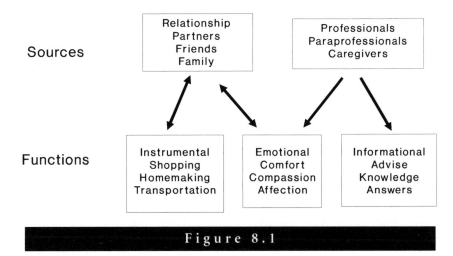

Figure 8.1

Sources and functions of social support.

strategies, these factors play an important role in the psychological adjustment to HIV infection.

Structurally, having a spouse or domestic partner, the frequency of social contacts, formal and informal group memberships, and sheer numbers of close friends influence adjustment (Berkman & Syme, 1979). Functionally, the content of social relationships affects health. Social support fosters a sense of purpose or meaning and promotes health behaviors, including treatment seeking and treatment compliance (House et al., 1988). Social support may also affect perceptions of stressful events and coping (Mulder & Antoni, 1992; O'Leary, 1990). Thus, there is considerable evidence that the structural and functional dimensions of support are important aspects of psychological adjustment to HIV–AIDS (Namir, Alumbaugh, Fawzy, & Wolcott, 1989).

STRUCTURE OF SOCIAL SUPPORT

Social networks vary across the HIV epidemic. However, like most aspects of the epidemic, information about the structure of social support has come from studies of primarily White, middle-class, gay and bisexual men. This bias in the literature may be particularly troublesome because social networks of gay men are qualitatively different from those of heterosexuals (Kurdek, 1988) and gay communities have organized to support people with AIDS. Gay men have historically migrated to large cities without their families and other potential sources of support (Turner et al., 1993). Well-defined gay communities are common in most U.S. cities and provide multiple sources of support (Britton, Zarski, & Hobfoll, 1993). Greater support is received by men more closely identified with gay communities, as opposed to bisexual men and men outside of gay social networks (W. D. Nicholson & Long, 1990; Ostrow et al., 1991). Although social networks within gay communities differ from those of other population segments, the benefits of social support do not differ (Kurdek, 1988).

Gay communities themselves are heterogeneous, with differences, for example, in social support among ethnic groups. Ostrow et al. (1991) found that African American gay men benefit less from social support and report less affirming social networks than their White counterparts. These differences may exist because social support networks vary in terms of ethnic composition and social classes (Green, 1993). For example, African Americans as a group exhibit social support structures that reflect cultural differences in help-seeking behaviors and informal support (Mays & Cochran, 1987). Factors related to accessing community resources influence ethnic and cultural differences in social support (Mays & Cochran, 1987). Similarly, Latin Americans and other ethnic minorities exhibit diverse patterns of social networks, and the social networks of women differ from those of men.

Injection drug users often lack support in their relationships. Opportunities for social support are reduced by unemployment, poverty, isolation, and other factors related to social disadvantage (Stowe et al., 1993). Social stigmas, loss of financial resources, changes in self-image, and alienation from peer groups are all aspects of HIV infection that affect the availability of and satisfaction with social support (Hays, Chauncey, & Tobey, 1990; Turner et al., 1993).

Depression and psychological distress, fear that others will discover one's condition, and concerns of transmitting the virus promote isolation (Namir et al., 1989). Even before learning they are HIV positive, however, many HIV-positive people compartmentalize their social networks (Hays, Chauncey et al., 1990). For example, gay men commonly have two sets of friends, gay and heterosexual, and two sets of family members, those who do and do not know their sexual orientation. Similar partitioned relationships also occur among injection drug users and low-income women

(Hays, Catania, McKusick, & Coates, 1990). Although segmentation may lead to reduced social contacts, the actual number of contacts per se is less important in psychological adjustment than is the quality of contacts (Hays, Chauncey et al., 1990; Namir et al., 1989). The most common sources of social support to people with HIV–AIDS include four types of caregivers: relationship partners, friends, family, and professional care-givers (Pearlin, Mullan, Aneshensel, Wardlaw, & Harrington, 1994).

Relationship Partners

Relationship partners are a primary source of social support (Bor et al., 1990; Hays, Chauncey et al., 1990; Kurdek, 1988). As in other chronic med-ical conditions (e.g., Medalie & Goldbourt, 1976), support from a spouse or long-term relationship partner is an important aspect of effective so-cial support systems in HIV infection (Wolcott et al., 1986). Unfortunately, support offered by relationship partners is often threatened by HIV in-fection. In particular, sexual relations and pair bonding can deteriorate when one or both partners are HIV positive (Gochros, 1992). For exam-ple, Agle, Gluck, and Pierce (1987) found that hemophiliacs suffer sexual relationship problems, with over half of those studied feeling concerned about potentially transmitting the virus to their partners. Similar issues arise for other subgroups of HIV-positive people (Green, 1993). Sexual re-lationships can become strained because of declines in health, as well as fears of transmitting HIV (Donlou et al., 1985; Green, 1993). Independent of caregiving, additional burdens are placed on partners who are them-selves HIV positive. Folkman, Chesney, Cooke, Boccellari, and Collette (1994) showed that depressed mood and life disruptions occur among HIV-positive gay men who provide care to their partner. The stress of HIV infection can cause an end to long-term relationships (Coates et al., 1987). Because many people with HIV infection live alone or outside of long-term relationships (Hart, Fitzpatrick, McLean, Dawson, & Boulton, 1990), friends and peers are often the primary source of social support.

Friends and Peers

Social support networks in HIV infection consist primarily of friendships and peer relationships. Friends are the main source of social support among gay and bisexual men and among injection drug users (Namir et al., 1989; Stowe et al., 1993). Friends offer empathy, accessibility, and shared values and culture, and friendships are associated with psychological adjustment among people with HIV infection (Hays, Catania et al., 1990).

Integration into a community that is sensitive to the needs of those with HIV infection increases the number of HIV-positive peers one has. As the HIV epidemic expands, numerous community-based organizations have emerged to bring people with HIV infection together. Relationships among people with HIV are grounded in common experiences that break down barriers of ignorance and stigmatization.

Family Support

Family relationships typically provide stable support during chronic illness despite the disruptions caused to family continuity (Sales, 1991). Stigmas that predate HIV infection create unfortunate barriers to family support (Frierson et al., 1987). For example, Donlou et al. (1985) found that gay men with HIV infection did not perceive their families as helpful in their efforts to cope with being HIV positive. Family estrangement can be closely related to a long history of rejection. Hays, Chauncey et al. (1990) found that HIV-negative as well as HIV-positive gay men perceived their parents and siblings as the least supportive people in their lives. However, Hays et al. also reported that 92% of gay men with AIDS sought help from family members, a higher number than both asymptomatic HIV-positive and HIV-negative gay men.

Families are being called on to assume greater responsibilities for caregiving, particularly at the later phases of infection (Takigiku, Brubaker, & Hennon, 1993). Caring for an ill person is a highly stressful role. Chronic illness has similar psychological affects on family caregivers as on patients themselves (Cassileth et al., 1985). Family caregivers report high levels of distress, with over 75% of parent caregivers experiencing symptoms of depression and 74% of siblings having repeated thoughts of death and dying (Bumbalo, Patsdaughter, & McShane, 1993; McShane, Bumbalo, & Patsdaughter, 1994). Parents of HIV-positive gay men (Takigiku et al., 1993) and hemophiliacs (Agle et al., 1987) worry about their child's health. Parents experience distress from the uncertainties of HIV disease and from witnessing its deteriorating effects over a long period of time (Siegl & Morse, 1994). Parental caregiver stress is obviously compounded when the parent himself or herself is HIV positive and he or she is caring for their HIV-infected child (Reidy, Taggart, & Asselin, 1991). Dual patient and caregiver roles are problematic in HIV infection because HIV-positive parents tend to be socially isolated (Hackl et al., 1995; Minkoff, Nanda, Menez, & Fikrig, 1987). Thus, family support can contribute to the adjustment of individuals with HIV infection, but caregiving involves considerable emotional costs to families (Greif & Porembski, 1988; Turner et al., 1993).

Professional Caregivers

Significant demands are placed on professional caregivers of people with chronic illnesses (Kiecolt-Glaser & Glaser, 1988b; Sales, Schulz, & Biegel, 1992). In addition to the usual stress of working with terminally ill patients, HIV infection involves social stigmas, prejudices, and biases (Adelman, 1989; J. M. George, Reed, Ballard, Colin, & Fielding, 1993; O'Dowd, 1988; Silverman, 1993). Like other chronically ill patients, people with HIV often express anger toward professional caregivers (Dilley, Ochitill, et al., 1985). Paraprofessionals and volunteers who offer support experience similar types of reactions (R. L. Miller, Holmes, & Auerbach, 1992). Thus, caregivers of HIV-infected loved ones require support themselves (Land & Harangody, 1990; Reidy et al., 1991).

Professional caregivers are crucial to social support systems in HIV infection. Although relationship partners, friends, and family provide emotional support and assistance with daily tasks, professional helpers are perceived by people with HIV as a critical link to health-related information resources and advice (Hays, Catania, et al., 1990). Access to information is an important feature of professional caregiver relationships. On the other hand, the nature of a professional caregiver relationship can restrict other types of support and usually does not allow for reciprocity of support (Hays, Catania, et al., 1990).

Disclosure, Reciprocity, and Loss

Social support can be available without disclosing HIV status, but to receive support related to HIV infection, individuals must disclose. Difficulties associated with HIV-status self-disclosure include fears of rejection and social isolation that can occur at times when needs for social support are greatest. Difficulty disclosing HIV status is common, even to sexual partners, where there is a moral obligation to do so (Marks et al., 1991, 1994; J. Peterson & Marin, 1988). Disclosures of HIV infection by parents to children are inhibited by fears of rejection and by the desire to protect the children (Pliskin et al., 1993). The potential costs of self-disclosure are therefore pitted against the benefits of gaining support (Turner et al., 1993).

Opportunities to reciprocate support are another important dimension to feeling supported. Providing social support can buffer stress to an even greater extent than receiving support. For example, reciprocity decreases hostility and depression among some people with HIV infection (Hays, Catania, et al., 1990). Many people with HIV infection seek opportunities to support others by joining support groups or volunteer organizations. The rewards of helping others with HIV infection have been reported in surveys of AIDS service volunteers (R. L. Miller et al., 1992).

Various sources of loss associated with HIV infection, including unemployment, rejection, and deaths of friends, attenuate social support by shrinking the size of social networks (Zich & Temoshok, 1990). Illness and death of relationship partners, friends, and acquaintances constrict social contacts and therefore reduce opportunities to gain and reciprocate support (Turner et al., 1993). Among population subgroups hit hardest by AIDS, relationship losses have been devastating. Entire branches of gay communities have been lost, resulting in a depletion of available support for individuals with HIV infection (Hays, Chauncey et al., 1990). Paradoxically, by becoming connected to a supportive network, such as through an AIDS service organization, an activist group, or a support group, a person increases their risk of losing relationships and constricting support that they have come to rely on (J. L. Martin & Dean, 1993a).

In summary, relationships with committed partners, friends, peers, family members, and professional helpers form a structure and context of social support. Ethnic, cultural, and gender differences in social networks, and social stigmas in HIV infection, create barriers to support, increasing isolation among people who most need support. To gain support and opportunities to reciprocate, HIV-positive individuals must overcome barriers and selectively self-disclose. Although numbers and frequencies of social contacts are related to the availability of support, the content of relationships and the actions of others determine the support that a person receives.

FUNCTIONAL DIMENSIONS OF SOCIAL SUPPORT

Feeling supported is determined by more than mere social contact (Lennon, Martin, & Dean, 1990; Siegel, Raveis, & Karus, 1994; Turner et al., 1993). Social interactions must address the demands of stressors if they are going to protect against emotional distress (Hays et al., 1992). Theories of social support traditionally encompass three functions that buffer stress and promote psychological well-being: emotional, informational, and instrumental support. Emotional support consists of affection, comforting, and encouragement that result in positive effects on self-esteem, feelings of self-worth, and a sense of belonging (Cohen & Willis, 1985; Turner et al., 1993). Informational support, such as advice or updated knowledge, may help people interpret, comprehend, or cope with HIV infection (Cohen & Willis, 1985). Finally, materials, assistance, and services have practical functions and constitute an instrumental dimension of support (Cohen & Willis, 1985). All three types of support are known to promote psychological adjustment among HIV-positive individuals (Hays et al., 1992; Rabkin et al., 1990).

Emotional Support

Relationships can establish and maintain emotional balance and are therefore considered a high priority in coping with HIV (Lennon et al., 1990; Wolcott et al., 1986). Emotional support, like emotion-focused coping, does not directly address matters that affect HIV progression or the symptoms of HIV infection. Emotional support does, however, enhance psychological well-being by building hope and optimism (Rabkin et al., 1990; Wolcott et al., 1986; Zich & Temoshok, 1990). One study of HIV-positive gay men found that emotionally supportive behaviors, such as expressing concern, providing encouragement, and serving as a confidant, were identified as the most helpful (Hays, Magee, & Chauncey, 1994).

One emotional support need identified by people with HIV infection is physical contact (Wolcott et al., 1986). Touch communicates not being afraid of casual HIV transmission and can be a symbol of acceptance and understanding. Having a confidant is another type of emotional support that promotes well-being (Ostrow, 1989; Ostrow et al., 1988; Remien et al., 1992). Emotional support can result from simply being with someone and enjoying his or her companionship. Thus, emotional support occurs when feelings are acknowledged, regardless of whether the contact is in close and intimate relationships, among friends, in support groups, or within a professional helping relationship (Wolcott et al., 1986).

Informational Support

Uncertainties of HIV infection can cause a strong need for information (Hays et al., 1992). Accurate information can lead to realistic expectations about the course of illness, which may in turn facilitate psychological adjustment (Linn et al., 1993). People with HIV infection may seek information about their prognosis, health care and treatment options, insurance coverage, and so forth (Hays et al., 1992). Gathering information contributes to a sense of control and contributes to problem-focused coping (Hays et al., 1992). The value of informational support has led to a proliferation of information networks and newsletters about HIV and AIDS. It is important to note that denial can interfere with the potential benefits of informational support by blocking interest and openness to information (Dew, Ragni, & Nimorwicz, 1991).

Instrumental Support

Practical assistance with everyday needs helps to reduce distress and increase positive health appraisals (Belkin et al., 1992; Namir et al., 1989). In some circumstances, instrumental support can have greater psychological benefits in HIV infection than either emotional or informational support (Namir et al., 1989). The availability of assistance can relieve stress caused by physical limitations. As has been the case with other psychological dimensions of HIV infection, the need for and availability of instrumental support, as well as other types of social support, changes over the course of HIV infection.

SOCIAL SUPPORT OVER THE COURSE OF HIV INFECTION

After initially testing HIV positive, individuals tend to be in crisis and benefit most from strong emotional and informational supports (Coleman & Harris, 1989), which are unfortunately often unavailable because of fears, stigmas, and attitudes toward sickness, death, and AIDS (Green, 1993). Initial responses from post-HIV antibody test counselors and AIDS service organizations usually offer assistance when there are few other sources. After the initial receipt of test results, and as HIV infection progresses, the need for multiple types of support from multiple sources increases (Lennon et al., 1990).

Fatigue, diminished self-esteem, physical disability, and illness reduce an individual's ability to maintain interpersonal relationships (Turner et al., 1993). Illness therefore brings dissatisfaction with support even when it is available (Green, 1993; Zich & Temoshok, 1987, 1990). Hays et al. (1992) found that satisfaction with informational support affected psychological adjustment but depended on the number of HIV symptoms a person had. Gay men with more symptoms and less informational support were most depressed relative to men with few symptoms and high informational support. Thus, informational support appeared to buffer the stress associated with developing symptoms (Hays et al., 1992). Relationships between social support and illness suggest that individuals who are most in need of support are therefore inclined to be dissatisfied with the support that they receive (Turner et al., 1993).

Decreased availability of social support at later phases of HIV infection contributes to anger, resentment, hopelessness, and depression (Zich & Temoshok, 1987, 1990). HIV infection invariably leads to hospitalizations, disabilities, unemployment, and fatigue, all of which contribute to social isolation. People in one's support networks may die from AIDS, others become emotionally exhausted, and still others turn away from sickness and anticipatory loss (Namir et al., 1989). People with AIDS therefore seek support from multiple sources, particularly when compared with their asymptomatic HIV-positive and HIV-negative counterparts (Hays, Catania, et al., 1990). Attempting to meet increased needs for support, AIDS service organizations, mental health and medical providers, and others have derived a host of social support interventions modeled after programs for other chronic and life-threatening illnesses.

SOCIAL SUPPORT INTERVENTIONS

Interventions for individuals affected by the HIV epidemic provide emotional, informational, and instrumental support. The most organized and accessible interventions have thus far included support groups, volunteer programs, and hospice services.

Support Groups

Support groups for people with HIV infection and their caregivers are similar to those for other medical patients (Newmark, 1984). Groups have been used to foster interpersonal relationships that benefit people with HIV infection and those who provide their care (Adelman, 1989; Di-Pasquale, 1990). To date, there has been only one published clinical trial that tested different models of support for HIV-positive therapy clients. Kelly, Murphy, Bahr, Kalichman, et al. (1993) randomly assigned 68 HIV-positive (non-AIDS) men with heightened depressed mood to one of three experimental treatment conditions: a cognitive–behavioral treatment group, a social support group, and an individual psychotherapy comparison condition. Kelly, Murphy, Bahr, Kalichman, et al. described the cognitive–behavioral condition as follows:

> The cognitive–behavioral groups focused on the use of cognitive and behavior strategies to reduce maladaptive anxiety and depression. Each session had a behavioral or skill training theme and the sessions involved teaching participants the skill, group discussion of potential uses and benefits of the skill, and weekly review of success in implementation. Skill areas included modification of cognitions that exacerbate anxiety or depression, progressive muscle relaxation, imaginal and cue-controlled relaxation, disclosure of serostatus and safer sex practices if sexually active, and establishment of a network of socially supportive relationships. Participant questions, concerns, and problems in implementation of change were handled from a cognitive problem-solving perspective. Most sessions also included at-home practice assignments.

In describing the social support group condition, Kelly, Murphy, Bahr, Kalichman, et al. (1993) stated that

> the support group condition was modeled after the type of social support groups commonly used in coping with other types of illness (such as cancer) and often offered to HIV-positive persons by community AIDS service programs. Leaders of the support groups encouraged members to describe their feelings about having HIV infection; to identify shared problems, concerns, fears, and hopes; to discuss how these issues are handled; and to adopt supportive and

encouraging roles toward others in the group. There was considerable member-initiated discussion of how problems related to HIV were handled, and participants were encouraged to share with, and learn from, experiences raised by others in the group. The group members generated the discussion topics of each session. Members often chose to talk generally about how it felt to have the group as a place to share with others their concerns about HIV. Skills training, behavior rehearsal, contracting, and practice assignments were not employed in this condition.

Results of the study showed that both support group models positively affected group members relative to the control group. However, the social support group appeared to have the greatest benefit over a 3-month follow-up period. Eighty-six percent of the social support group participants demonstrated clinically significant improvement on an index of distress severity, whereas two thirds of the comparison condition showed clinical deterioration, regressing below baseline levels during 3 months. Although members of the cognitive–behavioral group demonstrated a pattern of clinical change that was intermediate between the social support group and the control condition, cognitive–behavioral group participants did decrease their use of illicit substances to a greater degree than the other two groups.

Kelly, Murphy, Bahr, Kalichman, et al. (1993) concluded that the two group models provided different types of support with different outcomes. Whereas the social support group allowed more time for emotional support and therefore emotion-focused coping, the cognitive–behavioral group emphasized problem-focused and active coping skills training. Thus, emotional adjustment was greatest among the social support group members, whereas declines in maladaptive coping behaviors occurred among the skills training participants. Curiously, decreased illicit drug use did not seem to correspond to reductions in distress. These findings highlight the differential effects of emotional and informational support groups for people adjusting to HIV infection.

Emotional Support

Support groups can help people with HIV infection achieve a sense of emotional balance. Emotion-focused support groups emphasize hope, opportunities to gain insights from others, emotional catharsis, and interpersonal connectedness (Buck, 1991). Mathews and Bowes (1989) identified several dimensions of effective HIV-related support groups, including sharing common experiences, group cohesiveness, reinforcing hope, helping others, and learning from others' experiences. Sadovsky (1991) suggested that support groups deal with a client's fears and prejudices, coordinate community services, encourage independence and hope, allow for focusing on self, and promote informed choices. HIV-related support groups can facilitate emotional expression, promote acceptance, and reduce illness-related fears.

Bringing people with comparable life situations together creates a potentially supportive environment through a sense of mutual understanding (Adelman, 1989; O'Dowd, 1988; Siegel, 1986). Support groups also provide opportunities to deal with immediate crises. Psychosocial problem solving often occurs naturally in support groups (Adelman, 1989; Gamble & Getzel, 1989). The goals of another support group described in the literature were to provide an environment for exchanging coping strategies and reinforcing health management behaviors (Buck, 1991). Support groups allow for the sharing of concerns among peers and serve as a vehicle for developing and reinforcing coping strategies. However, for many people, support groups are most productive when they have tangible outcomes, such as when new friendships are formed or when new information is gained.

Informational Support

Support groups can include information dissemination pertinent to HIV infection and treatment. Alternatively, groups can focus exclusively on delivering and exchanging information, providing a forum for people with HIV infection to share experiences, knowledge, and ideas (Hedge & Glover, 1990). Knowledgeable group facilitators can become a primary source of information (Buck, 1991). Expert speakers may also be invited to provide specialized information to group members (Hedge & Glover, 1990), including infectious disease physicians, pharmacists, nutritionists, insurance agents, social welfare workers, and so on.

There are several examples of information-based support groups. Coleman and Harris (1989) conducted a psychoeducational support group to meet five specific information needs: information pertaining to HIV disease; management of health problems; health care and health insurance concerns; nutrition and its role in HIV infection; and issues of sexuality and intimate relationships. Similarly, Hedge and Glover (1990) described an informational support group that focused on general health, stress, diet, medications, the medical system, legal issues, relationships, safer sex, complementary therapies, and life-style changes brought about by HIV infection. The information content of sessions and the information needs of group members vary during the course of HIV infection. In the context of a support group, people receive information along with emotional support, as well as have the chance to share information with others, therefore reciprocating support.

Structure and Format of Support Groups

Support groups vary widely in structure and format. Groups may have limited numbers of sessions or go on indefinitely. Groups can have a set agenda or evolve over time (Land & Harangody, 1990). Support groups may be open with regard to allowing in new members (e.g., Coleman & Harris, 1989; D. Grant, 1988), or closed to new members for the life of the group (e.g., Hedge & Glover, 1990). Formatting groups as either open or closed requires choosing between the benefits of fresh perspectives in open groups or the benefits of trust and confidentiality fostered by closed groups (Hedge & Glover, 1990; Land & Harangody, 1990).

Another issue is group composition. Mixing clients who recently tested HIV positive with those who have been HIV positive for a long time, versus limiting groups to individuals at a particular phase of HIV infection, affects the issues addressed by the group. Certain types of support are needed after initial diagnosis compared with during symptomatic illness (Watson, 1983). Including recently diagnosed people and long-term survivors in the same group allows the newly diagnosed to gain emotional and informational support from those who have "been there" and survived HIV infection. On the other hand, the newly diagnosed can become distressed when confronted by AIDS. Decisions regarding group composition therefore shape many of the issues that arise in sessions. Other decisions include whether to mix groups or keep them homogeneous with respect to gender, sexual orientation, and modes of having contracted HIV infection (Land & Harangody, 1990). Although homogenous groups are often considered more effective (Buiss, 1989; S. H. Levine, Bystritsky, Baron, & Jones, 1991), there are benefits to diversity. Professional versus peer facilitators, cofacilitators versus a single facilitator, whether to invite outside speakers, and the degree to which group members and facilitators should be matched for sexes, ethnicity, and HIV status are issues that require careful consideration (Coleman & Harris, 1989; Gamble & Getzel, 1989). Unfortunately, there have been few empirical studies to guide these decisions.

One study reported interviews that focused on the experiences and perceptions of support groups for people with HIV infection (Kalichman, 1995). All of the interview participants who had known they were HIV positive for more than a few months had attended at least one support group offered by AIDS service organizations. It was almost universal that the emotional tone of support groups influenced participant satisfaction. Most desired groups focused on positive attitudes and hope, rather than expression of negative feelings and sharing the perils of HIV infection. Information exchange was another critical factor in the perceived effectiveness of support groups. Information, including that shared by fellow support group members, was considered among the greatest benefits. One woman illustrated this sentiment by stating,

> I can't sit in a group and listen to a lot of sadness. Some people do that; they would rather whine about it. When I get together with my HIV-positive friends, we talk about new drugs that have come out or something like that. I think it is a little more beneficial, hopeful that we can go out and do something.

Emotional support is gained from the feeling of not being alone. Groups can foster friendships and opportunities for activities or social events.

With respect to group composition, Kalichman (1995) found that the majority of gay men and heterosexual women felt comfortable coming to a mixed group and believed that diversity facilitated support. However, heterosexual men and injection drug users felt that their issues were different from those of gay men and heterosexual women and preferred separate groups. Perceptions of mixing different phases of HIV infection depended on stage of illness. Those early in the course of HIV infection felt that they could benefit from the experience of people who had been HIV positive longer. For example, one man who had been HIV positive for 5 years stated, "There is a lot of support in seeing someone who has survived a long time with HIV and hear their stories." On the other hand, those at later phases believed that the newly diagnosed could offer emotional support and encouragement, but to a lesser degree than other long-term survivors. For example, one man who had been HIV positive for 8 years stated,

> From newly diagnosed guys in the group I can learn about their fears, about their jobs, and about things they are going through. But I don't have to worry about a lot of that stuff anymore. I've been there. I get most of my support from other guys in the group who are at about the same stage of HIV. Learning what they do to cope with things on a daily basis, or maybe that their doctor is doing things a little different from my doctor allows me to take some new information to my doctor and say lets try this.

Support Groups for Caregivers and the Bereaved

Groups can meet the support needs of caregivers and people bereaved from AIDS. Caregiver support groups afford the opportunity to reflect, express, and reconcile feelings related to caring for the ill (Frost et al., 1991). Support groups for caregivers are therefore geared toward sustaining emotional well-being to enable caregivers to continue their care (Kelly & Sykes, 1989). Like groups for people with HIV infection, caregiver support groups require addressing multiple losses. Helping people with HIV infection means repeated exposure to death and dying (Bennett & Kelaher, 1993; Killeen, 1993). Goals for professional caregiver support groups may include stress reduction to prevent burnout, reinforcing values that promote continued work with HIV-positive clients, enhancing and maintaining compassionate care, and establishing professional boundaries with clients while fulfilling caregiver responsibilities (Grossman & Silverstein, 1993). Although there are few empirical studies of caregiver support groups, there is evidence that support provided to professionals who care for HIV-positive clients effectively buffers stress and improves the quality of care provided (J. M. George et al., 1993).

The death of a person to AIDS results in bereavement similar to that found in loss from other chronic illnesses. Support groups assist survivors in rebuilding their lives (Adelman, 1989). The need for support during bereavement is well recognized. Lennon et al. (1990) found that grief reactions were greatest among those who had cared for a friend dying of AIDS who did not have their own support system. In addition, 31% of the men in the Lennon et al. study indicated that they did not receive adequate instrumental support when providing care for their friend and were not receiving emotional support while grieving.

There have been few systematic studies of support groups for individuals who have suffered AIDS-related losses. In one small study, three men and four women who suffered a personal loss because of AIDS participated in a support group based on cognitive and behavioral coping strategies (Sikkema, Kalichman, Kelly, & Koob, in press). A nine-session support group focused on identifying and expressing emotions, developing adaptive coping strategies, increasing feelings of support, reducing psychological distress, and avoiding maladaptive coping behaviors. Sikkema et al. found that the support group significantly reduced depression, grief reactions, anxiety, somatization, and other signs of distress. The group participants benefitted from focusing on specific rather than global stressors, support offered by fellow group members, and their own emotional expression. Although it was based on a small sample without a control group, the study showed evidence for the potential value of support groups for those who suffer an AIDS-related loss.

Volunteer Programs

AIDS service organizations that provide support to people with HIV infection rely on volunteers, many of whom are HIV-positive themselves (Adelman, 1989; Siegel, 1986). For example, programs may designate a buddy to provide one-to-one support for a person with HIV infection. Buddy volunteer programs provide both companionship and physical assistance. Volunteers visit and telephone others with HIV infection as well as provide instrumental support by shopping, cleaning, cooking, and transportation (Lennon et al., 1990; Velentgas, Bynum, & Zierler, 1990). When individuals with HIV infection themselves volunteer to help others, they have the opportunity to gain support from a network of fellow volunteers as well as the reciprocity of support offered by these relationships. Volunteer experiences can increase self-esteem, enhance personal worth, and give a sense of meaning.

Terminal Care and Hospice

Hospice is an interdisciplinary approach to caring for patients with terminal illnesses, where recovery is unlikely and a prognosis is stated in months or weeks (V. Moss, 1990). Hospice care emphasizes the quality rather than quantity of life, holistic approaches to pain control that include psychological and spiritual pain, and the involvement of family and others in the care of the patient (Benjamin & Preston, 1993). Hospice care also supports caregivers by providing respite and convalescent care (Pinching, 1989). Another important aspect of hospice is its emphasis on palliative care. Palliation is a specialized form of care for patients with advanced progressive diseases where curative treatments are no longer feasible (E. Butters, Higginson, George, & McCarthy, 1993; Mansfield, Barter, & Singh, 1992). Thus, hospice care integrates psychological, social, and medical approaches to address the multidimensional issues of the terminally ill (Cassileth et al., 1985).

The progressive and terminal nature of HIV infection places it within the scope of the hospice mission. Unfortunately, many traditional hospices have been unwilling to accept AIDS patients into their services (Mansfield et al., 1992). The reluctance to care for people with AIDS has primarily been because of conflicts between aspects of HIV disease and eligibility criteria for hospice care. For example, people with AIDS often do not have a family member or friend willing to be designated as a primary caregiver, a necessity for hospice home care (Benjamin & Preston, 1993). Moreover, AIDS has a largely unpredictable course, with sudden changes and reversals of life-threatening conditions (V. Moss, 1990). Additional problems may occur in relation to characteristics of certain AIDS patients, such as the continued use of illicit drugs (Bulkin et al., 1988). These aspects of AIDS set the disease apart from other chronic illnesses serviced by most hospice agencies. Thus, hospices have been started to exclusively care for people with AIDS (Benjamin & Preston, 1993; Mansfield et al., 1992; Sadovsky, 1991). In general, the same hospice care is delivered, including an emphasis on pain control and quality of life, while also offering specialized care for AIDS. The same may be said for other psychosocial interventions, where the structure and mechanisms of care are not altered but the therapeutic context and treatment are tailored to address AIDS-related needs.

CONCLUSION

The first line of support after testing HIV positive usually comes from post-HIV antibody test counseling. The distress of testing HIV positive occurs even when a person suspects that he or she is HIV positive. Pre- and posttest counseling is considered essential and is required for federal support of testing programs (CDC, 1992j). Although counseling guidelines have been widely disseminated, many tests are taken with minimal counseling and support. Women may learn that they are HIV positive during routine prenatal screening, others may learn they are HIV positive after donating blood or selling plasma, and still others may get tested for a marriage license or to obtain health or life insurance. Thus, many start their journey with HIV infection with little information and emotional support.

AIDS service organizations play a critical role in supporting people after they test HIV positive. Community-based organizations typically address multiple support needs. Emotional support is addressed through support groups, buddy and other volunteer programs, and case management. Informational support is provided by case management, as well as hot lines, education programming, and library services. AIDS service organizations typically offer instrumental support through volunteers who provide home assistance and transportation, food banks, and legal assistance. Thus, formal structures of support have been established in many U.S. cities and can immediately benefit people after learning that they are HIV positive, as well as at later phases of HIV infection.

Meeting social support needs in HIV infection requires breaking down barriers and social stigmas. Support that was in place for a person before testing HIV positive can be threatened when the person discloses his or her HIV status. Mental health professionals provide a safe environment for clients with HIV infection to seek support and counseling.

9

Counseling and Psychotherapy

A s it is to the general public, AIDS is both familiar and mysterious to
many mental health professionals. Counselors and therapists tend to
doubt their ability to provide services to HIV-positive clients (Perry &
Markowitz, 1986). Because there is no formal specialization in the psychological treatment of people with HIV infection (Wofsy, 1988), mental
health professionals have little training and few sources of consultation in
HIV-related issues. Psychotherapy with HIV-positive clients relies on the
same techniques and processes as does therapy with HIV-negative clients.
However, treatment planning for HIV-positive clients requires consideration of medical and social aspects of the disease (Borden, 1989).

This chapter reviews the literature on HIV-related psychological assessment and psychotherapy and identifies themes of relevance to counseling HIV-positive clients. Issues of particular importance to treating
HIV-positive women are also discussed. Although there is little information available on these matters, practical suggestions for assessment and
intervention strategies are highlighted.

CLINICAL ASSESSMENT

Several characteristics of HIV disease should be considered when psychologically assessing HIV-positive clients. The overlap among illness symp-

toms, medication side effects, and vegetative symptoms of psychological distress have been well recognized, and tests of depression have been developed for specific use with medical patients and for the elderly (e.g., Zigmond & Snaith, 1983). Overlapping HIV symptoms and psychological distress pose particular problems when assessing depression and anxiety. For example, 7 of the 21 items on the Beck Depression Inventory (Beck & Steer, 1993) reflect symptoms of HIV infection. Overlap occurs for problems in concentration and decision making, negative changes in physical appearance, increased difficulty in social and occupational functioning, sleep disturbances, fatigue, loss of appetite, and excessive weight loss. Additional items reflect worries about physical health and physical attractiveness, declining sexual interests, and excessive guilt, all of which may be a part of HIV infection. Similarly, the *DSM-IV* (American Psychiatric Association, 1994) diagnostic criteria for major depression rely heavily on vegetative symptoms. For a diagnosis with major depression, a person must exhibit five of nine symptoms, five of which overlap with symptoms of HIV disease: significant weight loss, insomnia, fatigue, diminished ability to think or concentrate, and psychomotor retardation. Diagnostic criteria for dysthymia reflect similar overlapping physical symptoms. Thus, both paper-and-pencil and interactive diagnostic assessments of depression overlap with symptoms of HIV infection, as do other medical conditions.

Kalichman et al. (1995) found that people with HIV infection who scored above the clinical cutoff on the Beck Depression Inventory reported significantly more HIV symptoms than did nondepressed people, although depressed and nondepressed did not differ in their number of AIDS-defining conditions or T-helper cell counts. Specifically, 82% of depressed HIV positives had persistent fatigue and 57% reported night sweats, compared with 47% and 15% of nondepressed people, respectively. Neurovegetative signs of depression that overlap with HIV symptomatology are particularly important in clinical assessment because sleep disturbances and loss of appetite are among the most common symptoms of depression among people with HIV infection (Ritchie & Radke, 1992). Hintz et al. (1990) also found that HIV-positive individuals have greater sleep disturbance and appetite suppression than members of a depressed HIV-negative comparison group. Although potentially attributable to depression, physical symptoms cannot therefore be used as strong diagnostic indicators of depression without ruling out symptoms of HIV infection.

Similar problems exist in the assessment of anxiety. The Trait Anxiety Inventory (Spielberger, Gorsuch, & Lushene, 1970), for example, includes two items that reflect fatigue and cognitive confusion. In addition, the Hamilton Rating Scale for Anxiety reflects autonomic reactivity, including gastrointestinal distress and fatigue, symptoms that may also be indicative of progressing HIV infection. Table 9.1 summarizes HIV symptoms that overlap with symptoms of depression and anxiety commonly included in assessment instruments.

Assessment can be made more specific to psychological distress by decomposing assessment instruments into cognitive, affective, behavioral, and somatic domains. For example, Kertzner et al. (1993) modified the Hamilton Rating Scale for Anxiety in a study of HIV-positive people by omitting items pertaining to somatic distress. Unfortunately, alterations in standardized instruments limit their potential clinical usefulness because norms are rendered invalid and scores from idiosyncratically derived item subsets have unknown psychometric properties. An alternative strategy is to conduct a content analysis of scales. After scoring a scale according to standardized procedures and using available normative data, the scale can be inspected on an item-level basis to see how much scale elevation is accounted for by item subsets. This is a practice that many clinicians

Table 9.1

Overlapping Symptoms of Depression and Anxiety With HIV Infection

Distress symptom	HIV-related symptom
Fatigue/lethargy	Fatigue
Suppressed appetite	Weight loss
Muscle aches	Muscle aches
Insomnia, Increased sweating	Night sweats
Gastrointestinal distress	Diarrhea
Headaches/dizziness, Memory lapses	Neurological disturbances

routinely use with psychometric tests and that becomes essential in the evaluation of clients with HIV infection. The following example illustrates the importance of item-level analyses by focusing on the symptom co-morbidity of the Beck Depression Inventory.

Taken from a study of HIV-positive men and women (Kalichman et al., 1995), a participant scored 18 on the Beck Depression Inventory, where the clinical cutoff for depression is 15. As shown in Table 9.2, responses from this case indicate that 11 of the 18 points were accounted for by symptoms of depression that overlap with symptoms of HIV infection. Thus, an elevated depression score for this person was partially accounted for by physical and behavioral symptoms of depression that overlap with HIV infection. However, these physical symptoms did not, of course, occur in isolation of cognitive and affective symptoms of depression. On a separate index of HIV-related symptoms and illnesses, this same person indicated that he had persistent fatigue for at least 2 weeks, unintentionally lost at least 10 pounds, had diarrhea for at least 2 weeks, and had muscle aches and cramps. In addition, he had also been diagnosed with two AIDS-defining conditions, lymphoma and HIV wasting syndrome.

Clinical assessment of clients with HIV infection can reduce the potential problems of disease–distress symptom overlap by using tests that do not include physical symptoms as a benchmark for depression and anxiety. For example, the Hospital Anxiety and Depression Scale was developed to avoid physical symptom overlap in medical illnesses (Zigmond & Snaith, 1983). Another strategy is to assess clinical constructs that are closely associated with depression and anxiety but do not reflect physical symptomatology. For example, the Beck Hopelessness Scale correlates with measures of depression, predicts suicidal intentions, and does not include physical symptoms (Beck, Kovacs, & Weissman, 1975). Similarly, assessments of loneliness, guilt, and anger provide valuable information concerning negative affective states without reliance on concurrent HIV-related symptomatology. Corollary assessments may be used in combination with depression and anxiety inventories to support or call into question other test results.

Other psychological reactions to HIV infection require similar considerations in clinical assessment. Suicide risk fluctuates during HIV infection, and motivations to attempt suicide differ over the course of the disease. Hopelessness and despair are the most likely impetus for at-

Table 9.2

Item Responses on the Beck Depression Inventory by a Person
With Advanced HIV Infection

Beck Depression Inventory item	Scorable points
I feel sad	1
I feel discouraged about the future	1
I do not feel like a failure	0
I don't enjoy things the way I used to	1
I don't feel particularly guilty	0
I don't feel I am being punished	0
I am disappointed in myself	1
I don't feel I am any worse than anybody else	0
I don't have any thought of killing myself	0
I don't cry any more than usual	0
I get annoyed or irritated more easily than I used to	1
I am less interested in other people than I used to be	1
I make decisions about as well as I ever could	0
I am worried that I am looking old or unattractive	1
I have to push myself very hard to do anything	2
I don't sleep as well as I used to	1
I get tired from doing almost nothing	2
My appetite is not as good as it used to be	1
I have lost more than 10 pounds	2
I am worried about physical problems such as aches and pains, upset stomach, or constipation	1
I am less interested in sex than I used to be	1

NOTE: Items that overlap with HIV-related symptoms are in italics.

tempting suicide early in the course of HIV, and exerting personal control and avoiding pain may emerge as reasons for suicide later in infection. Periodic assessments of suicidal ideation, as well other dimensions of psychological distress, are therefore important in the clinical assessment of HIV-positive clients (Chuang et al., 1989).

When evaluating psychological adaptation to HIV infection, it is essential not to misattribute illness symptoms to distress reactions. Any symptoms of advancing HIV infection require medical evaluation and should not be dismissed as hypochondriasis, somatization, anxiety, or depression.

Another problem in clinical assessment involves evaluating scores against existing norms. Populations most affected by HIV have been the most underrepresented in normative samples. Culture and gender differences in symptom expression and subpopulation base rates may account for some observed distress. These issues underscore the importance of collecting convergent and divergent assessment data when evaluating clients with HIV infection, and they suggest that evaluations should be conducted with medical consultation. Caution is needed when screening for depression or anxiety on the basis of most standardized inventories because of the potential for false positives.

Assessment of HIV-positive clients almost necessarily demands integrative, multidimensional approaches. Biopsychosocial models are useful in conceptualizing evaluations of clients with HIV infection because of their emphasis on behavior as a function of the nervous system and various other organ systems that, in turn, reflect the functions of tissues, cells, and their components (Engel, 1980). Each biological and psychological system is interrelated to the others, so that experiences are tied to physiological processes and bodily systems are reciprocally affected by behavior. In psychological assessment it is therefore essential to inquire about health status, physical symptoms of illness, and, perhaps most important, what a person believes about his or her diagnosis and prognosis.

HIV-RELATED PSYCHOTHERAPY

Although the literature on psychotherapy with HIV-positive clients is sparse, available evidence suggests that psychological treatment for clients with HIV infection can be beneficial. For example, Markowitz and his colleagues (Markowitz, Klerman, & Perry, 1992, 1993; Markowitz, Klerman, Perry, Clougherty, & Josephs, 1993) reported treatment outcome for 23 HIV-positive clients who received an average of 16 sessions of individual, interpersonally oriented psychotherapy. Markowitz et al. focused on encouraging and supporting clients to take actions that included the following: becoming involved in their medical care, preventing HIV transmission, tailoring work and social activities to changes in physical functioning, and complying with medical treatment recommendations. Therapy also emphasized the here-and-now and framed illness as an opportunity to examine relationships and other issues of importance. Markowitz et al. emphasized exploring options and reinforcing hope. The results of evaluations taken over the course of therapy found that clients showed declines in depressed mood and other signs of emotional distress. Although the study was not a randomized, controlled treatment trial, it does provide data that encourage the use of individual psychotherapy with HIV-positive clients.

There is also evidence that clients with HIV infection and AIDS can benefit from group psychotherapy. Group therapy, however, should not be confused with support groups. By definition, therapy is conducted by trained therapists rather than peer facilitators, and therapeutic techniques are a part of the group experience (Beckett & Rutan, 1990). Group therapy does encompass similar features of traditional support groups, including disseminating information and fostering supportive relationships, but it goes beyond group experiences through therapeutic interventions. HIV-related group therapy can be based on models designed for other chronic illnesses (Yalom & Greaves, 1977). S. H. Levine et al. (1991) described a psychotherapy group that treated six clients with symptomatic HIV infection. The primary focus of the group was supportive psychotherapy, but it included giving accurate HIV-related information, instruction in adaptive coping strategies, and working through losses and anticipatory grief. Levine et al. stated that the treatment was centered around a supportive atmosphere that reduced HIV-related fears, addressed relationship issues, and built social supports, and they found that clients experienced reductions in psychological distress. Most of the current literature on therapy for HIV-positive clients relies upon a cognitive–behavioral therapy orientation.

Cognitive–Behavioral Approaches

Cognitive behavior therapy provides several techniques that have been successful in helping clients adjust to other chronic illnesses (e.g., Golden et al., 1992). Stress management, cognitive restructuring, and behavioral self-management skills have been the basis for most interventions with HIV-positive clients. For example, Coates et al. (1989) described a group intervention that consisted of eight 2-hour weekly sessions and emphasized instruction in systematic relaxation, health habit change such as smoking and alcohol reduction, increasing rest and exercise, and stress-management skills. Coates et al. found that participants benefitted from participating in the group. Similar cognitive–behavioral group therapies with HIV-positive clients have been effective in reducing psychological distress and enhancing quality of life (e.g., Emmot, 1991; Lamping et al., 1993; Mulder et al., 1992).

Two well-controlled clinical trials support the value of cognitive–behavioral techniques with HIV-positive clients. One study enrolled gay men into a cognitive–behavioral therapy intervention prior to notification of their HIV antibody test results. Antoni, Baggett, et al. (1991) based their treatment on cognitive–behavioral therapy that included the following: behavioral stress management, relaxation skills training, self-monitoring of environmental stressors, stress reappraisal, active coping, enhancing self-efficacy, and expanding social networks. This multicomponent intervention produced significant reductions in psychological distress among men who subsequently tested HIV positive. Antoni et al. concluded that therapy buffered post-HIV-test-notification depression and increased a sense of personal control among men who tested HIV positive.

Kelly, Murphy, Bahr, Kalichman, et al. (1993) also described an intensive cognitive–behavioral therapy group for depressed HIV-positive clients. As discussed earlier, the Kelly, Murphy, Bahr, Kalichman, et al. treatment consisted of an eight-session multicomponent group that relied on behavioral self-management and stress-reduction skills training. On the basis of the approaches described by Coates et al. (1989), Antoni, Baggett, et al. (1991), and Kelly, Murphy, Bahr, Kalichman, et al. (1993), the following cognitive–behavioral treatment components appear useful and may be incorporated into individual or group therapies for clients with HIV infection.

Relaxation and Stress Reduction

Standard relaxation exercises have been effective in reducing stress among HIV-positive clients (Antoni, Baggett, et al., 1991). Tension–relaxation procedures combine focused attention with neuromuscular tension reduction to produce a response incompatible with anxiety. Alternatively, guided imagery relaxation techniques can be used and may be preferable for clients with medical ailments. If imagery is used in relaxation training, however, it is important that clients not confuse it with spiritual or alternative healing imagery. Like all behavioral skills training, relaxation requires a thorough assessment, homework, self-monitoring, practice, and feedback. It is helpful to suggest that daily practice occur in a designated place and time. Audiotape recordings of relaxation instructions are often helpful, and scripts for relaxation skills instruction are available.

Cognitive Restructuring

Reframing and reappraising stressful life events can reduce distress and increase a sense of control. Techniques for cognitive restructuring are described by proponents of self-instruction training (Meichenbaum, 1977), Beck's (1976) cognitive therapy, and Ellis's (1962) rational–emotive therapy. In general, cognitive restructuring involves identifying maladaptive thoughts or self-statements, therapist modeling of adaptive behavior, and messages that guide adaptive behaviors. Cognitive restructuring can effectively reappraise current health status, reframe illness symptoms, and maintain a realistic outlook.

Communication Skills Building

Barriers to self-disclosing HIV infection can be addressed through assertiveness and social skills training and through behavioral problem-solving techniques. Issues of potential rejection and fear of isolation may be addressed using approaches outlined by cognitive–behavioral problem-solving instruction techniques (D'Zurilla & Goldfried, 1971). When self-disclosure of HIV status is desirable or necessary, clients can role-play disclosure in therapy and problem solve potential outcomes. Modeling, practice, and corrective feedback can increase client self-efficacy to self-disclose (Eisler, Miller, & Hersen, 1973; Kelly, 1982).

Health-Related Life-Style Changes

HIV-positive clients often require assistance to change health-related behaviors, including reducing practices that have adverse health effects (e.g., poor nutrition, tobacco use, alcohol and drug use, etc.), increasing behaviors that enhance fitness (e.g., rest, exercise, medication compliance, etc.), and eliminating sexual and drug-use behaviors that risk HIV transmission. Changes in life-style are broader than narrow behavior changes and include clusters of behaviors (Bruhn, 1988). Step-by-step planning in psychotherapy can set realistic goals. Clients benefit from encouragement and support, as well as from dissolving barriers that prohibit implementing changes. Self-monitoring progress, such as through the use of journals or diaries, is also helpful.

THEMES IN PSYCHOTHERAPY

HIV-positive clients represent a highly diverse population with a wide array of mental health challenges. Clients may seek services for the emotional turmoil of facing HIV and AIDS, to deal with loneliness and isolation, or to cope with fears of illness and death (Murphy, Bahr, Kelly, Bernstein, & Morgan, 1992). Counselors and therapists are called upon by HIV-positive clients for accurate information, clarification of medical treatment decisions, spiritual issues, financial concerns, and other immediate needs (Frierson & Lippmann, 1988; Winiarski, 1991). Figure 9.1 presents 14 themes in psychotherapy with HIV-positive clients, each of which is discussed below.

HIV-Related Information and Education

Although mental health professionals cannot provide detailed biomedical information or advice to clients, counselors and therapists can disseminate psychological information and can serve as a valuable information resource (D. Miller, 1990). Beliefs are often based on inaccurate information and can be altered simply by correcting misinformation (Schmaling & DiClementi, 1991). Therapists need a basic understanding of HIV disease to recognize misinformation when it is communicated by clients (Spector & Conklin, 1987). Numerous hotlines are readily available and can assist therapists in answering questions and clarifying concerns raised by their HIV-positive clients (see Appendix B). Physicians and public health officials can also serve as consultants. Mental health professionals may educate their clients about psychological issues related to HIV infection and psychological reactions to medical symptomatology. For example, educating clients about the overlap among symptoms of depression, HIV infection, and medication side effects can help lead to better understanding and improved psychological adjustment (Markowitz, Klerman, & Perry, 1993).

Themes in Psychotherapy

* Information and education

* Health promotion

* Disclosing HIV positive status

* Relationships

* Suicide / Hastened death

* Fear of cognitive decline

* Medical treatment issues

* Substance abuse

* Life planning

* Self-esteem and self-worth

* Spirituality

* Redefining quality of life

* Meaningful use of time

* Becoming attached and letting go

Figure 9.1

Common themes in psychotherapy with HIV-positive clients.

Behavior and Life-Style Changes

Altering health-compromising habits and adopting health-promoting behaviors can both improve overall fitness and enhance a sense of personal
control (Kelly, 1989). Psychotherapy can help clients alter behaviors with
potentially detrimental health effects. For example, cognitive and behavioral
techniques for smoking cessation are widely available and can be used as a
part of psychotherapy (Royce & Winkelstein, 1990). Aerobic exercise can
also promote fitness and a sense of control and can reduce depression and
anxiety and increase self-esteem (LaPerriere, Antoni, et al., 1990; Pfeiffer,

1992). Health psychology offers a rich literature to guide treatments for sleep disorders, nutritional and dietary changes, weight maintenance, medication compliance, and other problems that commonly occur in HIV infection.

The benefits of health-behavior change are many, but it is important that clients not be misled to believe that such changes reverse the course of HIV infection. There is no conclusive evidence that behavior changes have a clinically significant effect on HIV infection. A client who stops smoking or starts exercising only to decline in health should not blame him- or herself for "starting too late" or "not doing enough." However, because changes in health behavior cannot worsen HIV infection and can improve general health and fitness, clients should be encouraged to make such changes with realistic expectations.

Dealing With and Assisting in Self-Disclosure

Disclosing HIV seropositivity can be among the greatest challenges facing some HIV-positive clients. Disclosure can result in social sanctions but is necessary to gain certain types of support and to inform sexual and injection drug use partners (Perry, 1989; M. L. Smith & Martin, 1993), dentists, and others (Pinch, Brown, Dougherty, Allegretti, & McCarthy, 1993). In some cases, a therapist may be the only person that a client has told about their HIV status. Disclosure of HIV status can be approached with clients on a person-by-person, case-by-case basis. Clients may weigh the potential costs and benefits of disclosing their HIV status and evaluate their options for how and when to disclose. Role-playing and rehearsal can occur in therapy, where the therapist helps trouble-shoot potential responses to the disclosure (Landau-Stanton, Clements, & Stanton, 1993). When clients are unable to bring themselves to disclose to sexual and injecting partners, therapy can offer a vehicle for disclosure by way of couples sessions. Therapists then know that the partner has been told and can provide support to both the client and their partner. Therapists can also assist in problem solving, mediate interpersonal conflicts, and clarify relationship issues.

Interpersonal Relationships

Family conflicts often predate HIV infection and can become exacerbated after testing HIV positive (Bor, Perry, & Miller, 1989; Slowinski, 1989).

Fears and stigmas add to the isolation of HIV-positive clients. Long-term partnered relationships are also disrupted by HIV infection, and clients with HIV infection are often kept away from children. Issues of disclosing to partners, maintaining safer sexual relations, fears of future illness, and anticipatory loss can weaken relationship bonds (Slowinski, 1989). Therapy may therefore involve working through relationship issues and, when appropriate, include partners or family members.

Recurrent Suicide Risk

Risk for suicide among HIV-positive clients occurs within two distinct contexts. Suicidal ideations can occur in conjunction with hopelessness and clinical depression. Alternatively, clients may view suicide as a reasonable option in HIV infection (Perry & Markowitz, 1986). Thus, suicide interventions depend on the meaning of suicidal ideations and the motivation behind suicide intentions. Monitoring suicide risk is a continuous process. HIV-positive clients are reminded of their mortality by the deaths of others, the onset of symptoms, anniversaries of HIV testing, and the deaths of friends (Spector & Conklin, 1987). Therapists must have clear values on hastened death and partner-assisted hastened death so that they can remain nonjudgemental when dealing with these serious issues in therapy.

Neuropsychological Effects of HIV Infection

Perceptions of cognitive changes in relation to HIV infection require regular re-evaluation. Mental status can be monitored, and client attributions of changes should be assessed (Spector & Conklin, 1987). Because many do not experience neuropsychological impairment even late in the course of AIDS, clients can be reassured that cognitive limitations are not necessarily inevitable. If neuropsychological symptoms are confirmed by a neuropsychological consultant, therapists can assist clients in adapting to cognitive decline or vision impairment. Examples of interventions include maintaining home environment safety and consistency, use of time management techniques, and breaking difficult tasks down into smaller steps (Mapou & Law, 1994). Lapses in memory can be addressed by using reminders such as lists, notebooks, and calendars (Mapou & Law, 1994; Winiarski, 1991). Clients should be encouraged to be patient with themselves because completing complex tasks may require more time.

Counseling HIV-Positive Clients Within a Treatment Team

Mental health services occur within a broad spectrum of care for most HIV-positive clients (V. Moss, 1991; Pinching 1989). Communication among providers is therefore necessary because treatment components can be interactive. For example, antiretroviral drugs have behavior-related side effects such as fatigue and peripheral neuropathy, and certain antidepressant and cognitive performance-enhancing medications may interact with treatments of HIV infection. Permission to release and obtain information from other professionals involved in the care of HIV-positive clients should be routine. Multidisciplinary inpatient treatment teams can be emulated for outpatients by opening communication lines and building a network of cooperative relationships.

Psychotherapy can also help clients address medically related concerns, including treatment attitudes, compliance, and life-and-death issues. Mental health professionals can support clients who have selected a course of treatment and have been compliant. Clinicians can also help their HIV-positive clients clarify their wishes for terminal care, such as life support options and resuscitation. Haas et al. (1993) found that 62% of people with AIDS had not discussed preferences for life-sustaining care and advanced directives with their physicians even though 72% of them wanted to do so. Therapy can help clarify such issues for clients, and sessions can be used to problem solve barriers and role-play communicating desires for terminal care with physicians. Terminal care should be discussed early in the course of HIV infection to avoid later cognitive decline that will increase the difficulty of decision making (Dilley, Shelp, & Batki, 1985).

Substance Abuse Treatment

Substance abuse problems are common among HIV-positive clients and can become the focus of psychotherapy (O'Dowd et al., 1991). Clients with injection drug using histories can be particularly difficult to treat because of the strong addictive qualities of injected drugs and issues related to potential transmission of HIV to needle-sharing partners (Batki, Sorensen, Faltz, & Madover, 1988). All types of substance use, including alcohol, can serve as avoidance coping strategies and can raise the risk for engaging in

HIV-transmitting behaviors. Psychotherapy can assist HIV-positive clients who are motivated to stop using substances by helping them replace drug use with adaptive coping behaviors. However, specialized treatment may be necessary for substance abusive clients.

Planning for the Future

Clients with HIV infection become acutely aware of mortality and recognize that their time is limited. Goals for therapy therefore require attention to both short-term and long-term time lines (Winiarski, 1991). Clients should be encouraged to establish priorities for therapy and to identify a primary goal. Working with a therapist, clients can translate their primary goal into smaller, short-term goals (Landau-Stanton, et al. 1993). HIV-positive clients are often inclined to emphasize the near future and to cut short lifelong aspirations. A sense of realistic optimism, however, can allow clients to restore long-term goals, again stated in terms of concrete steps.

Self-Esteem and Self-Worth

Working through life issues and moving toward achieving goals is a self-enhancing process. Because clients with a life-threatening illness may have special needs to enhance their self-esteem (S. E. Taylor, 1983), therapy can work toward achieving greater self-acceptance. One therapeutic technique that is useful in this regard is the life review, where clients are guided through a self-examination of life transitions (Landau-Stanton et al., 1993). People with chronic illnesses commonly think about their past to gain a sense of closure. Therapy can therefore provide structure and support a life review process. For example, the life review may be framed along a time line, starting with an earliest memory and moving through one's life, recorded by the client in a journal. Life reviews can be useful in helping clients recognize their capacities and gain a sense of self-understanding (Borden, 1989).

Spirituality

Clients with HIV infection are often estranged from formal religious institutions and may therefore express unmet spiritual needs. Therapists can help clients clarify their values and identify spiritual needs in the context of psychotherapy. Therapy can also take the form of developing strategies for exploring traditional and nontraditional spiritual practices. Clients may wish to seek guidance from clergy and can use therapy as a means of problem solving barriers and evaluating options to meet their spiritual needs (Haburchak, Harrison, Miles, & Hannon, 1989).

Redefining Quality of Life

Needs and abilities change as a function of HIV infection. Adjustments in therapy goals, focus, and course are therefore required as HIV infection progresses (Corless et al., 1992; Perry & Markowitz, 1986). In particular, quality of life must be continuously evaluated and redefined over the course of illness. Pain, health status, physical functioning, social relationships, and energy level contribute to the quality of life (Cleary, Fowler, et al., 1993; Wachtel et al., 1992; Wu et al., 1991). When activities are disrupted and abilities are impaired, therapists can help find new activities that match current abilities and reframe quality of life along those lines.

Meaningful Use of Time

Unemployment, disability, and activity restrictions lead to boredom and other forms of discontent. Many HIV-positive clients state that quality use of their time is one of their primary concerns (Murphy et al., 1992). Counselors and therapists may help clients evaluate their physical capabilities and work through options to increase life satisfaction. Creativity and productivity can move HIV-positive clients out of passive victim roles (David & Sageman, 1987). Volunteering to help others, rediscovering hobbies and interests, taking time for oneself, and focusing on relationships are examples of ways to enhance a sense of meaning.

Becoming Attached and Letting Go

Professionals who treat patients suffering from life-threatening illnesses undergo a great deal of stress. Hopelessness, fear of death, spiritual crisis, and recognizing one's own mortality are common themes in terminal illness. As much as any area of psychotherapy, boundaries between the client and therapist can be blurred by the universality of death and mortality, issues that many therapists themselves have not worked through. A clear sense of one's own views on death and dying will enable clinicians to better serve their HIV-positive clients.

PSYCHOPHARMACOLOGICAL TREATMENTS

An emerging body of research suggests that medications are effective in treating HIV-positive clients, and the risk for adverse effects appear minimal (Mapou & Law, 1994; Rabkin & Harrison, 1990; Rabkin, Rabkin, Harrison, & Wagner, 1994; Rabkin, Rabkin, & Wagner, 1994). Markowitz, Rabkin, and Perry (1994) reviewed clinical trials of antidepressant medications in HIV infection and found that three controlled studies of imipramine demonstrated the efficacy of this drug with HIV-positive clients. Similar results were reported with other antidepressants as well as stimulants used to treat depression. Markowitz et al. concluded that the use of antidepressants with HIV-positive clients is supported by the available research. Unfortunately, studies evaluating antianxiety and other classes of psychiatric medications are not available. Infectious disease specialists should be consulted when psychiatric medications are considered because of potential immune system and drug interaction effects.

ISSUES FOR WOMEN

HIV-positive women experience the medical, social, and psychological aspects of HIV disease differently than men. Although HIV appears to take the same course in women as it does in men, immune-compromised women are susceptible to a number of gynecologic infections and cancers that have only recently been recognized. In addition, because most early studies of the natural history of HIV disease and the majority of treatment studies have only included gay men, less is known about HIV infection and effects of treatment among women. In terms of social aspects of HIV disease, women suffer more prejudices for sexually contracting HIV infection than do men. Sexual double standards contribute to shaming women for even being at risk for HIV infection and more so for being HIV positive.

Women are also subject to the stress of being a caretaker for an HIV-positive partner. Furthermore, the clinical picture for women is potentially complicated by pregnancy. Many women learn they are HIV positive through prenatal screening, a nearly routine test in most urban hospitals (Anderson, 1993; Nolan, 1989). If testing occurs early in pregnancy, women must decide whether to terminate in light of potential perinatal HIV transmission. Pregnant women must also consider the use of anti-retroviral medications that may help protect the fetus against infection but with risk of unknown teratogenic effects. Finally, women who already have children are burdened with assuring their care in anticipation of becoming disabled and ultimately dying.

Studies of psychological issues facing women with HIV infection have been few. Little information is therefore available to guide the treatment of women with HIV infection. The following case description illustrates several issues facing women with HIV infection. The case description is accurate with respect to all clinically relevant details, with identifiable characteristics altered to protect the client's identity.

> The client was a 23-year-old Mexican American woman diagnosed with HIV infection 3 months earlier through prenatal HIV screening. She was asymptomatic for HIV infection and was 8 months pregnant at the time of referral, but has since given birth. Maria has two children, including her newborn, and is engaged to be married. Her fiancé, however, tested HIV negative. She presented in therapy with symptoms of depression and anxiety related to her health and the uncertainty of her newborn's HIV status.
>
> Maria expressed great concern regarding potential perinatal transmission of HIV, providing care for her children after her death, disclosing her HIV status to others close to her, and issues of communication and support in her family and social relationships. She has disclosed her HIV status to her fiancé and best friend, the latter of whom she sees only infrequently. Her fiancé prefers not to discuss HIV-related issues. Maria fears her family's reaction to her HIV status and has not disclosed it to them.
>
> Maria reported the following symptoms of depression: decreased interest in activities, depressed mood, diurnal mood variation, tearfulness, loss of energy, feelings of hopelessness and being overwhelmed, diminished ability to concentrate, and recurrent thoughts of death. She denied sleep disturbance, changes in appetite, and suicidal ideation. Maria experienced an exacerbation in her depression

following the birth of her child and HIV-antibody screening conducted for her older son. Maria therefore met diagnostic criteria for a *DSM-IV* diagnosis of major depression. Her emotional reaction was related to her recent knowledge of her HIV status, perceived lack of social support, and concerns for her future and for her children.

Maria reported a history of depression and alcohol use during her adolescence. She received inpatient psychiatric treatment for depression and truancy. Maria was physically abused by her mother and reported an extensive family history of mental illness. Maria acknowledged previous maladaptive ways of coping and an attempted suicide during her adolescence. She described her previous psychological treatment as successful, through both psychotherapy and antidepressant medication.

The following short-term treatment goals were identified: (a) increasing the amount and quality of social support, including informing family members of HIV status and seeking an HIV-related support group; (b) developing adaptive coping strategies, initially through cognitive and behavioral approaches, to cope with her situation and to alleviate depression; and (c) increasing communication and support related to HIV issues with her partner. Following improved adjustment and adaptive coping, Maria identified a long-term therapy goal of addressing unresolved issues related to the future care of her children as her HIV infection progresses and to the physical abuse and perceived abandonment resulting from her mother's suicide.

Psychotherapeutic progress included an increase in social support through communication skills development and improved self-esteem, probably because of a supportive therapeutic relationship and successful experiences with assertiveness. Maria subsequently informed two family members of her HIV status and dealt effectively with their emotional reactions, which were initially supportive. Her older child tested negative for HIV antibodies, and she is waiting the testing period to confirm her newborn's HIV serostatus. Maria continues to feel anxious and depressed in relation to ongoing caregiving concerns and her children's welfare following her death. She is currently in good health and has received assistance from a community-based organization in the form of social services. Maria continues to have difficulty in communicating and receiving emotional support from her fiancé, as well as maintaining consistent safer sexual behaviors. Couples therapy was considered to deal with her complex relationship issues.

This case, although by no means representative, illustrates several salient issues that arise for women with HIV. The case involved a woman who was pregnant and who had a previous child and weak social supports. The case was also complicated because the client contracted HIV infection outside of her current relationship, a most difficult situation for women because of double standards for women's sexual behavior. Because most research has disprortionately sampled men, particularly White gay men, little is known about the interactions of these complex issues and how they affect therapy.

CONFIDENTIALITY

Privacy is a central element in effective psychotherapy. Therapists, however, are obligated to break confidentiality under certain circumstances. Issues of duty to protect are among the greatest HIV-related ethical and legal concerns among mental health professionals because of the role of confidentiality in professional relationships (Adler & Beckett, 1989; Ginzburg & Gostin, 1986; Melton, 1988; Sherer, 1988). Perceptions of dangerousness and identification of third parties who may be at risk have brought issues raised by the widely noted *Tarasoff v. Regents of California* (1976).

For *Tarasoff* to apply, there must be a foreseeable danger to an identifiable party as a result of a client's planned behavior (Knapp & Vande-Creek, 1990). The *Tarasoff* ruling involves an obligation for professionals to use reasonable care to protect intended victims when danger is reasonably predicted (Melton, 1988). The relationship between HIV risk and *Tarasoff* is highlighted by communicable diseases having long been considered a valid reason to break professional confidentiality to prevent the spread of illness (Silva, Leong, & Weinstock, 1989). In fact, *Tarasoff* itself was based on court decisions that ruled that physicians have a duty to act to protect when they know patients with infectious diseases threaten others (Knapp & VandeCreek, 1990).

The relationship between HIV risk and *Tarasoff* is not, however, as

clear as it may first seem. *Tarasoff* is usually associated with a direct verbal threat (Kermani & Weiss, 1989). However, HIV-positive clients are unlikely to use their infection to harm another person intentionally. Instead,
concerns revolve around the failure to take precaution. In addition, most
people at risk of exposure to HIV are not easy for clinicians to identify
(Perry, 1989). Duty to protect only extends to people who can be identified and who could reasonably be harmed (Knapp & VandeCreek, 1990).
Unlike in *Tarasoff*, potential victims of HIV transmission are probably already aware of the risks associated with their own behavior, given that
high-risk practices are well known and everyone is advised to protect
themselves (Perry, 1989). Nevertheless, certain cases may require breaking
confidentiality to warn a third party. For example, an HIV-positive client
who states that he or she refuses to use condoms during sexual intercourse
with his or her spouse involves a statement of intentional harm toward an
identifiable third person who is known to be at risk. Thus, several professional associations have developed ethical policy statements regarding
these cases.

The American Medical Association recommends that when physicians
know that an HIV-positive patient is endangering a third party, they should
be persuaded to stop engaging in risk behaviors. If the person fails to
comply, the physician should notify public health authorities, and if the
authorities do not act, the physician should notify the endangered party
him- or herself (Kermani & Weiss, 1989). Similarly, the Canadian Medical
Association states that physicians can ethically disclose a patient's HIV status to a spouse when the patient is unwilling to inform him or her
(I. Kleinman, 1991). Following these general parameters, the American
Psychiatric Association (1992, 1993a) has proposed its own guidelines. A
policy statement recommends that psychiatrists work with all patients to
reduce their risk for HIV transmission, regardless of serostatus, and be
competent in counseling about HIV testing (American Psychiatric Association, 1992). In terms of protecting third parties, the policy statement
(1993a) reads as follows:

> In a situation where a psychiatrist received convincing clinical in-
> formation that the patient is infected with HIV, the psychiatrist
> should advise and work with the patient either to obtain agreement
> to cease behavior that places others at risk of infection or to notify

individuals who may be at continuing risk of exposure. If a patient refuses to agree to change behavior or to notify the person(s) at ongoing risk or if the psychiatrist has good reason to believe that the patient has failed to or is unable to comply with this agreement, it is ethically permissible for the psychiatrist to notify identifiable persons who the psychiatrist believes to be in danger of contracting the virus, or to arrange for public health authorities to do so. (p. 721)

The American Psychiatric Association (1993a) also states that it is ethically permissible to notify public health authorities when a patient's behavior constitutes a risk to people who cannot be identified, as well as to past sexual or drug-injecting partners. Similar guidelines were established for psychiatric inpatients (American Psychiatric Association, 1993b), as well by other professions, including social workers (Reamer, 1991).

When clinicians feel they must breach confidentiality to warn a third party, they are advised to take prudent action (Melton, 1988). Protective actions can include interventions to stop their client's risk behavior and therefore eliminate potential harm. When clients are noncompliant, therapists may notify public health authorities of the danger rather than directly warn the third party. Partner notification falls within the professional role of public health workers rather than that of psychotherapists and counselors (Melton, 1988). Certain clients, such as those who are sexually impulsive, manic, psychotic, or antisocial, may require involuntary hospitalization, in effect isolating them from potential victims (Knapp & VandeCreek, 1990; Winiarski, 1991). Hospitalization should, however, only be used to treat mental illness; decisions to quarantine again fall within professional roles of public health authorities, not mental health professionals (Melton, 1988). Finally, clients should be informed of the limits of confidentiality before they start treatment as a part of routine informed consent procedures. Informing clients that information pertaining to potential harm to others must be reported to appropriate authorities provides clinicians with a stated basis for disclosing otherwise confidential information (Boyd, 1992; Kermani & Weiss, 1989).

SEXUAL RISK-REDUCTION COUNSELING

Cessation of all fluid-exchanging sexual and drug-using behaviors is essential among persons with HIV infection to protect others from infection, as well as to protect themselves from reinfection and contracting other sexually transmitted pathogens (Filice & Pomeroy, 1991; Gellert, Page, Weismuller, & Ehling, 1993). Behaviors that confer high risk for HIV transmission are difficult to change because they are highly reinforcing, sustained over long periods of time, driven by biological needs, and interwoven with aspects of self-concept, affection, and belongingness. Abstinence from sexual intercourse or consistent practice of safer sex is difficult to achieve and can require support. In many cases, psychotherapy provides an environment for modifying high-risk behavioral practices (I. Kleinman, 1991). Trust and commitment in psychotherapy facilitates behavior change and can do so with HIV risk reduction (Grace, 1994).

According to the Centers for Disease Control and Prevention (CDC, 1993c), personalized risk-reduction counseling should include accurate information about HIV transmission, addressing personal needs and life circumstances related to risk behaviors; skills to reduce risk effectively; and a realistic, feasible plan of risk reduction. Counseling should also be culturally competent, developmentally appropriate, and sensitive to issues of sexual orientation and gender (CDC, 1993a; Doll & Kennedy, in press).

Strategies that have to date demonstrated reductions in high-risk sexual behaviors among HIV-risk populations have been based on principles of social cognitive theory. Components of effective interventions include providing accurate information pertaining to HIV transmission, personal risk sensitization, instructing individuals in self-management skills to reduce risk, instruction in identifying antecedent cues to risk-producing situations, identifying and managing behavior-change barriers, instruction in proper condom use and needle cleaning, and training in interpersonal assertiveness and other communication skills necessary to develop and maintain lower-risk relationships. Cognitive–behavioral interventions are known to decrease rates of unprotected sexual intercourse among homosexually active men, inner-city women, chronic mentally ill adults, African American adolescent males, and runaway adolescents (Kelly, Murphy, Sikkema, & Kalichman, 1993). In most studies, multisession group interventions produce substantial reductions in high-risk sexual practices.

Cognitive–behavioral skills training interventions have used principles based on social cognitive theory (Bandura, 1986, 1989, 1994) and cognitive–behavioral skills training techniques (Kelly, 1982), including risk and behavior-change education, modeling relationship skills related to risk reduction, generating behavioral self-management strategies, providing problem-solving skills for risk-producing situations, emphasizing the importance of practice for effective behavior change, and providing opportunities for guided practice with corrective feedback. Intervention participants increase HIV-risk-related knowledge, increase personal sensitization to risk, increase rates of condom use, and reduce high-risk sexual practices. Intervention outcomes have been highly encouraging, and the principles of effective behavior change can be applied to counseling and therapy with HIV-positive clients (Kelly, in press). The following components included in HIV-risk-reduction training can be adapted for use in individual and group psychotherapy.

Basic HIV Education and Risk Sensitization

HIV-positive clients must possess accurate and up-to-date information about HIV risk behaviors (Morokoff, Holmes, & Weisse, 1987). An evaluation of the client's knowledge of HIV risk transmission factors can be guided by using an objective test of AIDS knowledge (see Appendix C for an AIDS knowledge test). Going over specific knowledge areas in sessions can help clarify information needs. Therapists may consult with local health departments and AIDS service organizations for educational materials. Numerous pamphlets and videotapes are available and can support therapy-based education. Counselors should be able to clarify misconceptions, dispel myths about AIDS, and supply correct information to replace misinformation.

Personal Risk Assessment

Clients should be guided through a personal assessment of their own behavioral risk histories and identify individual life situations that contribute to risk. Sexual intercourse (vaginal, anal, and oral) and sharing injection equipment are the absolute highest risk behaviors for contracting HIV infection. It is most important that these behaviors be the target for risk-behavior change. A comprehensive sexual history is therefore necessary and should include questions about sexual experimentation, sexual trade, previous sexually transmitted diseases, perceived risk of sexual partners, and use of condoms. A useful tool for guiding a client through a personal risk assessment is to have them place their behavior on a risk continuum, indicating the degree to which their behavior has placed them at risk. An assessment of the client's readiness to change is also necessary, and motivational counseling may be needed before instituting a program for behavior change.

Condom Use and Needle-Cleaning Instructions

Many clients can benefit from instruction in the proper use of condoms and needle cleaning. The greatest obstacles to condom use are attitudes regarding reduced sensation and inconvenience. Cognitive restructuring where clients focus on sensations and total sexual acts to increase sexual satisfaction with condoms can effectively change attitudes. Acknowledging benefits of condoms, such as protection from sexually transmitted diseases and increased duration of penile erection, can also help reframe condom attitudes. The proper use of condoms should be instructed using the following steps: (a) carefully opening the package and not damaging the latex, (b) pinching the tip of the condom to assure a reservoir and remove air, (c) rolling the condom from the tip of the head of the penis all of the way back to the base, (d) removing the condom immediately after intercourse and disposing of it after one use. It is also important to educate clients that latex condoms with water-based, not water-soluble, lubricants protect against infections. Information and instruction in the now-available condom-like barriers for women should also be discussed. The female condom, although more expensive than penile condoms, offers women more control in safer sex decisions.

Clients who use injection drugs should also be instructed in cleaning injection equipment, following these steps: (a) prepare a bleach–water solution using one part bleach to nine parts water, (b) syphon in the solution through the needle to fill the syringe, (c) flush all of the solution through the needle, (d) repeat this action twice, (e) rinse in water twice after cleaning. Of course, it is best not to share needles at all. The use of clean needles relies heavily on policy regarding injection equipment availability and needle exchange. Studies show that needle exchange reduces HIV infection rates, and people should be encouraged to use sterile needles whenever possible (Compton, Cottler, Decker, Mager, & Stringfellow, 1992).

Behavior Self-Management Skills

Clients can be instructed to identify environmental and cognitive–affective cues that serve as "triggers" for high-risk situations, including mood states, substance use, settings, and sexual partner characteristics. Strategies for handling risk-related cues and situations may include avoiding certain partners, places, or substance use in relation to sexual situations. Rearranging the environment to reduce risk in specific situations can also be achieved by instruction in performing certain acts, such as redirecting sexual activities toward safer sex alternatives, carrying condoms, avoiding sex after drinking, and remembering relevant risk information.

Another important aspect of behavioral self-management is the use of self-monitoring techniques. Journals, diaries, and logs of personal risk behavior as well as risk behavior triggers can have reactive effects and reduce risk. Self-monitoring also provides a useful assessment technique and can help identify particularly difficult risk situations, which may then be addressed through problem solving and action planning.

Dissolving Barriers to Sustaining Safer Sexual Behaviors

Identification of barriers to risk reduction can be achieved in therapy. Behavioral self-management of barriers can be placed in the context of a problem-solving model in which clients (a) identify personal problem situations, (b) gather information for possible solutions, (c) evaluate options, and (d) plan a course of action. Step-by-step plans developed with clients should be realistic and feasible. Homework can be used for achieving short-term goals and evaluated at subsequent sessions.

Sexual Communication Skills

Therapy can focus on the role of sexual negotiation, assertiveness, and refusal skills to reduce risk for HIV infection. Increasing skills for disclosing HIV serostatus, resisting partner coercion to engage in sexual intercourse without condoms, and increasing comfort in discussing safer sex with partners in advance of sexual activity can be accomplished through instruction, role-play modeling, practice in communicating sexual decisions, and discussing individual limits to behavior change. Clients can identify past situations of high risk and generate statements that would have led to a lower risk. Emphasis can be placed on effective communication of feelings and sexual behavior limits prior to entering sexual situations. Practice sessions can increase communication skills, self-efficacy, and comfort discussing sexual alternatives with partners. Basic skills in (a) interpersonal assertiveness, (b) refusal to engage in risk-related sexual behaviors, and (c) negotiating safer sexual activities with partners can be modeled by therapists and practiced with feedback.

Using communication techniques to reduce risk may have special implications for women because of sexual double standards placed on talking about sex. Women are often punished for taking an assertive role in sexual situations. It is important that efforts by women to protect themselves not inadvertently result in endangerment. Negotiating safer sex may therefore be placed in the context of health and reproductive needs, reducing the possibility of suspicion and angry reactions to initiating safer sex discussions.

Although these intervention components have been effective in group formats, they can be instituted in individual therapy. Kelly (1991) described a case of a young HIV-positive gay man who had lapsed into unsafe sex. Kelly applied skills training in the context of eight sessions of individual therapy. First, a detailed history was conducted to identify the functional relationships between risk behaviors and specific settings, feelings, moods, situations, partners, and anything else the client associated with his behavior. Kelly stated that it is necessary to conduct intensive reviews of circumstances surrounding recent risk-taking activities to determine the skills needed to handle situations in the future. Once these were identified, Kelly used skills instruction techniques similar to those described in group interventions, including role-playing and behavioral rehearsal.

Research continues to identify new and effective strategies for HIV risk reduction that vary for men and women, sexual orientation groups, ethnic groups, age groups, and types of relationships. As new intervention approaches for HIV prevention emerge, there will be additional procedures available to therapists. Methods of adapting these procedures to psychotherapy are evolving and should become available to clinicians.

CONCLUSION

Mental health professionals are providing increasingly more services in the HIV epidemic. Unfortunately, professionals are unlikely to have training or previous experience in treating HIV-positive clients (Campos, Brasfield, & Kelly, 1989; Kinderman, Matteo, & Morales, 1993). Werth and Carney (1994) suggested that psychologists receive training in confidentiality, issues of hastened death, assessment, and counseling diverse populations. Training in this area is particularly important given the potential for attitudes to interfere with the therapeutic process (Corless et al., 1992). Issues of sexuality, intimacy, death, disease, spirituality, and caretaking occur with HIV-positive clients and require particular sensitivity (McKusick, 1988).

A number of sources are now available to train mental health professionals in HIV–AIDS-related issues. Local health departments and AIDS service organizations provide educational programming on a regular basis. HIV-positive guest speakers are usually available to share insights into their experiences. Workshops and seminars are offered through conferences, conventions, and other forums. Finally, the American Psychological Association's HIV Office on Psychology Education (HOPE) program offers training seminars conducted by local psychologists with expertise in treating HIV-positive clients. Education in human sexuality and HIV disease, familiarity with HIV-related issues, and awareness of sexual orientation and gender increases the ability of mental health professionals to provide effective services for their HIV-positive clients.

References

Abrams, D. I. (1992). Dealing with alternative therapies for HIV. In M. A. Sande & P. A. Volberding (Eds.), *The medical management of AIDS* (3rd ed., pp. 111–128). Philadelphia: Saunders.

Adelman, M. (1989). Social support and AIDS. *AIDS & Public Policy Journal, 4,* 31–39.

Adjorlolo-Johnson, G., De Cock, K. M., Ekpini, E., Vetter, K. M., Sibailly, T., Brattegaard, K., Yavo, D., Doorly, R., Whitaker, J. P., Kestens, L., Ou, C. Y., George, J. R., & Gayle, H. D. (1994). Prospective comparison of mother-to-child transmission of HIV-1 and HIV-2 in Abidjan, Ivory Coast. *Journal of the American Medical Association, 272,* 462–466.

Adler, G., & Beckett, A. (1989). Psychotherapy of the patient with an HIV infection: Some ethical and therapeutic dilemmas. *Psychosomatics, 30,* 203–208.

Affleck, G., Tennen, H., Pfeiffer, C., & Fifield, J. (1987). Appraisals of control and predictability in adapting to a chronic disease. *Journal of Personality and Social Psychology, 53,* 273–279.

Agle, D., Gluck, H., & Pierce, G. F. (1987). The risk of AIDS: Psychologic impact on the hemophilic population. *General Hospital Psychiatry, 9,* 11–17.

Allen, J. R., & Setlow, V. P. (1991). Heterosexual transmission of HIV: A view of the future. *Journal of the American Medical Association, 266,* 1695–1696.

American Psychiatric Association. (1987). *Diagnostic and statistical manual of mental disorders* (3rd ed., rev.). Washington, DC: Author.

American Psychiatric Association. (1992). AIDS Policy: Guidelines for outpatient psychiatric services. *American Journal of Psychiatry, 149,* 721.

American Psychiatric Association. (1993a). AIDS Policy: Position statement on confidentiality, disclosure, and protection of others. *American Journal of Psychiatry, 150,* 852.

American Psychiatric Association. (1993b). AIDS Policy: Guidelines for inpatient psychiatric services. *American Journal of Psychiatry, 150,* 853.

American Psychiatric Association (1994). *Diagnostic and statistical manual of mental disorders* (4th ed.). Washington, DC: Author.

Anders, K. H., Guerra, W. F., Tomiyasu, U., Verity, M. A., & Vinters, H. V. (1986). The neuropathology of AIDS: UCLA experience and review. *American Journal of Pathology, 124,* 537–558.

Anderson, J. R. (1993). Early intervention for HIV infection in a gynecologic setting. *Journal of Women's Health, 2,* 343–346.

Anderson, R. M., & May, R. M. (1992). Understanding the AIDS pandemic. *Scientific American, 266,* 58–66.

Andrulis, D. P., Weslowski, V. B., Hintz, E., & Spolarich, A. W. (1992). Comparisons of hospital care for patients with AIDS and other HIV-related conditions. *Journal of the American Medical Association, 267,* 2482–2486.

Antoni, M., August, S., LaPerriere, A., Baggett, H. L., Klimas, N., Ironson, G., Schneiderman, N., & Fletcher, M. (1990). Psychological and neuroendocrine measures related to functional immune changes in anticipation of HIV-1 serostatus notification. *Psychosomatic Medicine, 52,* 496–510.

Antoni, M. H., Baggett, L., Ironson, G., LaPerriere, A., August, S., Klimas, N., Schneiderman, N., & Fletcher, M. A. (1991). Cognitive–behavioral stress management intervention buffers distress responses and immunologic changes following notification of HIV-1 seropositivity. *Journal of Consulting and Clinical Psychology, 59,* 906–915.

Antoni, M. H., Schneiderman, N., Fletcher, M. A., Goldstein, D. A., Ironson, G., & LaPerriere, A. (1990). Psychoneuroimmunology of HIV-1. *Journal of Consulting and Clinical Psychology, 58,* 38–49.

Antoni, M., Schneiderman, N., Klimas, N., LaPerriere, A., Ironson, G., & Fletcher, M. (1991). Disparities in psychological, neuroendocrine, and immunologic patterns in asymptomatic HIV-1 seropositive and seronegative gay men. *Biological Psychiatry, 29,* 1023–1041.

Antonucci, T. C. (1989). Social support influences on the disease process. In L. L. Carstensen & J. M. Neale (Eds.), *Mechanisms of psychological influence on physical health, with special attention to the elderly* (pp. 23–41). New York: Plenum Press.

Aral, S. O., & Holmes, K. K. (1991). Sexually transmitted diseases in the AIDS era. *Scientific American, 264,* 62–69.

Aral, S. O., & Wasserheit, J. (in press). Interactions among HIV, other sexually transmitted diseases (STDs), socioeconomic status and poverty in women. In A. O'Leary & L. S. Jemmott (Eds.), *Women at risk: Issues in the primary prevention of AIDS.* New York: Plenum Press.

Araneta, M. R. G., Weisfuse, I. B., Greenberg, B., Schultz, S., & Thomas, P. A. (1992). Abortions and HIV-1 infection in New York City, 1987–1989. *AIDS, 6,* 1195–1201.

Aronow, H. A., Brew, B. J., & Price, R. W. (1988). The management of the neurological complications of HIV infection and AIDS. *AIDS, 2*(Suppl.), S151–S159.

Atkinson, J. H., Grant, I., Kennedy, C. J., Richman, D. D., Spector, S. A., & McCutchan, J. A. (1988). Prevalence of psychiatric disorders among men infected with human immunodeficiency virus. *Archives of General Psychiatry, 45,* 859–864.

Baba, T. W., Sampson, J. E., Fratazzi, C., Greene, M. F., & Ruprecht, R. M. (1993). Maternal transmission of the human immunodeficiency virus: Can it be prevented? *Journal of Women's Health, 2,* 231–242.

Bacchetti, P., Osmond, D., Chaisson, R. E., Dritz, S., Rutherford, G. W., Swig, L., & Moss, A. R. (1988). Survival patterns of the first 500 patients with AIDS in San Francisco. *Journal of Infectious Diseases, 157,* 1044–1047.

Bacchetti, P., Osmond, D., Chaisson, R. E., & Moss, A. R. (1988). Survival with AIDS in New York [Letter]. *New England Journal of Medicine, 318,* 1464.

Bacellar, H., Munoz, A., Miller, E. N., Cohen, B., Besley, D., Selnes, O., Becker, J., & McArthur, J. (1994). Temporal trends in the incidence of HIV-1-related neurologic diseases: Multicenter AIDS Cohort Study, 1985–1992. *Neurology, 44,* 1892–1900.

Bagdades, E. K. (1991). Current treatment of opportunistic infections in HIV disease. *AIDS Care, 3,* 461–466.

Bakal, D. A. (1992). *Psychology and health* (2nd ed.). New York: Springer.

Bandura, A. (1986). *Social foundations of thought and action: A social cognitive theory.* Englewood Cliffs, NJ: Prentice-Hall.

Bandura, A. (1989). Perceived self–efficacy in the exercise of control over AIDS infection. In V. M. Mays, G. W. Albee, & S. F. Schneider (Eds.), *Primary prevention of AIDS: Psychological approaches* (pp. 128–141). Newbury Park, CA: Sage.

Bandura, A. (1994). Social cognitive theory and exercise of control over HIV infection. In R. DiClemente & J. Peterson (Eds.), *Preventing AIDS: Theories, methods, and behavioral interventions* (pp. 25–60). New York: Plenum Press.

Barsky, A. J., Cleary, P. D., Sarnie, M. K., & Klerman, G. L. (1993). The course of transient hypochondriasis. *American Journal of Psychiatry, 150,* 484–488.

Barsky, A. J., Wyshak, G., & Klerman, G. L. (1990). Transient Hypochondriasis. *Archives of General Psychiatry, 47,* 746–752.

Bartlett, J. G. (1993a). *The Johns Hopkins Hospital guide to medical care of patients with HIV infection* (3rd ed.). Baltimore, MD: Williams & Wilkins.

Bartlett, J. G. (1993b). Zidovudine now or later? *New England Journal of Medicine,* *329,* 351–352.

Bartrop, R. W., Luckhurst, E., Lazarus, L., Kiloh, L., & Penny, R. (1977). Depressed lymphocyte function after bereavement. *Lancet,* 834–836.

Batki, S. L., Sorensen, J. L., Faltz, B., & Madover, S. (1988). Psychiatric aspects of treatment of IV drug abusers with AIDS. *Hospital and Community Psychiatry,* *39,* 439–441.

Beck, A. T. (1976). *Cognitive therapy and emotional disorders.* New York: International Universities Press.

Beck, A. T., Kovacs, M., & Weissman, A. (1975). Hopelessness and suicidal behavior: An overview. *Journal of the American Medical Association, 234,* 1146–1149.

Beck, A. T., & Steer, R. A. (1993). *BDI: Beck Depression Inventory manual.* New York: Psychological Corporation.

Becker, M., & Joseph, J. (1988). AIDS and behavioral change to reduce risk: A review. *American Journal of Public Health, 78,* 394–410.

Beckett, A., & Rutan, J. S. (1990). Treating persons with ARC and AIDS in group psychotherapy. *International Journal of Group Psychotherapy, 40,* 19–29.

Bednarik, D. P., & Folks, T. M. (1992). Mechanisms of HIV-1 latency. *AIDS, 6,* 3–16.

Beevor, A. S., & Catalan, J. (1993). Women's experience of HIV testing: The views of HIV positive and HIV negative women. *AIDS Care, 5,* 177–186.

Belkin, G. S., Fleishman, J. A., Stein, M. D., Piette, J., & Mor, V. (1992). Physical symptoms and depressive symptoms among individuals with HIV infection. *Psychosomatics, 33,* 416–427.

Benjamin, A. E., & Preston, S. D. (1993, Spring). A comparative perspective on hospice care for persons with AIDS. *AIDS & Public Policy Journal,* 36–43.

Bennett, L., & Kelaher, M. (1993). Variables contributing to experiences of grief in HIV/AIDS health care professionals. *Journal of Community Psychology, 21,* 210–217.

Beral, V., Bull, D., Darby, S., Weller, I., Carne, C., Beecham, M., & Jaffe, H. (1992). Risk of Kaposi's sarcoma and sexual practices assocaited with faecal contact in homosexual or bisexual men with AIDS. *Lancet, 339,* 632–635.

Berkman, L. F., & Syme, S. L. (1979). Social networks, host resistance, and mortality: A nine-year follow-up study of Alameda county residents. *American Journal of Epidemiology, 109,* 186–204.

Berrios, D. C., Hearst, N., Coates, T. J., Stall, R., Hudes, E. S., Turner, H., Eversley, R., & Catania, J. (1993). Human immunodeficiency virus antibody testing among those at risk for infection: The national acquired immune deficiency syndrome behavioral survey. *Journal of the American Medical Association, 270,* 1576–1580.

Biggar, R.J ., Pahwa, S., Minkoff, H., Mendes, H., Willoughby, A., Landesman, S., & Goedert, J. J. (1989). Immunosuppression in pregnant women infected with human immunodeficiency virus. *American Journal of Obstetrics and Gynecology, 161,* 1239–1244.

Billings, A. G., & Moos, R. H. (1981). The role of coping resources in attenuating the stress of life events. *Journal of Behavioral Medicine, 7,* 139–157.

Billings, A. G., & Moos, R. H. (1984). Coping, stress, and social resources among adults with unipolar depression. *Journal of Personality and Social Psychology, 46,* 877–891.

Billy, J. O. G., Tanfer, K., Grady, W., & Klepinger, D. H. (1993).The sexual behavior of men in the United States. *Family Planning Perspectives, 25,* 52–60.

Bliwise, N. G., Grade, M., Irish, T. M., & Ficarrotto, T. J. (1991). Measuring medical and nursing students' attitudes toward AIDS. *Health Psychology, 10,* 289–295.

Blumenfield, M., Smith, P. J., Milazzo, J., Seropian, S., & Wormser, G. P. (1987). Survey of attitudes of nurses working with AIDS patients. *General Hospital Psychiatry, 9,* 58–63.

Bolan, G. (1992). Management of syphilis in HIV-infected persons. In M. A. Sande & P. A. Volberding, *The medical management of AIDS* (3rd ed., pp. 383–398). Philadelphia: Saunders.

Bollinger, R. C., & Siliciano, R. (1992). Immunodeficiency in HIV-1 infection. In G. P. Wormser (Ed.), *AIDS and other manifestations of HIV infection* (2nd ed., pp. 145–164). New York: Raven Press.

Booth, R. E., Watters, J. K., & Chitwood, D. D. (1993). HIV risk-related sex behaviors among injection drug users, crack smokers, and injection drug users who smoke crack. *American Journal of Public Health, 83,* 1144–1148.

Booth, W. (1988). AIDS and drug abuse: No quick fix. *Science, 239,* 717–719.

Bor, R., Perry, L., & Miller, R. (1989). A systems approach to AIDS counselling. *Journal of Family Therapy, 11,* 77–86.

Bor, R., Prior, N., & Miller, R. (1990). Complementarity in relationships of couples affected by HIV. *Counselling Psychology Quarterly, 3,* 217–220.

Borden, W. (1989). Life review as a therapeutic frame in the treatment of young adults with AIDS. *Health and Social Work, 14,* 253–259.

Borden, W. (1991). Beneficial outcomes in adjustment to HIV seropositivity. *Social Service Review, 65,* 434–450.

Bornstein, R. A. (1993, April). *Neuropsychological function in the course of HIV infection.* Paper presented at the meeting of the Michigan Psychiatric Society.

Bornstein, R. A., Nasrallah, H. A., Para, M. G., Whitacre, C. C.,Rosenberger, P., Fass, R. J., & Rice, R. (1992). Neuropsychological performance in asymptomatic HIV infection. *The Journal of Neuropsychiatry and Clinical Neurosciences, 4,* 386–394.

Bornstein, R. A., Pace, P., Rosenberger, P., Nasrallah, H., Para, M., Whitacre, C., & Fass, R. (1993). Depression and neuropsychological performance in asymptomatic HIV infection. *American Journal of Psychiatry, 150,* 922–927.

Bottomley, P. A., Hardy, C. J., Cousins, J. P., Armstrong, M., & Wagle, W. A. (1990). AIDS dementia complex: Brain high-energy phosphate metabolite deficits. *Radiology, 176,* 407–411.

Boyd, K. M. (1992). HIV infection and AIDS: The ethics of medical confidentiality. *Journal of Medical Ethics, 18,* 173–179.

Bozovich, A., Cianelli, L., Johnson, J., Wagner, L., Chrash, M., & Mallory, G. (1992). Assessing community resources for rural PWAs. *AIDS Patient Care, 6,* 229–231.

Bredesen, D. E., Levy, R. M., & Rosenblum, M. L. (1988). The neurology of human immunodeficiency virus infection. *Quarterly Journal of Medicine, 68,* 665–677.

Brennan, T. A. (1991). Transmission of the human immunodeficiency virus in the health care setting—time for action. *New England Journal of Medicine, 324,* 1504–1509.

Brettle, R. P., & Leen, L. S. (1991). The natural history of HIV and AIDS in women. *AIDS, 5,* 1283–1292.

Brew, B. J., Bhalla, R. B., Fleisher, M., Paul, M., Khan, A., Schwartz, M. K., & Price, R. W. (1989). Cerebrospinal fluid beta 2 microglobulin in patients infected with human immunodeficiency virus. *Neurology, 39,* 830–840.

Britton, P. J., Zarski, J. J., & Hobfoll, S. E. (1993). Psychological distress and the role of significant others in a population of gay/bisexual men in the era of HIV. *AIDS Care, 5,* 43–54.

Broadhead, W. E., Kaplan, B. H., James, S. A., Wagner, E. H., Schoenbach, V. J., Grimson, R., Heyden, S., Tibblin, G., & Gehlbach (1983). Reviews and commentary: The epidemiologic evidence for a relationship between social support and health. *American Journal of Epidemiology, 117,* 521–537.

Broder, S., Merigan, T. C., & Bolognesi, D. (1994). *Textbook of AIDS medicine.* Baltimore: Williams & Wilkins.

Brooner, R., Greenfield, L., Schmidt, C., & Bigelow, G. (1993). Antisocial personality disorder and HIV infection among intravenous drug abusers. *American Journal of Psychiatry, 150,* 53–58.

Brown, G. R., & Rundell, J. R. (1989). Suicidal tendencies in women with human immunodeficiency virus infection. *American Journal of Psychiatry, 146,* 556–557.

Brown, G., & Rundell, J. (1990). Prospective study of psychiatric amorbidity in HIV-seropositive women without AIDS. *General Hospital Psychiatry, 12,* 30–35.

Bruhn, J. G. (1988). Life-style and health behavior. In D. S. Gochman (Ed.), *Health behavior: Emerging research perspectives* (pp. 71–86). New York: Plenum Press.

Buck, B. A. (1991, October). Support groups for hospitalized AIDS patients. *AIDS Patient Care,* 255–258.

Buehler, J. W., & Ward, J. W. (1993). A new definition for AIDS surveillance. *Annals of Internal Medicine, 118,* 390–392.

Buiss, A. (1989). A peer counselling program for persons testing HIV antibody positive. *Canadian Journal of Counseling, 23,* 127–132.

Bulkin, W., Brown, L., Fraioli, D., Giannattasio, E., McGuire, G., Tyler, P., & Friedland, G. (1988). Hospice care of the intravenous drug user AIDS patient in a skilled nurse facility. *Journal of Acquired Immune Deficiency Syndromes, 1,* 375–380.

Bumbalo, J. A., Patsdaughter, C. A., & McShane, R. E. (1993, January). Impact of AIDS on the family: Family functioning and symptoms among family members. *Wisconsin AIDS/HIV Update,* 15–18.

Burgess, A. P., Irving, G., & Riccio, M. (1993). The reliability and validity of a symptom checklist for use in HIV infection: A preliminary analysis. *International Journal of STD & AIDS, 4,* 333–338.

Burish, T., Carey, M., Wallston, K., Stein, M., Jamison, P., & Lyles, J. (1984). Health locus of control and chronic disease: An external orientation may be advantageous. *Journal of Social and Clinical Psychology, 2,* 326–332.

Burns, B. H. & Howell, J. B. L. (1969). Disproportionately severe breathlessness in chronic bronchitis. *Quarterly Journal of Medicine, 38,* 277–294.

Burrack, J. H., Barrett, D. C., Stall, R., Chesney, M. A., Ekstrand,M. L., & Coates, T. J. (1993). Depressive symptoms and CD4 lymphocyte decline among HIV-infected men. *Journal of the American Medical Association, 270,* 2568–2573.

Butters, E., Higginson, I., George, R., & McCarthy, M. (1993). Palliative care for people with HIV/AIDS: Views of patients, carers and providers. *AIDS Care, 5,* 105–116.

Butters, N., Grant, I., Haxby, J., Judd, L. L., Martin, A.,McClelland, J., Pequegnat, W., Schacter, D., & Stover, E. (1990). Assessment of AIDS-related cognitive changes: Recommendations of the NIMH workshop on neuropsychological assessment approaches. *Journal of Clinical and Experimental Neuropsychology, 12,* 963–978.

Calabrese, J., Kling, M., & Gold, P. (1987). Alterations in immunocompetence during stress, bereavement, and depression: Focus on neuroendocrine regulation. *American Journal of Psychiatry, 144,* 1123–1134.

Campbell, C. A. (1990). Prostitution and AIDS. In D. G. Ostrow (Ed.), *Behavioral aspects of AIDS* (pp. 121–138). New York: Plenum Press.

Campos, P. E., Brasfield, T. L., & Kelly, J. A. (1989). Psychology training related to AIDS: Survey of doctoral graduate programs and predoctoral internship programs. *Professional Psychology: Research and Practice, 20,* 214–220.

Camus, A. (1948). *The plague* (S. Gilbert, Trans.). New York: Vintage.

Cao, Y., Qin, L., Zhang, L., Safrit, J., & Ho. D. D. (1995). Virologic and immunologic characterization of long-term survivors of human immunodeficiency virus type-1 infection. *New England Journal of Medicine, 332,* 201–208.

Capitanio, J. (1994, January). *Variability in HIV disease: Toward an animal model of psychosocial influences.* Paper presented at the NIMH Neuroscience Findings in AIDS Research, Rockville, MD.

Carey, M. A., Jenkins, R. A., Brown, G. R., Temoshok, L., & Pace, J. (1991, June). *Gender differences in psychosocial functioning in early stage HIV patients.* Paper presented at the Seventh International Conference on AIDS, Florence, Italy.

Carmen, E., & Brady, S. (1990). AIDS risk and prevention for the chronic mentally ill. *Hospital and Community Psychiatry, 41,* 652–657.

Carpenter, C. C. J., Mayer, K. H., Stein, M. D., Leibman, B. D.,Fisher, A., & Fiore, T.C. (1991). Human immunodeficiency virus infection in North American women: Experience with 200 cases and a review of the literature. *Medicine, 70,* 307–325.

Carr, J. N. (1975). Drug patterns among drug-addicted mothers: Incidence, variance in use, and effects on children. *Pediatric Annals, 4,* 65–77.

Carson, V. (1990). Hope and spiritual well-being: Essentials for living with AIDS. *Perspectives in Psychiatric Care, 26,* 28–34.

Cassens, B. (1985). Social consequences of the acquired immunodeficiency syndrome. *Annals of Inernal Medicine. 103,* 768–771.

Cassileth, B. R., Lusk, E. J., Strouse, T. B., Miller, D. S., Brown, L. L., Cross, P. A., & Tenaglia, A. N. (1984). Psychosocial status in chronic illness: A comparative analysis of six diagnostic groups. *The New England Journal of Medicine, 311,* 506–511.

Cassileth, B. R., Lusk, E. J., Strouse, T. B., Miller, D.S ., Brown, L. L., & Cross, P. A. (1985). A psychological analysis of cancer patients and their next-of-kin. *Cancer, 55,* 72–76.

Castro, K. G., Lieb, S., Jaffe, H. W., Narkunas, J. P., Calisher, C. H., Bush, T. J., & Witte, J. J. (1988). Transmission of HIV in Belle Clade, Florida: Lessons for other communities in the United States. *Science, 239,* 193–197.

Castro, K. G., Lifson, A. R., White, C. R., Bush, T. J., Chamberland, M. E., Lekatsas, A. M., & Jaffe, H. W. (1988). Investigations of AIDS patients with no previously identified risk factors. *Journal of the American Medical Association, 259,* 1338–1342.

Catalan, J. (1988). Invited review: Psychosocial and neuropsychiatric aspects of HIV infection: Review of their extent and implications for psychiatry. *Journal of Psychosomatic Research, 32,* 237–248.

Catalan, J., & Burgess, A. (1991). Neuroscience of HIV infection: Basic and clinical frontiers. *AIDS Care, 3,* 467–471.

Catalan, J., & Thornton, S. (1993). Editorial review: Whatever happened to HIV dementia? *International Journal of STD & AIDS, 4,* 1–4.

Catania, J. A., Coates, T. J., Stall, R., Turner, H., Peterson, J., Hearst, N., Dolcini, M. M., Hudes, E., Gagnon, J., Wiley, J., & Groves, R. (1992). Prevalence of AIDS-related risk factors and condom use in the United States. *Science, 258,* 1101–1106.

Catania, J. A., Turner, H. A., Choi, K., & Coates, T. J. (1992). Coping with death anxiety: Help-seeking and social support among gay men with various HIV diagnoses. *AIDS, 6,* 999–1005.

Catania, J. A., Turner, H., Kegeles, S. M., Stall, R., Pollack, L., & Coates, T. J. (1989). Older Americans and AIDS: Transmission risks and primary prevention research needs. *The Gerontologist, 29,* 373–381.

CDC. (1981a). Kaposi's sarcoma and *Pneumocystis* pneumonia among homosexual men—New York City and California. *Morbidity and Mortality Weekly Report, 30,* 305–308.

CDC. (1981b). *Pneumocystis* pneumonia—Los Angeles. *Morbidity and Mortality Weekly Report, 30,* 250–252.

CDC. (1986). Classification system for Human T-Lymphocyte virus Type III/lymphadenopathy-associated virus infections. *Morbidity and Mortality Weekly Report, 35,* 334–339.

CDC. (1987a). Antibody to human immunodeficiency virus in female prostitutes. *Morbidity and Mortality Weekly Report, 36,* 157–161.

CDC. (1987b). Recommendations for prevention of HIV transmission in health-care settings. *Morbidity and Mortality Weekly Report, 36*(2-S), 3–18.

CDC. (1987c). Revision of the CDC surveillance case definition for acquired immunodeficiency syndrome. *Morbidity and Mortality Weekly Report, 36,* 3s–15s.

CDC. (1988). Number of sex partners and potential risk of sexual exposure to human immunodeficiency virus. *Morbidity and Mortality Weekly Report, 37,* 565–568.

295

CDC. (1991a). Characteristics and risk behaviors of homeless Black men seeking services from the community homeless assistance plan—Dade County, Florida, August 1991. *Morbidity and Mortality Weekly Report, 40,* 865–868.

CDC. (1991b). Drug use and sexual behaviors among sex partners of injecting-drug users—United States, 1988–1990. *Morbidity and Mortality Weekly Report, 40,* 855–860.

CDC. (1991c). HIV/AIDS knowledge and awareness of testing and treatment—behavioral risk factors surveillance system, 1990. *Morbidity and Mortality Weekly Report, 40,* 794–805.

CDC. (1991d). Mortality attributable to HIV infection/AIDS—United States, 1981–1990. *Morbidity and Mortality Weekly Report, 40,* 41–44.

CDC. (1991e). Update: Transmission of HIV infection during an invasive dental procedure—Florida. *Morbidity and Mortality Weekly Report, 40,* 21–33.

CDC. (1992a). Condom use among male injecting-drug users—New York City, 1987–1990. *Morbidity and Mortality Weekly Report, 41,* 617–620.

CDC. (1992b). Heterosexual transmission of HIV—Puerto Rico, 1981–1991. *Morbidity and Mortality Weekly Report, 41,* 899–906.

CDC. (1992c). HIV counseling and testing services from public and private providers—United States, 1990. *Morbidity and Mortality Weekly Report, 41,* 743, 749–752.

CDC. (1992d). HIV infection, syphilis, and tuberculosis screening among migrant farm workers—Florida, 1992. *Morbidity and Mortality Weekly Report, 41,* 723–725.

CDC. (1992e). HIV prevention in the U.S. correctional system, 1991. *Morbidity and Mortality Weekly Report, 41,* 389–392.

CDC. (1992f). HIV seroprevalence among adults treated for cardiac arrest before reaching a medical facility—Seattle, Washington, 1989–1990. *Morbidity and Mortality Weekly Report, 41,* 381–383.

CDC. (1992g). Mortality patterns—United States, 1989. *Morbidity and Mortality Weekly Report, 41,* 121–125.

CDC. (1992h). 1993 revised classification system for HIV infection and expanded surveillance case definition for AIDS among adolescents and adults. *Morbidity and Mortality Weekly Report, 41*(RR-17), 1–19.

CDC. (1992i). Patient exposures to HIV during nuclear medicine procedures. *Morbidity and Mortality Weekly Report, 41,* 575–578.

CDC. (1992j). Publicly funded HIV counseling and testing—United States, 1991. *Morbidity and Mortality Weekly Report, 41,* 613–617.

CDC. (1992k). Selected behaviors that increase risk for HIV infection among high school students—United States, 1990. *Morbidity and Mortality Weekly Report, 41*, 231–240.

CDC. (1992l). Selected behaviors that increase risk for HIV infection, other sexually transmitted diseases, and unintended pregnancy among high school students—United States, 1991. *Morbidity and Mortality Weekly Report, 41*, 945–950.

CDC. (1992m). Sexual behavior among high school students—United States, 1990. *Morbidity and Mortality Weekly Report, 41*, 885–888.

CDC. (1992n). Surveillance for occupationally acquired HIV infection—United States, 1981–1992. *Morbidity and Mortality Weekly Report, 41*, 823–825.

CDC. (1992o). Testing for antibodies to human immunodeficiency virus Type-2 in the United States. *Morbidity and Mortality Weekly Report, 41*, 259–262.

CDC. (1992p). Unexplained CD4+ T-lymphocyte depletion in persons without evident HIV infection—United States. *Morbidity and Mortality Weekly Report, 41*, 541–545.

CDC. (1992q). Update: Acquired immunodeficiency syndrome—United States, 1991. *Morbidity and Mortality Weekly Report, 41*, 463–468.

CDC. (1992r). Update: CD4+ T-lymphocytopenia in persons without evident HIV infection—United States. *Morbidity and Mortality Weekly Report, 41*, 578–579.

CDC. (1992s). Update: Investigations of patients who have been treated by HIV-infected health care workers. *Morbidity and Mortality Weekly Report, 41*, 344–346.

CDC. (1992t). Update: Serological testing for human T-lymphotropic virus type I—United States, 1989–1990. *Morbidity and Mortality Weekly Report, 41*, 259–262.

CDC. (1993a). Condom use and sexual identity among men who have sex with men—Dallas, 1991. *Morbidity and Mortality Weekly Report, 42*, 7, 13–14.

CDC. (1993b). Impact of the expanded AIDS surveillance case definition on AIDS case reporting—United States, first quarter, 1993. *Morbidity and Mortality Weekly Report, 42*, 308–310.

CDC. (1993c). Recommendations for HIV testing services for inpatients and outpatients in acute-care hospital settings and technical guidance on HIV counseling. *Morbidity and Mortality Weekly Report, 42*(RR-2), 1–6.

CDC. (1993d). Recommendations on prophylaxis and therapy for disseminated mycobacterium avium complex for adult and adolescents infected with human immunodeficiency virus. *Morbidity and Mortality Weekly Report, 42*(RR-9), 17–20.

CDC. (1993e). Self-reported HIV-antibody testing among persons with selected risk behaviors—Southern Los Angeles County, 1991–1992. *Morbidity and Mortality Weekly Report, 42*, 786–789.

CDC. (1993f). Update: Acquired immunodeficiency syndrome—United States, 1992. *Morbidity and Mortality Weekly Report, 42,* 547–557.

CDC. (1993g). Update: Barrier protection against HIV infection and other sexually transmitted diseases. *Morbidity and Mortality Weekly Report, 42,* 589–591, 597.

CDC. (1993h). Update: Investigations of persons treated by HIV-infected health-care workers—United States. *Morbidity and Mortality Weekly Report, 42,* 329–331, 337.

CDC. (1994a). *Cryptosporidium* infections associated with swimming pools—Dane County, Wisconsin, 1993. *Morbidity and Mortality Weekly Report, 43,* 561–563.

CDC. (1994b). *HIV/AIDS surveillance report: Provisional 1993 year end report.* Atlanta: Author.

CDC. (1994c). Human immunodeficiency virus transmission in household settings—United States. *Morbidity and Mortality Weekly Report, 43,* 347–356.

CDC. (1994d). Recommendations of the U.S. Public Health Service Task Force on the use of zidovudine to reduce perinatal transmission of human immunodeficiency virus. *Morbidity and Mortality Weekly Report, 43*(RR–11), 1–20.

CDC. (1994e). Update: Trends in AIDS diagnosis and reporting under expanded surveillance definition for adolescents and adults—United States, 1993. *Morbidity and Mortality Weekly Report, 43,* 826–831.

CDC. (1994f). Zidovudine for the prevention of HIV transmission from mother to infant. *Morbidity and Mortality Weekly Report, 43,* 285–287.

CDC. (1994g). 1994 revised classification system for human immunodeficiency virus infection in children less than 13 years of age. *Morbidity and Mortality Weekly Report, 43*(RR-12) 1–10.

Ceballos-Capitaine, A., Szapocznik, J., Blaney, N., Morgan, R., Millon, C., & Eisdorfer, C. (1990). Ethnicity, emotional distress, stress-related disruption, and coping among HIV seropositive gay males. *Hispanic Journal of Behavioral Sciences, 12,* 135–152.

Cello, J. P. (1992), Gastrointestinal tract manifestations of AIDS. In P. A. Volberding (Ed.), *The medical management of AIDS* (3rd ed., pp. 176–192). Philadelphia: Saunders.

Chaisson, R. E. (1992). Bacterial infections in HIV disease. In M. A. Sande & P. A. Volberding (Eds.), *The medical management of AIDS* (3rd ed., pp. 346–358). Philadelpia: Saunders.

Chang, S. W., Katz, M. H., & Hernandez, S. R. (1992). The new AIDS case definition: Implications for San Francisco. *Journal of the American Medical Association, 267,* 973–975.

Chang, Y., Cesarman, E., Pessin, M. S., Lee, F., Culpepper, J., Knowles, D. M., & Moore, P. S. (1994). Identification of herpes virus-like DNA sequences in AIDS-associated Kaposi's sarcoma. *Science, 266*, 1865–1869.

Chiasson, M. A., Stoneburner, R. L., Hildebrandt, D. S., Ewing, W. E., Telzak, E. E., & Jaffe, H. W. (1991). Heterosexual transmission of HIV-1 associated with the use of smokable freebase cocaine (crack). *AIDS, 5*, 1121–1126.

Chitwood, D. D., McCoy, C. B., Inciardi, J. A., McBride, D. C., Comerford, M., Trapido, E., McCoy, V., Page, J. B., Griffin, J., Fletcher, M. A., & Ashman, M. A. (1990). HIV seropositivity of needles from shooting galleries in South Florida. *American Journal of Public Health, 80*, 150–152.

Chmiel, J. S., Detels, R., Kaslow, R. A., Van Raden, M., Kingsley, L. A., & Brookmeyer, R. (1987). Factors associated with prevalent human immunodeficiency virus (HIV) infection in the Multicenter AIDS Cohort Study. *American Journal of Epidemiology, 126*, 568–575.

Chorba, T. L., Holman, R. C., & Evatt, B. L. (1993). Heterosexual and mother-to-child transmission of AIDS in the hemophilia community. *Public Health Reports, 108*, 99–105.

Chow, Y., Hirsch, M., Merrill, D., Bechtel, L., Eron, J., Kaplan, J., & D'Aquila, R. (1993). Use of evolutionary limitations of HIV-1 multidrug resistance to optimize therapy. *Nature, 361*, 650–654.

Christ, G. H., & Wiener, L. S. (1985). Psychosocial issues in AIDS. In V. T. DeVita, S. Hellman, & S. A. Rosenberg (Eds.), *AIDS: Etiology, diagnosis, treatment and prevention* (pp. 275–297). Philadelphia: Lippincott.

Christ, G. H., Wiener, L. S., & Moynihan, R. T. (1986). Psychosocial issues in AIDS. *Psychiatric Annals, 16*, 173–179.

Chu, S. Y., Buehler, J. W., & Berkelman, R. L. (1990). Impact of the human immunodeficiency virus epidemic on mortality in women of reproductive age, United States. *Journal of the American Medical Association, 264*, 225–229.

Chu, S. Y., Buehler, J. W., Fleming, P. L., & Berkelman, R. L.(1990). Epidemiology of reported cases of AIDS in lesbians. *American Journal of Public Health, 80*, 1380–1381.

Chu, S. Y., Conti, L., Schable, B., & Diaz, T. (1994). Female-to-female sexual contact and HIV transmission. *Journal of the American Medical Association, 272*, 443.

Chuang, H. T., Devins, G., Hunsley, J., & Gill, M. J. (1989). Psychosocial distress and well-being among gay and bisexual men with human immunodeficiency virus infection. *American Journal of Psychiatry, 146*, 876–880.

Chuang, H. T., Jason, G., Pajurkova, E., & Gill, J. (1992). Psychiatric morbidity in patients with HIV infection. *Canadian Journal of Psychaitry, 37*, 109–115.

Cleary, P. D., Fowler, F. J., Weissman, J., Massagli, M. P., Wilson, I., Seage, G. R., Gatsonis, C., & Epstein, A. (1993). Health-related quality of life in persons with acquired immune deficiency syndrome. *Medical Care, 31,* 569–580.

Cleary, P. D., Van Devanter, N., Rogers, T., Sinwer, E., Shipton-Levy, R., Steilen, M., Stuart, A., Avorn, J., & Pindyck, J. (1993). Depressive symptoms in blood donors notified of HIV infection. *American Journal of Public Health, 83* 534–539.

Clement, M., & Hollander, H. (1992). Natural history and management of the seropositive patient. In M. A. Sande & P. A. Volberding (Eds.), *The medical management of AIDS* (3rd ed., pp. 87–96). Philadelphia: Saunders.

Clifford, D. B., Jacoby, R. G., Miller, J. P., Seyfried, W. R., & Glicksman, M. (1990). Neuropsychometric performance of asymptomatic HIV-infected subjects. *AIDS, 4,* 767–774.

Clumeck, N., Taelman, H., Hermans, P., Piot, P., Schoumacher, M., & De Wit, S. (1989). A cluster of HIV infection among heterosexual people without apparent risk factors. *New England Journal of Medicine, 321,* 1460–1462.

Coates, T., McKusick, L., Kuno, R., & Stites, D. (1989). Stress reduction training changed number of sexual partners but not immune function in men with HIV. *American Journal of Public Health, 79,* 885–886.

Coates, T., Moore, S., & McKusick, L. (1987). Behavioral consequences of AIDS antibody testing among gay men. *Journal of the American Medical Association, 258,* 1889.

Coates, T. J., Temoshok, L., & Mandel, J. (1984). Psychosocial research is essential to understanding and treating AIDS. *American Psychologist, 39,* 1309–1314.

Cobb, S. (1976). Social support as a moderator of life stress. *Psychosomatic Medicine, 38,* 300–314.

Cochran, S. D. & Mays, V. M. (1988). Women and AIDS-related concerns. *American Psychologist, 44,* 529–535.

Cochran, S. D., & Mays, V. M. (1994). Depressive distress among homosexually active African American men and women. *American Journal of Psychiatry, 151,* 524–529.

Cockerell, C. J. (1992). Cutaneous and histologic signs of HIV infection other than Kaposi's sarcoma. In G.P. Wormser (Ed.), *AIDS and other manifestations of HIV infection* (2nd ed., pp. 463–476). New York: Raven Press.

Cohen, F. L. & Nehring, W. M. (1994). Foster care of HIV-positive children in the United States. *Public Health Reports, 109,* 60–67.

Cohen, S. (1988). Psychosocial models of the role of social support in the etiology of physical disease. *Health Psychology, 7,* 269–297.

Cohen, S., & Williamson, G. (1991). Stress and infectious disease in humans. *Psychological Bulletin, 109,* 5–24.

Cohen, S., & Willis, T. A. (1985). Stress, social support, and the buffering hypothesis. *Psychological Bulletin, 98,* 310–357.

Coleman, V. E., & Harris, G. N. (1989). Clinical notes: A support group for individuals recently testing HIV positive: A psycho-educational group model. *Journal of Sex Research, 26,* 539–548.

Collier, A. C., Marra, C., Coombs, R. W., Claypoole, K., Cohen, W., Longstreth, W. T., Townes, B. D., Maravilla, K. R., Critchlow, C., Murphy, V. L., & Handsfield, H. H. (1992). Central nervous system manifestations in human immunodeficiency virus infection without AIDS. *Journal of Acquired Immune Deficiency Syndrome, 5,* 229–241.

Compton, W. M., Cottler, L. B., Decker, S. H., Mager, D., & Stringfellow, R. (1992). Legal needle buying in St. Louis. *American Journal of Public Health, 82,* 595–596.

Conant, M., Hardy, D., Sernatinger, J., Spicer, D., & Levy, J. A.(1986). Condoms prevent transmission of AIDS-associated retrovirus. *Journal of the American Medical Association, 255,* 1706.

Connor, E. M., Sperling, R. S., Gelber, R., Kiselev, P., Scott, G., O'Sullivan, M. J., VanDyke, R., Bey, M., Shearer, W., Jacobson, R. L., Jimenez, E., O'Neill, E., Bazin, B., Delfraissy, J. F., Culnane, M., Coombs, R., Elkins, M., Moye, J., Stratton, P., & Balsley, J. (1994). Reduction of maternal–infant transmission of human immunodeficiency virus type 1 with zidovudine treatment. *The New England Journal of Medicine, 331,* 1173–1180.

Cooper, D. A. (1994). Early antiretroviral therapy. *AIDS, 8*(Suppl. 3), S9–S14.

Corless, I. B., Fulton, R., Lamers, E. P., Bendiksen, R., Hysing-Dahl, B., MacElveen-Hoehn, P., O'Connor, P., Harvei, U., Schjolberg, T., & Stevenson, E. (1992). Assumptions and principles concerning care for persons affected by HIV disease. *AIDS & Public Policy Journal, 7,* 28–31.

Cournos, F., Empfield, M., Horwath, E., McKinnon, K., Meyer, I., Phil, M., Schrage, H., Currie, C., & Agosin, B. (1991). HIV seroprevalence among patients admitted to two psychiatric hospitals. *American Journal of Psychiatry, 148,* 1225–1230.

Cournos, F., Horwath, E., Guido, J. R., McKinnon, K., & Hopkins, N. (1994). HIV-1 infection at two public psychiatric hospitals in New York City. *AIDS Care, 6,* 443–452.

Crandall, C. S. (1991). Multiple stigma and AIDS: Illness stigma and attitudes toward homosexuals and IV drug users in AIDS-related stigmatization. *Journal of Community & Applied Social Psychology, 1,* 165–172.

Crandall, C. S. & Coleman, R. (1992). AIDS-related stigmatization and the disruption of social relationships. *Journal of Social and Personal Relationships, 9,* 163–177.

Crawford, I., Humfleet, G., Ribordy, S. C., Ho, F. C., & Vickers, V. L. (1991). Stigmatization of AIDS patients by mental health professionals. *Professional Psychology: Research and Practice, 5,* 357–361.

Creagh, T., Doi, P., Andrews, E., Nusinoff-Lehrman, S., Tilson, H., Hoth, D., & Barry, D. W. (1988). Survival experience among patients with AIDS receiving zidovudine. *Journal of the American Medical Assocaition, 260,* 3009–3015.

Crystal, S., & Jackson, M. M. (1989). Psychosocial adaptation and economic circumstances of persons with AIDS and ARC. *Family and Community Health, 12,* 77–88.

Curtis, J. R., & Patrick, D. L. (1993). Race and survival time with AIDS: A synthesis of the literature. *American Journal of Public Health, 83,* 1425–1428.

David, I. R., & Sageman, S. (1987). Psychological aspects of AIDS as seen in art therapy. *American Journal of Art Therapy, 26,* 3–10.

Davis, K. A., Cameron, B., & Stapleton, J. T. (1992). The impact of HIV patient migration to rural areas. *AIDS Patient Care, 6,* 225–228.

Dawson, J. M., Fitzpatrick, R. M., Reeves, G., Boulton, M., McLean, J., Hart, G. J., & Brookes, M. (1994). Awareness of sexual partners' HIV status as an influence upon high-risk sexual behaviour among gay men. *AIDS, 8,* 837–841.

Dax, E. M., Adler, W. H., Nagel, J. E., Lange, W. R., & Jaffe, J. H. (1991). Amyl nitrite alters human in vitro immune function. *Immunopharmacology and Immunotoxicology, 13*(4), 577–587.

Deicken, R. F., Hubesch, B., Jensen, P. C., Marinier, D. S., Krell, P., Wisniewski, A., Vanderburg, D., Parks, R., Fein, G., & Weiner, M. W. (1991). Alterations in brain phosphate metabolite concentrations in patients with human immunodeficiency virus infection. *Archives of Neurology, 48,* 203–209.

Derix, M. M. A., de Gans, J., Stam, J., & Portegies, P. (1990). Mental changes in patients with AIDS. *Clinical Neurology and Neurosurgery, 92,* 215–222.

Derogatis, L. R., Abeloff, M. D., & Melisaratos, N. (1979). Psychological coping mechanisms and survival time in metastatic breast cancer. *Journal of the American Medical Association, 242,* 1504–1508.

Derogatis, L. R., Morrow, G. R., Fetting, J., Penman, D., Piasetsky, S., Schmale, A. M., Henrichs, M., & Carnicke, C. L. M. (1983). The prevalence of psychiatric disorders among cancer patients. *Journal of the American Medical Association, 249,* 751–757.

Des Jarlais, D. C., Friedman, S. R., & Casriel, C. (1990). Target groups for preventing AIDS among intravenous drug users: 2. The "hard" data studies. *Journal of Consulting and Clinical Psychology, 58,* 50–56.

Des Jarlais, D. C., Friedman, S. R., & Stoneburner, R. L. (1988). HIV infection and intravenous drug use: Critical issues in the transmission dynamics, infection outcomes, and prevention. *Reviews of Infectious Diseases, 10,* 151–158.

Dew, M. A., Ragni, M. V., & Nimorwicz, P. (1990). Infection with human immunodeficiency virus and vulnerability to psychiatric distress. *Archives of General Psychiatry, 47,* 737–744.

Dew, M. A., Ragni, M. V., & Nimorwicz, P. (1991). Correlates of psychiatric distress among wives of hemophilic men with and without HIV infection. *American Journal of Psychiatry, 148,* 1016–1022.

Dhooper, S. S., Royse, D. D., & Tran, T. V. (1987–1988). Social work practitioners' attitudes towards AIDS victims. *The Journal of Applied Social Sciences, 12,* 109–123.

Dilley, J. W, Faltz, B., Macks, J., & Madover, S. (1986, April). Brief guide to office practice: Psychological complications of AIDS. *Medical Aspects of Human Sexuality,* 55–56.

Dilley, J. W., Ochitill, H., Perl, M., & Volberding, P. (1985). Findings in psychiatric consultations with patients with acquired immune deficiency syndrome. *American Journal of Psychiatry, 142,* 82–86.

Dilley, J. W., Shelp, E. E., & Batki, S. L. (1985, November). *Psychiatric and ethical issues in the care of patients with AIDS: An overview.* Paper presented at the annual meeting of American Academy of Psychosomatic Medicine, San Francisco, California.

Dimond, M. (1979). Social support and adaptation to chronic illness: The case of maintenance hemodialysis. *Research in Nursing and Health, 2,* 101–108.

DiPasquale, J. A. (1990). The psychological effects of support groups on individuals infected by the AIDS virus. *Cancer Nursing, 13,* 278–285.

Doll, L. S., & Kennedy, M. B. (in press). HIV counseling and testing: What is it and how well does it work? In G. Schochetman & J. R. George (Eds.), *AIDS Testing.* New York: Springer-Verlag.

Donegan, E., Stuart, M., Niland, J. C., Sacks, H., Azen, S., Dietrich, S., Faucett, C., Fletcher, M. A., Kleinman, S., Operskalski, E., Perkins, H, Pindyck, J., Schiff, E., Stites, D., Tomasulo, P., Mosely, J., & The Transfusion Study Group. (1990). Infection with human immunodeficency virus type-1 (HIV-I) among recipients of antibody-positive blood donations. *Annals of Internal Medicine, 113,* 733–739.

Donlou, J. N., Wolcott, D., Gottlieb, M., & Landsverk, J. (1985). Psychosocial aspects of AIDS and AIDS-related complex: A pilot study. *Journal of Psychosocial Oncology, 3*, 39–55.

Drebing, C. E., Van Gorp, W. G., Hinkin, C., Miller, E. N., Satz, P., Kim, D. S., Holston, S., & D'Elia, L. F. (1994). Confounding factors in the measurement of depression in HIV. *Journal of Personality Assessment, 62*, 68–83.

Drew, W. L., Buhles, W., & Erlich, K. S. (1992). Management of herpes virus infections (CMV, HSV, VZV). In M. A. Sande & P. A. Volberding (Eds.), *The medical management of AIDS* (3rd ed., pp. 359–382). Philadelphia: Saunders.

Duesberg, P. (1988). HIV is not the cause of AIDS. *Science, 241*, 514, 517.

Duesberg, P. H. (1989). Human immunodeficiency virus and acquired immunodeficiency syndrome: Correlation but not causation. *Proceedings of the National Academy of Science, 86*, 755–764.

Dunkel-Schetter, C., Feinstein, L. G., Taylor, S. E., & Falke, R. L. (1992). Patterns of coping with cancer. *Health Psychology, 11*, 79–87.

Dwyer, J., Wood, C., McNamara, J., & Kinder, B. (1987). Transplantation of thymic tissue into patients with AIDS. *Archives of Internal Medicine, 147*, 513–517.

D'Zurilla, T. J., & Goldfried, M. R. (1971). Problem solving and behavior modification. *Journal of Abnormal Psychology, 78*, 107–126.

Egan, V. (1992). Neuropsychological aspects of HIV infection. *AIDS Care, 4*, 3–10.

Egan, V., Brettle, R. P., & Goodwin, G. M. (1992). The Edinburgh cohort of HIV-positive drug users: Pattern of cognitive impairment in relation to progression of disease. *British Journal of Psychiatry, 161*, 522–531.

Egan, V. G., Chiswick, A., Brettle, R. P., & Goodwin, G. M. (1993). The Edinburgh cohort of HIV-positive drug users: The relationship between auditory P3 latency, cognitive function and self-rated mood. *Psychological Medicine, 23*, 1–10.

Eisler, R. M., Miller, P. M., & Hersen, M. (1973). Components of assertive behavior. *Journal of Clinical Psychology, 29*, 295–299.

Elford, J., Bor, R., & Summers, P. (1991). Research into HIV and AIDS between 1981 and 1990: The epidemic curve. *AIDS, 5*, 1515–1519.

Ellis, A. (1962). *Reason and emotion in psychotherapy.* New York: Lyle Stuart.

Emmot, S. (1991, June). *Cognitive group therapy for coping with HIV infection.* Paper presented at the VII International Conference on AIDS, Florence, Italy.

Empfield, M., Cournos, F., Meyer, I., Phil, M., McKinnon, H., Horworth, E., Silver, M., Schrage, H., & Herman, R. (1993). HIV seroprevalence among homeless patients admitted to a psychiatric inpatient unit. *American Journal of Psychiatry, 150*, 47–52.

Engel, G. L. (1980). The clinical application of the biopsychosocial model. *American Journal of Psychiatry, 137,* 535–544.

Ericksen, K. P., & Trocki, K. F. (1992). Behavioral risk factors for sexually transmitted diseases in American households. *Social Science Medicine, 34,* 843–853.

Esterling, B. A., Antoni, M. H., Schneiderman, N., Carver, C. S.,LaPerriere, A., Ironson, G., Klimas, N. G., & Fletcher, M. A. (1992). Psychosocial modulation of antibody to Epstein-Barr viral capsid antigen and human herpes virus type-6 in HIV-1 infected and at-risk gay men. *Psychosomatic Medicine, 54,* 354–371.

Esterling, B. A., Kiecolt–Glaser, J. K., Bodnar, J. C., & Glaser, R. (1994). Chronic stress, social support, and persistent alterations in the natural killer cell response to cytokines in older adults. *Health Psychology, 13,* 291–298.

Evans, R. L., & Northwood, L. K. (1983). Social support needs in adjustment to stroke. *Archives of Physical and Medical Rehabilitation, 64,* 61–64.

Fahey, J. L., Prince, H., Weaver, M., Groopman, J., Visscher, B., Schwartz, K., & Detels, R. (1984). Quantitative changes in T helper or T suppressor/cytotoxic lymphocyte subsets that distinguish acquired immune deficiency syndrome from other immune subset disorders. *The American Journal of Medicine, 76,* 95–100.

Farrer, L. (1986). Suicide and attempted suicide in Huntington disease: Implications for preclinical testing of persons at risk. *American Journal of Medical Genetics, 24,* 305–311.

Fauci, A. S. (1986). Current issues in developing a strategy for dealing with the acquired immunodeficieny syndrome. *Proceedings of the National Academy of Sciences, 83,* 9278–9283.

Fauci, A. S. (1988). The human immunodeficiency virus: Infectivity and mechanisms of pathogenesis. *Science, 239,* 617–622.

Fauci, A., & Dale, D. (1975). Alternate-day prednisone therapy and human lymphocyte subpopulations. *The Journal of Clinical Investigation, 55,* 22–32.

Fauci, A. S., Macher, A. M., Longo, D. L., Lane, H. C., Rook, A. H., Masur, H., & Gelmann, E. P. (1984). Acquired immunodeficiency syndrome: Epidemiologic, clinical, immunologic, and therapeutic considerations. *Annals of Internal Medicine, 100,* 92–106.

Faulstich, M. (1987). Psychiatric aspects of AIDS. *American Journal of Psychiatry, 144,* 551–555.

Feifel, H., Strack, S., & Nagy, V. T. (1987). Coping strategies and associated features of medically ill patients. *Psychosomatic Medicine, 49,* 616–625.

Feldblum, P. J., & Fortney, J. A. (1988). Condoms, spermicides and the transmission of human immunodeficieny virus. *Amercian Journal of Public Health, 78,* 52–54.

Felton, B. J., & Revenson, T. A. (1984). Coping with chronic illness: A study of illness controllability and the influence of coping strategies on psychological adjustment. *Journal of Consulting and Clinical Psychology, 52*, 343–353.

Filice, G. A., & Pomeroy, C. (1991). Preventing secondary infections among HIV-positive persons. *Public Health Reports, 106*, 503–517.

Fink, R., Shapiro, S., & Lewison, J. (1968). The reluctant participant in a breast cancer screening program. *Public Health Reports, 83*, 479–490.

Finley, J. L., Joshi, V. V., & Neill, J. S. A. (1992). General pathology of HIV infection. In G. P. Wormser (Ed.), *AIDS and other manifestations of HIV infection* (2nd ed.). New York: Raven Press.

Fischl, M. A. (1992). Treatment of HIV infection. In M. A. Sande & P. A. Volberding (Eds.), *The medical management of AIDS* (3rd ed., pp. 97–110). Philadelphia: Saunders.

Fischl, M. A. (1995). Treatment of HIV infection. In M. A. Sande & P. A. Volberding (Eds.), *The medical management of AIDS* (4th ed., pp. 141–160). Philadelphia: Saunders.

Fischl, M. A., Dickenson, G. M., Scott, G. B., Klimas, N., Fletcher, M. A., & Parks, W. (1987). Evaluation of heterosexual partners, children, and household contacts of adults with AIDS. *Journal of the Amercian Medical Association, 257*, 640–644.

Fischl, M. A., Richman, D. D., Grieco, M. H., Gottlieb, M. S., Volberding, P. A., Laskin, O., Leedom, J., Groopman, J., Mildvan, D., Schooley, R., Jackson, G., Durack, D., Phil, D., King, D., & AZT Collaborative Group. (1987). The efficacy of azidothymidine (AZT) in the treatment of patients with AIDS and AIDS-related complex. *New England Journal of Medicine, 317*, 185–191.

Fisher, A. G., Ensoli, B., Looney, D., Rose, A., Gallo, R., Saag, M., Shaw, G., Hahn, B., & Wong-Staal, F. (1988). Biologically diverse molecular variants within a single HIV-1 isolate. *Nature, 334*, 444–447.

Fisher, S. (1967). Motivation for patient delay. *Archives of General Psychiatry, 16*, 676–678.

Fleishman, J. A., & Fogel, B. (1994). Coping and depressive symptoms among people with AIDS. *Health Psychology, 13*, 156–169.

Flemming, D. W., Cochi, S. L., Steece, R. S., & Hull, H. F. (1987). Acquired immunodeficiency syndrome in low-incidence areas: How safe is unsafe sex? *Journal of the American Medical Association, 258*, 785–787.

Fogel, B. S., & Mor, V. (1993). Depressed mood and care preferences in patients with AIDS. *General Hospital Psychiatry, 15*, 203–207.

Folkman, S. (1994). *The San Francisco AIDS Bereavment and Coping Project update.* Paper presented at the meeting of NIMH prevention centers, New York.

Folkman, S., Chesney, M. A., Cooke, M., Boccellari, A., & Collette, L. (1994). Caregiver burden in HIV-positive and HIV-negative partners of men with AIDS. *Journal of Consulting and Clinical Psychology, 62,* 746–756.

Folkman, S., Chesney, M., Pollack, L., & Coates, T. (in press). Stress, control, coping, and depressive mood in HIV+ and HIV− gay men in San Francisco. *Journal of Nervous and Mental Disorders.*

Folkman, S., Chesney, M., Pollack, L., & Phillips, C. (1992). Stress, coping, and high-risk sexual behavior. *Health Psychology, 11,* 218–222.

Folkman, S., Lazarus, R., Dunkel-Schetter, C., DeLongis, A., & Gruen, R. (1986). Dynamics of a stressful encounter: Cognitive appraisal, coping, and encounter outcomes. *Journal of Personality and Social Psychology, 50,* 571–579.

Forstein, M. (1984). The psychosocial impact of the acquired immunodeficiency syndrome. *Seminars in Oncology, 11,* 77–83.

Fox, R., Odaka, N., Brookmeyer, R., & Polk, B. F. (1987). Effect of HIV antibody disclosure on subsequent sexual activity in homosexual men. *AIDS, 1,* 241–246.

Frankl, V.E. (1963). *Man's search for meaning.* New York: Pocket Books.

Friedland, G. H., Saltzman, B. R., Rogers, M. F., Kahl, P. A., Lesser, M. L., Mayers, M. M., & Klein, R. S. (1986). Lack of transmission of HTLV-III/LAV infection to household contacts of patients with AIDS or AIDS-related complex with oral candidasis. *New England Journal of Medicine, 314,* 344–349.

Friedman, Y., Franklin, C., Freels, S., & Weil, M. H. (1991). Long-term survival of patients with AIDS, *Pneumocystis* carinii pneumonia, and respiratory failure. *Journal of the American Medical Association, 266,* 89–92.

Frierson, R. L., & Lippmann, S. B. (1987). Psychologic implications of AIDS. *American Family Physician, 35,* 109–116.

Frierson, R. L., & Lippmann, S. B. (1988). Suicide and AIDS. *Psychosomatics, 29,* 226–231.

Frierson, R. L., Lippmann, S. B., & Johnson, J. (1987). AIDS: Psychological stresses on the family. *Psychosomatics, 28,* 65–68.

Frost, J. C., Makadon, H. J., Judd, D., Lee, S., O'Neill, S. F., & Paulsen, R. (1991). Care for caregivers: A support group for staff caring for AIDS patients in hospital-based primary care practice. *General Internal Medicine, 6,* 162–167.

Gallo, R.C. (1986). The first human retrovirus. *Scientific American, 255,* 88–98.

Gallo, R. C. (1987). The AIDS virus. *Scientific American, 256,* 46–56.

Gallo, R. C. (1988). HIV—the cause of AIDS: An overview on its biology, mechanisms of disease induction, and our attempts to control it. *Journal of Acquired Immune Deficiency Syndromes, 1,* 521–535.

Gallo, R. C. (1991). *Virus hunting AIDS, cancer, & the human retrovirus: A story of scientific discovery.* New York: Basic Books.

Gallo, R. C., & Montagnier, L. (1988). AIDS in 1988. *Scientific American, 259,* 41–48.

Gallop, R. M., Lancee, W. J., Taerk, G., Coates, R. A., & Fanning, M. (1992). Fear of contagion and AIDS: Nurses' perception of risk. *AIDS Care, 4,* 103–109.

Gallop, R. M., Lancee, W. J., Taerk, G., Coates, R. A., Fanning, M., & Keatings, M. (1991). The knowledge, attitudes and concerns of hospital staff about AIDS. *Canadian Journal of Public Health, 82,* 409–412.

Gallop, R. M., Taerk, G., Lancee, W. J., Coates, R. A., & Fanning, M. (1992). A randomized trial of group interventions for hospital staff caring for persons with AIDS. *AIDS Care, 4,* 177–185.

Gamble, R., & Getzel, G. S. (1989, March). Group work with gay men with AIDS. *Social Casework: The Journal of Contemporary Social Work,* pp. 172–179.

Garber, G. E., Cameron, D. W., Hawley–Foss, N., Greenway, D., & Shannon, M. E. (1991). The use of ozone-treated blood in the therapy of HIV infection and immune disease: A pilot study of safety and efficacy. *AIDS, 5,* 981–984.

Gardner, W., & Wilcox, B. (1993). Political intervention in scientific peer review: Research on adolescent sexual behavior. *Amercian Psychologist, 48,* 972–983.

Gayle, H. D., & D'Angelo, L. J. (1991). Epidemiology of acquired immunodeficiency syndrome and human immunodeficiency virus infection in adolescents. *Pediatric Infectious Disease Journal, 10,* 322–328.

Gellert, G. A., Page, B., Weismuller, P. C., & Ehling, L.R. (1993). Managing the non-compliant HIV-infected individual: Experiences from a local health department. *AIDS & Public Policy Journal, 8,* 20–26.

Gelman, D. (1993, November 29). A resistance to reason. *Newsweek,* p. 79.

George, J. M., Reed, T., Ballard, K., Colin, J., & Fielding, J. (1993). Contact with AIDS patients as a source of work-related distress: Effects of organizational and social support. *Academy of Management Journal, 36,* 157–171.

George, R. J. D. (1992). Coping with death anxiety—trying to make sense of it all? *AIDS, 6,* 1037–1038.

Gerberding, J. L. (1992). HIV transmission to providers and their patients. In M. A. Sande & P. A. Volberding (Eds.), *The medical management of AIDS* (3rd ed., pp. 54–64). Philadelphia: Saunders.

Gerberding, J. L., Littell, C., Brown, A., & Schecter, W. P. (1990). Risk of exposure of surgical personnel to patients' blood during surgery at San Francisco General Hospital. *Journal of the American Medical Association, 322,* 1788–1793.

Gerbert, B., Maguire, B. T., Bleecker, T., Coates, T. J., & McPhee, S. J. (1991). Primary care physicians and AIDS: Attitudinal and structural barriers to care. *Journal of the American Medical Association, 266,* 2837–2842.

Gerbert, B., Maguire, B. T., & Coates, T. J. (1990). Are patients talking to their physicians about AIDS? *American Journal of Public Health, 80,* 467–469.

Gerbert, B., Sumser, J., & Maguire, B. (1991). The impact of who you know and where you live on opinions about AIDS and health care. *Social Science and Medicine, 32,* 677–681.

Gilmore, N., Orkin, A. J., Duckett, M., & Grover, S. A. (1989). International travel and AIDS. *AIDS, 3*(Suppl. 1), S225–S230.

Ginzburg, H. M., & Gostin, L. (1986). Legal and ethical issues associated with HTLV-III diseases. *Psychiatric Annals, 16,* 180–185.

Giulian, D., Vaca, K., & Noonan, C. A. (1990). Secretion of neurotoxins by mononuclear phagocytes infected with HIV-1. *Science, 250,* 1593–1596.

Glaser, J. B., Strange, T. J., & Rosati, D. (1989). Heterosexual human immundeficiency virus transmission among the middle class. *Archives of Internal Medicine, 149,* 645–649.

Glaser, R., & Kiecolt-Glaser, J. (1987). Stress-associated depression in cellular immunity: Implications for acquired immune deficiency syndrome (AIDS). *Brain, Behavior and Immunity, 1,* 107–112.

Glaser, R., Kiecolt-Glaser, J., Speicher, C., & Holliday, J. (1985). Stress, loneliness, and changes in herpes virus latency. *Journal of Behavioral Medicine, 8,* 249–260.

Glasner, P. D., & Kaslow, R. A. (1990). The epidemiology of human immunodeficiency virus infection. *Journal of Consulting and Clinical Psychology, 58,* 13–21.

Glass, R. M. (1988). Editorial: AIDS and suicide. *Journal of the American Medical Association, 259,* 1369–1370.

Gochros, H. L. (1992). The sexuality of gay men with HIV infection. *Social Work, 37,* 105–109.

Goffman, E. (1963). *Stigma: Notes on the management of spoiled identity.* Englewood Cliffs, NJ: Prentice-Hall.

Golden, W. L., Gersh, W. D., & Robbins, D. M. (1992). *Psychological treatment of cancer patients: A cognitive–behavioral approach.* Needham Heights, MA: Allyn & Bacon.

Gollub, E. L., & Stein, Z. A. (1993). Commentary: The new female condom—Item 1 on a women's AIDS prevention agenda. *American Journal of Public Health, 83,* 498–500.

Golombok, S., Sketchley, J., & Rust, J. (1989). Condom failure among homosexual men. *Journal of Acquired Immune Deficiency Syndromes, 2,* 404–409.

Goodenow, C., Reisine, S. T., & Grady, K. E. (1990). Quality of social support and associated social and psychological functioning in women with rheumatoid arthritis. *Health Psychology, 9,* 266–284.

Goodkin, K., Blaney, N. T., Feaster, D., Fletcher, M. A., Baum, M. K., Atienza, E. M., Klimas, N. G., Millon, C., Szapocznik, J., & Eisdorfer, C. (1992). Active coping style is associated with natural killer cell cytotoxicity in asymptomatic HIV-1 seropositive homosexual men. *Journal of Psychosomatic Research, 36,* 635–650.

Gordon, J. H., Ulrich, C., Feeley, M., & Pollack, S. (1993). Staff distress among haemophilia nurses. *AIDS Care, 5,* 359–367.

Gorman, J. M. & Kertzner, R. (1990). Psychoneuroimmunology and HIV infection. *Journal of Neuropsychiatry, 2,* 241–252.

Gorman, J., Kertzner, R., Cooper, T., Goetz, R., Lagomasino, I., Novacenko, H., Williams, J., Stern, Y., Mayeux, R., & Ehrhardt, A. (1991). Glucocorticoid level and neuropsychiatric symptoms in homosexual men with HIV infection. *American Journal of Psychiatry, 148,* 41–45.

Gostin, L. O. (1989). Public health strategies for confronting AIDS: Legislative and regulatory policy in the United States. *Journal of the American Medical Association, 261,* 1621–1630.

Grace, W. C. (1994). HIV counseling research needs suggested by psychotherapy process and outcome studies. *Professional Psychology: Research and Practice, 25,* 403–409.

Grady, W. R., Klepinger, D. H., Billy, J. O., & Tanfer, K. (1993). Condom characteristics: The perspectives and preferences of men in the United States. *Family Planning Perspectives, 25,* 67–73.

Graham, N., Zeger, S., Park, L., Vermund, S., Detels, R., Rinaldo, C., & Phair, J. (1992). The effects on survival of early treatment of human immunodeficiency virus infection. *The New England Journal of Medicine, 326,* 1037–1042.

Grant, D. (1988). Support groups for youth with the AIDS virus. *International Journal of Group Psychotherapy, 38,* 237–251.

Grant, D., & Anns, M. (1988). Counseling AIDS antibody-positive clients: Reactions and treatment. *American Psychologist, 18,* 72–74.

Grant, I., Atkinson, J. H., Hesselink, J. R., Kennedy, C. J.,Richman, D. D., Spector, S. A., & McCutchan, J. A. (1987). Evidence for early central nervous system involvement in the acquired immunodefiency syndrome (AIDS) and other human immunodeficiency virus (HIV) infections. *Annals of Internal Medicine, 107,* 828–836.

Grant, I., & Heaton, R. K. (1990). Human immunodeficiency virus—type 1 (HIV-1) and the brain. *Journal of Consulting and Clinical Psychology, 58*, 22–30.

Grant, I., Olshen, R. A., Atkinson, H., Heatong, R. K., Nelson, J., McCutchan, J. A., & Weinrich, J. D. (1993). Depressed mood does not explain neuropsychological deficits in HIV-infected persons. *Neuropsychology, 7*, 53–61.

Green, G. (1993). Editorial review: Social support and HIV. *AIDS Care, 5*, 87–104.

Greenberg, A. E., Thomas, P., Landesman, S., Mildvan, D., Seidlin, M., Friedland, G., Holzman, R., Starrett, B., Braun, J., Bryan, E., & Evans, R. F. (1992). The spectrum of HIV-1-related disease among outpatients in New York City. *AIDS, 6*, 849–859.

Greenblatt, R. M., Hollander, H., McMaster, J. R., & Henke, C. J. (1991). Polypharmacy among patients attending an AIDS clinic: Utilization of prescribed, unorthodox, and investigational treatments. *Journal of Acquired Immune Deficiency Syndromes, 4*, 136–143.

Greenspan, J. S., & Greenspan, D. (1992). Oral lesions associated with HIV infection. In G. P. Wormser (Ed.), *AIDS and other manifestations of HIV infection* (2nd ed., pp. 489–498). New York: Raven Press.

Greenspan, J. S., Greenspan, D., & Winkler, J. (1992). Oral complications of HIV infection. In M. A. Sande & P. A. Volberding (Eds.), *The medical management of AIDS* (3rd ed., pp. 161–175). Philadelpia: Saunders.

Greenwood, D. U. (1991). Neuropsychological aspects of AIDS dementia complex: What clinicians need to know. *Professional Psychology: Research and Practice, 22*, 407–409.

Greer, S., Morris, T., & Pettingale, K. W. (1979). Psychological responses to breast cancer: Effect on outcome. *Lancet, 2*(8146), 785–787.

Greif, G .L., & Porembski, E. (1988). AIDS and significant others: Findings from a preliminary exploration of needs. *Health and Social Work, 13*, 259–265.

Griffiths, K., & Wilkins, E. G. L. (1993, June). *Patterns of coping with an HIV+ diagnosis: Psychological responses, threat appraisal, and stress mediation.* Paper presented at the IX International AIDS Conference, Berlin.

Grossman, A. H. (1991). Gay men and HIV/AIDS: Understanding the double stigma. *Journal of the Association of Nurses in AIDS Care, 2*, 28–32.

Grossman, A. H., & Silverstein, C. (1993). Facilitating support groups for professionals working with people with AIDS. *Social Work, 38*, 144–151.

Guccione, B. (1993, September). Interview with Peter Duesberg. *Spin*, pp. 95–108.

Gupta, S., Anderson, R., & May, R. (1989). Networks of sexual contacts: Implications for the pattern of spread of HIV. *AIDS, 3*, 807–817.

Gwinn, M., Pappaioanou, M., George, R., Hannon, H., Wasser, S. C., Redus, M. A., Hoff, R., Grady, G. F., Willoughby, A., Novello, A. C., Peterson, L. R., Dondero, T. J., & Curran, J. W. (1991). Prevalence of HIV infection in childbearing women in the United States. *Journal of the American Medical Association, 265,* 1704–1708.

Haas, J. S., Weissman, J. S., Cleary, P. D., Goldberg, J., Gatsonis, C., Seage, G. R., Fowler, F. J., Massagli, M. P., Makadon, H. J., & Epstein, A. M. (1993). Discussion of preferences for life-sustaining care by persons with AIDS. *Archives of International Medicine, 153,* 1241–1248.

Haburchak, D. R., Harrison, S. M., Miles, F. W., & Hannon, R. N. (1989). Resolving patient feelings of guilt: A need for physician–chaplain liaison. *AIDS Patient Care, 3,* 42–43.

Hackl, K., Kalichman, S. C., & Somlai, A. (1995, February). *Women with HIV/AIDS: The dual challenges of patient and primary caregiver.* Paper presented at the Conference on HIV Infection in Women, Washington, DC.

Halstead, S., Riccio, M., Harlow, P., Oretti, R., & Thompson, C. (1988). Psychosis associated with HIV infection. *British Journal of Psychiatry, 153,* 618–623.

Hamburg, M. A., Koenig, S., & Fauci, A.S. (1990). Immunology of AIDS and HIV infection. In G.L. Mandell, R. G. Douglas, & J. E. Bennett (Eds.). *Principles and practice of infectious diseases* (pp. 1046–1059). New York: Churchill Livingstone.

Haney, C. A. (1984). Psychosocial factors in the management of patients with cancer. In C. L. Cooper (Ed.), *Psychosocial Stress and Cancer* (pp. 201–227). Sommerset, NJ: Wiley.

Hankins, C. A., Gendron, S., Handley, M. A., Richard, C., Tung, M. T. L., & O'Shaughnessy, M. (1994). HIV infection among women in prison: An assessment of risk factors using a nonnominal methodology. *American Journal of Public Health, 84,* 1637–1640.

Hanson M., Kramer, T. H., Gross, W., Quintana, J., Li, P. W., & Asher, R. (1992). AIDS awareness and risk behaviors among dually disordered adults. *AIDS Education and Prevention, 4,* 1–51.

Hardy, A. (1991). Long-term survivor collaborative study group: Characterization of long-term survivors of AIDS. *Journal of Acquired Immune Deficiency Syndromes, 4,* 386–391.

Hardy, A., & Dawson, D. (1990). HIV antibody testing among adults in the United States: Data from 1988 NHIS. *American Journal of Public Health, 80,* 586–589.

Harker, J. O., Satz, P., Jones, F. D.-L., Verma, R. C., Gan, M. P., Mathisen, G., Poer,

H. L., Gould, B. D., & Chervinsky, A. (1993). *Measurement of depression and neuropsychological impairment in HIV-1 infection.* Manuscript submitted for publication.

Hart, G., Fitzpatrick, R., McLean, J., Dawson, J., & Boulton, M. (1990). Gay men, social support and HIV disease: A study of social integration in the gay community. *AIDS Care, 2,* 163–170.

Hartgers, C., Buning, E. C., van Santen, G. W., Verster, A. D., & Coutinho, R. A. (1989).The impact of the needle and syringe-exchange programme in Amsterdam on injecting risk behavior. *AIDS, 3,* 571–576.

Hatcher, R. A., Guest, F., Stewart, F., Stewart, G. K., Trussell, J., Bowen, S. C., & Cates, W. (1988). *Contraceptive technology 1988–1989* (14th rev. ed.). New York: Irvington.

Hawkins, C., Gold, J., Whimbey, E., Kiehn, T., Brannon, P., Cammarata, R., Brown, A., & Armstrong, D. (1986). *Mycobacterium avium* complex infections in patients with the acquired immunodeficiency syndrome. *Annals of Internal Medicine, 105,* 184–188.

Hays, R. B., Catania, J. A., McKusick, L., & Coates, T. J. (1990). Help-seeking for AIDS-related concerns: A comparison of gay men with various HIV diagnoses. *American Journal of Community Psychology, 18,* 743–755.

Hays, R. B., Chauncey, S., & Tobey, L. A. (1990). The social support networks of gay men with AIDS. *Journal of Community Psychology, 18,* 374–385.

Hays, R. B., Magee, R. H., & Chauncey, S. (1994). Identifying helpful and unhelpful behaviours of loved ones: The PWA's perspective. *AIDS Care, 6,* 379–392.

Hays, R. B., Turner, H., & Coates, T. J. (1992). Social support, AIDS-related symptoms, and depression among gay men. *Journal of Consulting and Clinical Psychology, 60,* 463–469.

Hedge, B., & Glover, L. F. (1990). Group intervention with HIV seropositive patients and their partners. *AIDS Care, 2,* 147–154.

Hein, K. (1990). Lessons from New York City on HIV/AIDS in adolescents. *New York State Journal of Medicine, 90,* 143–145.

Hellinger, F. (1990). Updated forecasts of the costs of medical care for persons with AIDS, 1989–93. *Public Health Reports, 105,* 1–12.

Hellinger, F. J. (1993). The lifetime cost of treating a person with HIV. *Journal of the American Medical Association, 270,* 474–478.

Henderson, D. K., Saah, A. J., Zak, B. J., Kaslow, R. A., Lane, H. C.,Folks, T., Blackwelder, W. C., Schmitt, J., LaCamera, D. J., Masur, H., & Fauci, A. S. (1986). Risk of nosocomial infection with human T-cell lymphocyte virus type-III/lymphadenopathy-associated virus in a large cohort of intensively exposed health caer workers. *Annals of Internal Medicine, 104,* 644–647.

Henry, K., Maki, M., & Crossley, K. (1988). Analysis of the use of HIV antibody testing in a Minnesota hospital. *Journal of the American Medical Association, 259,* 229–232.

Herbert, T. B., & Cohen, S. (1993). Depression and immunity: A meta-analytic review. *Psychological Bulletin, 113,* 472–486.

Herek, G. (1990). Illness, stigma, and AIDS. In G. M. Herek, S. M. Levy, S. Maddi, S. Taylor, & D. Wertlieb (Eds.), *Psychological aspects of chronic illness: Chronic conditions, fatal diseases, and clinical care* (pp. 7–60). Washington, DC: American Psychological Association.

Herek, G. M. & Capitanio, J. P. (1993). Public reactions to AIDS in the United States: A second decade of stigma. *American Journal of Public Health, 83,* 574–577.

Herek, G. M. & Glunt, E. K. (1988). An epidemic of stigma: Public reactions to AIDS. *American Psychologist, 43,* 886–891.

Herndier, B. G., Kaplan, L. D., & McGrath, M. S. (1994). Pathogenesis of AIDS lymphomas. *AIDS, 8,* 1025–1049.

Hinkin, C. H., van Gorp, W. G., Satz, P., Weisman, J. D., Thommes, J., & Buckingham, S. (1992). Depressed mood and its relationship to neuropsychological test performance in HIV-1 seropositive individuals. *Journal of Clinical and Experimental Neuropsychology, 14,* 289–297.

Hintz, S., Kuck, J., Peterkin, J. J., Volk, D. M., & Zisook, S. (1990). Depression in the context of human immunodeficiency virus infection: Implications for treatment. *Journal of Clinical Psychiatry, 51,* 497–501.

Hirsch, M. S., & D'Aquila, R. T. (1993). Therapy for human immunodeficiency virus infection. *New England Journal of Medicine, 328,* 1686–1695.

Hirsch, M., Schooley, R., Ho, D., & Kaplan, J. (1984). Possible viral interactions in the acquired immunodeficiency syndrome (AIDS). *Reviews of Infectious Diseases, 6,* 726–731.

Hirsch, M. S., Wormser, G. P., Schooley, R. T., Ho, D. D., Felsenstein, D., Hopkins, C. C., Joline, C., Duncanson, F., Sarngadharan, M. G., Saxinger, C., & Gallo, R. C. (1985). Risk of nosocomial infection with human T-cell lymphotropic virus III (HTLV-III). *New England Journal of Medicine, 312,* 1–4

Ho, D. D., Bredesen, D. E., Vinters, H. V., & Daar, E. S. (1989). The acquired immunodeficiency syndrome (AIDS) dementia complex. *Annals of Internal Medicine, 111,* 400–410.

Hoff, R., Berardi, V. P., Weiblen, B. J., Mahoney-Trout, L., Mitchell, M. L., & Grady,

G. F. (1988). Seroprevalence of human immunodeficiency virus among child-bearing women. *The New England Journal of Medicine, 318,* 525–530.

Hogg, R. S., Strathdee, S. A., Craib, K. J., O'Shaughnessy, M. V., Montaner, J. S., & Schechter, M. T. (1994). Lower socioeconomic status and shorter survival following HIV infection. *The Lancet, 344,* 1120–1124.

Holland, H. K., Saral, R., Rossi, J., Donnenberg, A., Burns, W., Beschorner, W., Farzadegan, H., Jones, R., Quinnan, G., Vogelsang, G., Vriesendorp, H., Wingard, J., Zaia, J., & Santos, G. (1989). Allogeneic bone marrow transplantation, zidovudine, and human immunodeficiency virus type 1 (HIV-1) infection. *Annals of Internal Medicine, 111,* 973–981.

Holland, J. (1982). Psychological aspects of cancer. In J. Holland & E. Frei (Eds.), *Cancer Medicine* (2nd ed., pp. 1175–1203). Philadelphia: Lea & Febiger.

Holland, J. C., & Tross, S. (1985). The psychosocial and neuropsychiatric sequelae of the acquired immunodeficiency syndrome and related disorders. *Annals of Internal Medicine, 103,* 760–764.

Hollerman, J. J., Bernstein, M. A., & Beute, G. H. (1987). Thoracic manifestations of AIDS. *American Family Practice, 35,* 109–118.

Hoover, D. R., Saah, A. J., Bagellar, H., Phair, J., Detels, R., Anderson, R., & Kaslow, R. A. (1993). Clinical manifestations of AIDS in the era of pneumocystis prophylaxis. *The New England Journal of Medicine, 329,* 1922–1926.

Hopewell, P. C. (1992). Pneumocystis Carinii pneumonia: Current concepts. In M. A. Sande & P. A. Volberding (Eds.), *The medical management of AIDS* (3rd ed., pp. 261–283). Philadelpia: Saunders.

Horsburgh, C. R. (1991). *Mycobacterium avium* complex infection in the acquired immunodeficiency syndrome. *The New England Journal of Medicine, 324,* 1332–1338.

Horstman, W. R., & McKusick, L. (1986). The impact of AIDS on the physician. In L. McKusick (Ed.), *What to do about AIDS: Physicians and mental health professionals discuss the issues* (pp. 63–74). Berkeley: University of California Press.

House, J. S., Landis, K. R., & Umberson, D. (1988). Social relationships and health. *Science, 241,* 540–545.

Howe, J. E., Minkoff, H. L., & Duerr, A. C. (1994). Contraceptives and HIV. *AIDS, 8,* 861–871.

Huggins, J., Elman, N., Baker, C., Forrester, R., & Lyter, D. (1991). Affective and behavioral responses of gay and bisexual men to HIV antibody testing. *Social Work, 36,* 61–66.

Humphry, D. (1991). *Final exit: The practicalities of self-deliverance and assisted suicide for dying patients*. Secaucus, NJ: Carol.

Hutchinson, C. M., Wilson, C., Reichart, C. A., Marsiglia, V. C., Zenilman, J. M., & Hook, E. W. (1991). CD4 lymphocyte concentrations in patients with newly identified HIV infection attending STD clinics: Potential impact on policy funded health care resources. *Journal of the American Medical Association, 266,* 253–256.

Ickovics, J. R., Morrill, A. C., Beren, S. E., Walsh, U., & Rodin, J. (1994). Limited effects of HIV counseling and testing for women: A prospective study of behavioral and psychological consequences. *Journal of the American Medical Association, 272,* 443–448.

Ickovics, J. R., & Rodin, J. (1992). Women and AIDS in the United States: Epidemiology, natural history, and mediating mechanisms. *Health Psychology, 11,* 1–16.

Imagawa, D. T., Lee., M., Wolinsky, S., Sano, K., Morales, F., & Kwok, S. (1989). Human immunodeficiency virus type 1 infection in homosexual men who remain seronegative for prolonged periods. *New England Journal of Medicine, 320,* 1458–1462.

Imam, N., Carpenter, C. C. J., Mayer, K. H., Fisher, A., Stein, M., & Dansforth, S. B. (1990). Hierarchical pattern of mucosal candida infections in HIV-seropositive women. *American Journal of Medicine, 89,* 142–146.

Imperato, P. J., Feldman, J. G., Nayeri, K., & DeHovitz, J. A. (1988). Medical students' attitudes towards caring for patients with AIDS in a high incidence area. *New York State Journal of Medicine, 88,* 223–227.

Ironson, G., LaPerriere, A., Antoni, M., O'Hearn, P., Schneiderman, N., Klimas, N., & Fletcher, M. (1990). Changes in immune and psychological measures as a function of anticipation and reaction to news of HIV-1 antibody status. *Psychosomatic Medicine, 52,* 247–270.

Israel, B. A., & Antonucci, T. C. (1987). Social network characteristics and psychological well-being: A replication and extension. *Health Education Quarterly, 14,* 461–481.

Israelski, D. M., & Remington, J. S. (1992). AIDS-associated Toxoplasmosis. In M. A. Sande & P. A. Volberding (Eds.), *The medical management of AIDS* (3rd ed., pp. 319–345). Philadelpia: Saunders.

Jackson, G., Perkins, J., Rubenis, M., Paul, D., Knigge, M., Despotes, J., & Spencer, P. (1988). Passive immunoneutralisation of human immunodeficiency virus in patients with advanced AIDS. *Lancet, 8612,* 647–652.

Jacobsen, P., Perry, S., & Hirsch, D. A. (1990). Behavioral and psychological responses to HIV antibody testing. *Journal of Consulting and Clinical Psychology, 58*, 31–37.

Jacobson, M. (1992). Mycobacterial diseases: Tuberculosis and disseminated Mycobacterial avium complex infection. In M.A. Sande & P. A. Volberding (Eds.), *The medical management of AIDS* (3rd ed., pp. 284–296). Philadelpia: Saunders.

Jacobson, M. A., Bacchetti, P., Kolokathis, A., Chaisson, R. E., Szabo, S., Polsky, B., Valainis, G. T., Mildvan, D., Abrams, D., Wilber, J., Winger, E., Sacks, H. S., Hendrickson, C., & Moss, A. (1991). Surrogate markers for survival in patients with AIDS and AIDS related complex treated with zidovudine. *British Medical Journal, 302*, 73–78.

Jacobson, M., Hopewell, P., Yajko, D., Hadley, W. K., Lazarus, E., Mohanty, P., Modin, G., Feigal, D., Cusick, P., & Sande, M. (1991). Natural history of disseminated mycobacterium avium complex infection in AIDS. *The Journal of Infectious Diseases, 164*, 994–998.

James, J. S. (1994). *AIDS treatment news: Vol. 3. Issues 126–189.* Boston, MA: Alyson.

Janssen, R. S., Cornblath, D. R., Epstein, L. G., Foa, R. P., McArthur, J. C., & Price, R. W. (1991). Nomenclature and research case definitions for neurologic manifestations of human immunodeficiency virus—type 1 (HIV-1) infection. *Neurology, 41*, 778–785.

Jemmott, J., & Locke, S. (1984). Psychosocial factors, immunologic mediation, and human susceptibility to infectious diseases: How much do we know? *Psychological Bulletin, 95*, 78–108.

Jenike, M. A. & Pato, C. (1986). Case report: Disabling fear of AIDS responsive to imipramine. *Psychosomatics, 27*, 143–144.

Jenkins, R. A., & Pargament, K. I. (1988). Cognitive appraisals in cancer patients. *Social Science and Medicine, 26*, 625–633.

Jensen, P. S. (1983). Risk, protective factors, and supportive interventions in chronic airway obstruction. *Archives of General Psychiatry, 40*, 1203–1207.

Jillson-Boostrom, I. (1992). The impact of HIV on minority populations. In P. I. Ahmed & N. Ahmed (Eds.), *Living and dying with AIDS* (pp. 235–254). New York: Plenum Press.

Johnson, J. P., Nair, P., Hines, S. E., Seiden, S. W., Alger, L., Revie, D. R., O'Neil, K. M., & Hebel, R. (1989). Natural history and serologic diagnosis of infants born to human immunodeficiency virus-infected women. *American Journal of Diseases of Children, 143*, 1147–1153.

Joseph, J. G. Caumartin, S., Tal, M., Kirscht, J., Kessler, R., Ostrow, D., & Wortman,

C. (1990). Psychological functioning in a cohort of gay men at risk for AIDS. *Journal of Nervous and Mental Disease, 178*, 607–615.

Joseph, J., Montgomery, S., Emmons, C., Kirscht, J., Kessler, R., Ostrow, D., Wortman, C., O'Brien, K., Eller, M., & Eshleman, S. (1987). Perceived risk of AIDS: Assessing the behavioral and psychosocial consequences in a cohort of gay men. *Journal of Applied Social Psychology, 17*, 231–250.

Kalichman, S. C. (1994). Magic Johnson and public attitudes towards AIDS: A review of empirical findings. *AIDS Education and Prevention, 6*, 542–557.

Kalichman, S. C. (1995). *Coping and support needs among persons with HIV infection: An exploratory study.* Unpublished manuscript.

Kalichman. S. C., Adair, V., Somlai, A., & Weir, S. (in press). The perceived social context of AIDS: Study of inner-city sexually transmitted disease clinic patients. *AIDS Education and Prevention.*

Kalichman, S. C., & Hunter, T. (1993). AIDS-related risk and HIV antibody testing: An urban community survey. *AIDS Education and Prevention, 5*, 234–243.

Kalichman, S. C., Hunter, T. L., & Kelly, J. A. (1992). Perceptions of AIDS risk susceptibility among minority and nonminority women at risk for HIV infection. *Journal of Consulting and Clinical Psychology, 60*, 725–732.

Kalichman, S. C., Kelly, J. A., Johnson, J., & Bulto, M. (1994). Factors associated with risk for human immunodeficiency virus (HIV) infection among chronic mentally ill adults. *American Journal of Psychiatry, 151*, 221–227.

Kalichman. S. C., Somlai, A., Adair, V., & Weir, S. (in press). Psychological and social factors associated with HIV testing among sexually transmitted disease clinic patients. *Psychology and Health.*

Kalichman, S. C., & Sikkema, K. J. (1994). Psychological sequelae of HIV infection and AIDS: Review of empirical findings. *Clinical Psychology Review, 14*, 611–632.

Kalichman, S. C., Sikkema, K., & Somlai, A. (1995). Assessing persons with human immunodeficiency virus (HIV) infection using the Beck Depression Inventory: Disease processes and other potential confounds. *Journal of Personality Assessment, 64*, 86–100.

Kalish, R. A. (Ed.). (1985). *Death, grief, and caring relationships* (2nd. ed.). Monterey, CA: Books/Cole.

Kandel, E. R., Schwartz, J. H., & Jessell, T. M. (1991). *Principles of neural science* (3rd ed.). Norwalk, CT: Appelton & Lange.

Kane, S. (1991). HIV, heroin and heterosexual relations. *Social Science Medicine, 9*, 1037–1050.

Kaplan, E. H., Khoshnood, K., & Heimer, R. (1994). A decline in HIV-infected needles returned to New Haven's needle exchange program: Client shift or needle exchange? *American Journal of Public Health, 84,* 1991–1994.

Kaplan, L. D., & Northfelt, D. W. (1992). Malignancies associated with AIDS. In M. A. Sande & P. A. Volberding (Eds.), *The medical management of AIDS* (3rd ed., pp. 399–429). Philadelphia: W. B. Saunders.

Kappel, S., Vogt, R. L., Brozicevic, M., & Kutzko, D. (1989). AIDS knowledge and attitudes among adults in Vermont. *Public Health Reports, 104,* 388–391.

Karasu, T. B., Docherty, J. P., Gelenberg, A., Kupfer, D. J., Merriam, A. E., & Shadoan, R. (1993). Practice guideline for major depressive disorder in adults. *American Journal of Psychiatry, 150*[S], 1–26.

Karon, J. M., Dondero, T. J., & Curran, J. W. (1988). The projected incidence of AIDS and estimated prevalence of HIV infection in the United States. *Journal of Acquired Immune Deficiency Syndromes, 1,* 542–550.

Kaslow, R. A., Blackwelder, W. C., Ostrow, D. G., Yerg, D., Palenicek, J., Coulson, A. H., & Valdiserri, R. O. (1989). No evidence for a role of alcohol or other psychoactive drugs in accelerating immunodeficiency in HIV-1-positive individuals: A report from the multicenter AIDS cohort study. *Journal of the American Medical Association, 261,* 3424–3429.

Kaslow, R., Ostrow, D., Detels, R., Phair, J., Polk, B. F., & Rinaldo, C. (1987). The multicenter AIDS cohort study: Rationale, organization, and selected characteristics of the participants. *American Journal of Epidemiology, 126,* 310–318.

Kaslow, R. A., Phair, J. P., Friedman, H. B., Lyter, D., Solomon, R. E., Dudley, J., Polk, F., & Blackwelder, W. (1987). Infection with the human immunodeficiency virus: Clinical manifestations and their relationship to immune deficiency. *Annals of Internal Medicine, 107,* 474–480.

Keet, I. P. M., van Lent, N.A., Sandfort, T. G. M., Coutinho, R. A., & van Griensven, J. P. (1992). Orogenital sex and transmission of HIV among homosexual men. *AIDS, 6,* 223–226.

Kegeles, S. M., Coates, T. J., Christopher, T. A., & Lazarus, J. L. (1989). Perceptions of AIDS: The continuing saga of AIDS-related stigma. *AIDS, 3*(Suppl.), S253–S258.

Kegeles, S. M., Coates, T. J., Lo, B., & Catania, J. A. (1989). Mandatory reporting of HIV testing would deter men from being tested. *Journal of the American Medical Association, 261,* 1275–1276.

Kelly, J. A. (1982). *Social skills training: A practical guide for interventions.* New York: Springer.

Kelly, J. A. (1989). Helping patients cope with AIDS and other HIV conditions. *Comprehensive Therapy, 15,* 56–62.

Kelly, J. A. (1991). Changing the behavior of an HIV-seropositive man who practices unsafe sex. *Hospital and Community Psychiatry, 42*, 239–240, 264.

Kelly, J. A. (1992). Psychosocial aspects of AIDS. *Current Opinion in Psychiatry, 5*, 820–824.

Kelly, J. A. (in press). *Helping people change HIV/AIDS risk behavior: Practical strategies for risk reduction counseling.* New York: Guilford Press.

Kelly, J. A., & Kalichman, S. C. (1995). *Increased attention to human sexuality can improve HIV/AIDS prevention efforts: Key research issues and directions.* Manuscript submitted for publication.

Kelly, J. A., Murphy, D. A., Bahr, G. R., Kalichman, S. C., Morgan, M. G., Stevenson, L. Y., Koob, J. J., Brasfield, T. L., & Bernstein, B. M. (1993). Outcome of cognitive–behavioral and support group brief therapies for depressed, HIV-infected persons. *American Journal of Psychiatry, 150*, 1679–1686.

Kelly, J. A., Murphy, D. A., Bahr, G. R., Koob, J., Morgan, M., Kalichman, S. C., Stevenson, L. Y., Brasfield, T. L.,Bernstein, B., & St. Lawrence, J. (1993). Factors associated with severity of depression and high-risk sexual behavior among persons diagnosed with human immunodeficiency virus (HIV) infection. *Health Psychology, 12*, 215–219.

Kelly, J. A., Murphy, D. A., Roffman, R. A., Solomon, L. J., Winnett, R. A., Stevenson, L. Y., Koob, J., Ayotte, D., Flynn, B., Desiderato, L., Hauth, A., Lemke, A., Lombard, D., Morgan, M., Norman, A., Sikkema, K., Steiner, S., & Yaffe, D. (1992). Acquired immunodeficiency syndrome/human immunodeficiency virus risk behavior among gay men in small cities. *Archives of Internal Medicine, 152*, 2293–2297.

Kelly, J. A., Murphy, D., Sikkema, K., & Kalichman, S. (1993). Psychological interventions are urgently needed to prevent HIV infection: New priorities for behavioral research in the second decade of AIDS. *American Psychologist, 48*, 1023–1034.

Kelly, J. A., St. Lawrence, J. S., Smith, S., Hood, H. V., & Cook, D. J. (1987a). Medical students' attitudes toward AIDS and homosexual patients. *Journal of Medical Education, 62*, 549–556.

Kelly, J. A., St. Lawrence, J. S., Smith, S., Hood, H. V., & Cook, D. J. (1987b). Stigmatization of AIDS patients by physicians. *American Journal of Public Health, 77*, 789–791.

Kelly, J., & Sykes, P. (1989, May). Helping the helpers: A support group for family members of persons with AIDS. *Social Work*, pp. 239–242.

Kemeny, M. E. (1991). Psychological factors, immune processes, and the course of herpes simplex and human immunodeficiency virus infection. In N. Plotnikoff,

A. Murgo, R. Faith, & J. Wybran (Eds.), *Stress and immunity* (pp. 199–210). Boca Raton, FL: CRC Press.

Kemeny, M. E. (in press). Stressful events, psychological responses and progression of HIV infection. In R. Glaser & J. Kiecolt-Glaser (Eds.), *Handbook on stress and immunity*. New York: Academic Press.

Kemeny, M. E., Cohen, F., Zegans, L. S., & Conant, M. A. (1989). Psychological and immunological predictors of genital herpes recurrence. *Psychosomatic Medicine, 51*, 195–208.

Kemeny, M. E., Weiner, H., Taylor, S. E., Schneider, S., Visscher, B., & Fahey, J. L. (1994). Repeated bereavement, depressed mood, and immune parameters in HIV seropositive and seronegative gay men. *Health Psychology, 13*, 14–24.

Kermani, E. J., & Weiss, B. A. (1989). AIDS and confidentiality: Legal concept and its application in psychotherapy. *American Journal of Psychotherapy, 43*, 25–31.

Kertzner, R. M., Goetz, R., Todak, G., Cooper, T., Lin, S., Reddy, M., Novacenko, H., Williams, J., Ehrhardt, A., & Gorman, J. (1993). Cortisol levels, immune status and mood in homosexual men with and without HIV infection. *American Journal of Psychiatry, 150*, 1674–1678.

Kessler, R. C., Foster, C., Joseph, J., Ostrow, D., Wortman, C., Phair, J., & Chmiel, J. (1991). Stressful life events and symptom onset in HIV infection. *American Journal of Psychiatry, 148*, 733–738.

Kessler, R. C., O'Brien, K., Joseph, J. G., Ostrow, D. G., Phair, J. P., Chmiel, J. S., Wortman, C. B., & Emmons, C. A. (1988). Effects of HIV infection, perceived health and clinical status on a cohort at risk for AIDS. *Society of Science and Medicine, 27*, 569–578.

Kessler, S. (1987). Psychiatric implications of presymptomatic testing for Huntington's disease. *American Journal of Orthopsychiatry, 57*, 212–219.

Kessler, S., Field, T., Worth, L., & Mosbarger, H. (1987). Attitudes of persons at risk for Huntington disease toward predictive testing. *American Journal of Medical Genetics, 26*, 259–270.

Kiecolt-Glaser, J., Fisher, L., Ogrocki, P., Stout, J., Speicher, C., & Glaser, R. (1987). Marital quality, marital disruption, and immune function. *Psychosomatic Medicine, 49*, 13–34.

Kiecolt-Glaser, J., Garner, W., Speicher, C., Penn, G., Holliday, J., & Glaser, R. (1984). Psychosocial modifiers of immunocompetence in medical students. *Psychosomatic Medicine, 46*, 7–14.

Kiecolt-Glaser, J., & Glaser, R. (1988a). Psychological influences on immunity. *American Psychologist, 43*, 892–898.

Kiecolt-Glaser, J., & Glaser, R. (1988b). Major life changes, chronic stress, and immunity. In T. P. Bridge (Ed.), *Psychological, neuropsychiatric, and substance abuse aspects of AIDS* (pp. 217–224). New York: Raven Press.

Kiecolt-Glaser, J., Glaser, R., Shuttleworth, E., Dyer, C., Ogrocki, P., & Speicher, C. (1987). Chronic stress and immunity in family caregivers of Alzheimer's disease victims. *Psychosomatic Medicine, 49*, 523–535.

Kiecolt-Glaser, J., Kennedy, S., Malkoff, S., Fisher, L., Speicher, C., & Glaser, R. (1988). Marital discord and immunity in males. *Psychosomatic Medicine, 50*, 213–229.

Killeen, M. E. (1993, September–October). Getting through our grief: For caregivers of persons with AIDS. *The American Journal of Hospice & Palliative Care*, pp. 18–24.

Kinderman, S. S., Matteo, T. M., & Morales, E. (1993). HIV training and perceived competence among doctoral students in psychology. *Professional Psychology: Research and Practice, 24*, 224–227.

Kingsley, L. A., Detels, R., Kaslow, R., Polk, B. F., Rinaldo, C. R., & Chmiel, J. (1987). Risk factors for seroconversion to human immunodeficiency virus among male homosexuals. *Lancet, 1*(8529), 345–349.

Kirby, M. (1988). AIDS—legal issues. *AIDS, 2*(Suppl. 1), S209–S215.

Kishlansky, M., Geary, P., & O'Brien, P. (1991). *Civilization in the West.* New York: Harper-Collins.

Kizer, K. W., Green, M., Perkins, C. I., Doebbert, G., & Hughes, M. J. (1988). AIDS and suicide in California. *Journal of the American Medical Association, 260*, 1881.

Kleck, R. E. (1968). Self-disclosure patterns of the nonobviously stigmatized. *Psychological Reports, 23*, 1239–1248.

Kleinman, A. (1988). *The illness narratives: Suffering, healing and the human condition.* New York: Basic Books.

Kleinman, I. (1991). HIV transmission: Ethical and legal considerations in psychotherapy. *Cancer Journal of Psychiatry, 36*, 121–123.

Kloser, P., & Craig, J. (1994). *The woman's HIV sourcebook: A guide to better health and well-being.* Dallas, TX: Taylor.

Knapp, S., & VandeCreek, L. (1990). Application of the duty to protect to HIV-positive patients. *Professional Psychology: Research and Practice, 21*, 161–166.

Knox, M. D., & Dow, M. G. (1989). Staff discomfort in working with HIV spectrum patients. *International Conference on AIDS, 5*, 720. (Abstract No. M.C.P. 60)

Koenig, H. G., Meador, K. G., Cohen, H., & Blazer, D. (1988). Depression in elderly hospitalized patients with medical illness. *Archives of Internal Medicine, 148*, 1929–1936.

Kokkevi, A., Hatzakis, G., Maillis, A., Pittadaki, J., Zalonis, J., Samartzis, D., Touloumi, G., Mandalaki, T., & Stefanis, C. (1991). Neuropsychological assessment of HIV-seropositive haemophiliacs. *AIDS, 5,* 1223–1229.

Koppel, B. S. (1992). Neurological complications of AIDS and HIV infection. In G. P. Wormser (Ed.), *AIDS and other manifestations of HIV infection* (2nd ed., pp. 315–348). New York: Raven Press.

Krikorian, R., & Worbel, A. J. (1991). Cognitive impairment in HIV infection. *AIDS, 5,* 1501–1507.

Krupp, L., Belman, A., & Schneidman, P. (1992). Progressive multifocal leukoencephalopathy and HIV-1 infection. In G. P. Wormser (Ed.), *AIDS and other manifestations of HIV infection* (2nd ed., pp. 3409–418). New York: Raven Press.

Kubler-Ross, E. (1969). *On death and dying.* New York: MacMillan.

Kubler-Ross, E. (1975). *Death: The final stage of growth.* Englewood Cliffs, NJ: Prentice-Hall.

Kubler-Ross, E. (1981). *Living with death and dying.* New York: MacMillan.

Kurdek, L. A. (1988). Perceived social support in gays and lesbians in cohabitating relationships. *Journal of Personality and Social Psychology, 54,* 504–509.

Kurdek, L. A., & Siesky, G. (1990). The nature and correlates of psychological adjustment in gay men with AIDS-related conditions. *Journal of Applied Social Psychology, 20,* 846–860.

Lagakos, S., Fischl, M. A., Stein, D. S., Lim, L., & Volberding, P. (1991). Effects of zidovudine therapy in minority and other subpopulations with early HIV infection. *Journal of the American Medical Association, 266,* 2709–2712.

Lakey, B., & Cassady, P. B. (1990). Cognitive processes in perceived social support. *Journal of Personality and Social Psychology, 59,* 337–343.

Lamping, D. L., Abrahamowicz, M., Gilmore, N., Edgar, L., Grover, S. A., Tsoukas, C., Falutz, J., Lalonde, R., Hamel, M., & Darsigny, R. (1993, June). *A randomized, controlled trial to evaluate a psychosocial intervention to improve quality of life in HIV infection.* Paper presented at the IX International Conference on AIDS, Berlin.

Land, H., & Harangody, G. (1990, October). A support group for partners of persons with AIDS. *Families in Society: The Journal of Contemporary Human Services,* pp. 471–481.

Landau-Stanton, J., Clements, C. D., & Stanton, M. D. (1993). Psychotherapeutic intervention: From individual through group to extended network. In J. Landau-Stanton & C. D. Clements (Eds.), *AIDS, health, and mental health: A primary sourcebook* (pp. 214–266). New York: Brunner/Mazel.

Lane, H. C. (1994). Interferons in HIV and related diseases. *AIDS, 8*(Suppl. 3), S19–S23.

LaPerriere, A. R., Antoni, M. H., Schneiderman, N., Ironson, G., Klimas, N., Caralis, P., & Fletcher, M. A. (1990). Exercise intervention attenuates emotional distress and natural killer cell decrements following notification of positive serologic status for HIV-1. *Biofeedback and Self-Regulation, 15,* 229–242.

LaPerriere, A., Schneiderman, N., Antoni, M., & Fletcher, M. (1990). Aerobic exercise and psychoneuroimmunology in AIDS research. In L. Temoshok & A. Baum (Eds.), *Psychological perspectives on AIDS: Etiology, prevention, and treatment* (pp. 259–286). Hillsdale, NJ: Erlbaum.

Latif, A. S., Katzenstein, D. A., Bassett, M. T., Houston, S., Emmanuel, J. C., & Marowa, E. (1989). Genital ulcers and transmission of HIV among couples in Zimbabwe. *AIDS, 3,* 519–523.

Laurence, J. (1992). Viral cofactors in the pathogenesis of HIV disease. In G. P. Wormser (Ed.), *AIDS and other manifestations of HIV infection* (2nd ed.). New York: Raven Press.

Lazarus, R. S., & Folkman, S. (1984). *Stress, appraisal, and coping.* New York: Springer.

LeBlanc, A. J. (1993). Examining HIV-related knowledge among adults in the U.S. *Journal of Health and Social Behavior, 34,* 23–36.

Lemp, G. F., Hirozawa, A. M., Givertz, D., Nieri, G. N., Anderson, L., Lindegren, M. L., & Janssen, R. S. (1994). Seroprevalence of HIV and risk behaviors among young homosexual and bisexual men. *Journal of the American Medical Association, 272,* 449–454.

Lemp, G. F., Payne, S. F., Neal, D., Temelso, T., & Rutherford, G. W. (1990). Survival trends for patients with AIDS. *Journal of the American Medical Association, 263,* 402–406.

Lennon, M. C., Martin, J. L., & Dean, L. (1990). The influence of social support on AIDS-related grief reaction among gay men. *Social Science and Medicine, 31,* 477–484.

Leonard, A. S. (1985). Employment discrimination against persons with AIDS. *University of Dayton Law Review, 10,* 681–703.

Leserman, J., Perkins, D., & Evans, D. (1992). Coping with the threat of AIDS: The role of social support. *American Journal of Psychiatry, 149.* 1514–1520.

Levenson, J. L. (1989). Treatable causes of CNS dysfunction in AIDS patients. *Journal of Clinical Psychiatry, 50,* 147–148.

Levine, A., Gill, P., & Salahuddin, S. (1992). Neoplastic complications of HIV infection. In G. P. Wormser (Ed.), *AIDS and other manifestations of HIV infection* (2nd ed., pp. 443–454). New York: Raven Press.

Levine, S. H., Bystritsky, A., Baron, D., & Jones, L. D. (1991). Group psychotherapy for HIV-seropositive patients with major depression. *American Journal of Psychotherapy, 45*, 413–424.

Levy, J. A. (1992). Viral and immunolgic factors in HIV infection. In M. A. Sande & P. A. Volberding (Eds.), *The medical management of AIDS* (3rd ed., pp. 18–32). Philadelphia: Saunders.

Levy, J. A., Kaminsky, R. M., & Bredesen, D. E. (1988). Central nervous system dysfunction in acquired immunodeficiency syndrome. *Journal of Acquired Immune Deficiency Syndromes, 1*, 41–64.

Levy, J. A., Kaminsky, L. S., Morrow, W. J., Steimer, K., Luciw, P., Dina, D., Hoxie, J., & Oshiro, L. (1985). Infection by the retrovirus associated with the acquired immunodeficiency syndrome: Clinical, biological, and molecular features. *Annals of Internal Medicine, 103*, 694–699.

Levy, J. A., Shimabukuro, J., Hollander, H., Mills, J., & Kaminsky, L. (1985). Isolation of AIDS-associated retroviruses from cerebrospinal fluid and brain of patients with neurological symptoms. *Lancet, 2*, 586–588.

Levy, R. M., & Bredesen, D. E. (1988). Central nervous system dysfunction in acquired immunodeficiency syndrome. *Journal of Acquired Immune Deficiency Syndromes, 1*, 41–64.

Lifson, A. R. (1988). Do alternative modes of transmission of human immunodeficiency virus exist? *Journal of the American Medical Association, 259*, 1353–1356.

Lifson, A. R., Hessol, N.A., Buchbinder, S. P., & Holmberg, S. D. (1991). The association of clinical conditions and serological tests with CD4+ lymphocyte counts in HIV-infected subjects without AIDS. *AIDS, 5*, 1209–1215.

Lindsay, M. K., Peterson, H. B., Boring, J., Gramling, J., Willis, S., & Klein, L. (1992). Crack cocaine: A risk factor for human immunodeficiency virus infection type 1 among inner-city patients. *Obstetrics & Gynecology, 80*, 981–984.

Linn, J. G., Lewis, F. M., Cain, V. A., & Kimbrough, G. A. (1993). HIV-illness, social support, sense of coherence, and psychosocial well-being in a sample of help-seeking adults. *AIDS Education and Prevention, 5*, 254–262.

Lipowski, Z. J. (1988). Somatization: The concept and its clinical application. *American Journal of Psychiatry, 145*, 1358–1368.

Lipsitz, J. D., Williams, J., Rabkin, J., Remien, R., Bradbury, M., Sadr, W., Goetz, R., Sorrell, S., & Gorman, J. (1994). Psychopathology in male and female intravenous drug users with and without HIV infection. *American Journal of Psychiatry, 151*, 1662–1668.

Littlefield, C. H., Rodin, G. M., Murray, M. A., & Craven, J. L. (1990). Influence of functional impairment and social support on depressive symptoms in persons with diabetes. *Health Psychology, 9,* 737–749.

Loftus, R., & Gold, D. (1995). Protease inhibitors: Where are they now? *GMHC Treatment Issues, 9*(1), 1–5. (Available from the Gay Men s Health Crisis, New York City)

Longo, M., Spross, J., & Locke, A. (1990). Identifying major concerns of persons with acquired immunodeficiency syndrome: A replication. *Clinical Nurse Specialist, 4,* 21–26.

Lui, K. J., Darrow, W. W., & Rutherford, G. W. (1988). A model-based estimate of the mean incubation period for AIDS in homosexual men. *Science, 240,* 1333–1335.

Lundgren, J. D., Phillips, A. N., Pedersen, C., Clumeck, N., Gatell, J. M., Johnson, A. M., Ledergerber, B., Vella, S., Nielsen, J. O., & The AIDS in Europe Study Group. (1994). Comparison of long-term prognosis of patients with AIDS treated and not treated with zidovudine. *Journal of the American Medical Association, 271,* 1088–1092.

Lyketsos, C., Hanson, A., Fishman, M., Rosenblatt, A., McHugh, P., & Treisman, G. (1993). Manic syndrome early and late in the course of HIV. *American Journal of Psychiatry, 150,* 326–327.

Lyketsos, C. C. G., Hoover, D., Guccione, M., Senterfitt, W., Dew, A., Wesch, J., Van-Raden, M., Treisman, G., & Morgenstern, H. (1993). Depressive symptoms as predictors of medical outcomes in HIV infection. *Journal of the American Medical Association, 270,* 2563–2567.

Lyter, D., Valdiserri, R., Kingsley, L., Amoroso, W., & Rinaldo, C. (1987). The HIV antibody test: Why gay and bisexual men want or do not want to know their results. *Public Health Reports, 102,* 468–474.

MacDonell, K. B., Chmiel, J. S., Poggensee, L., Wu, S., & Phair, J. P. (1990). Predicting progression of AIDS: Combined usefulness of CD4 lymphocyte counts and p24 antigenemia. *The American Journal of Medicine, 89,* 706–712.

Maddox, J. (1993, March 25). Where the AIDS virus hides away. *Nature, 362,* p. 287.

Magura, S., Grossman, J. I., Lipton, D. S., Siddiqi, Q., Shapiro, J., Marion, I., & Amann, K. R. (1989). Determinants of needle sharing among intravenous drug users. *American Journal of Public Health, 79,* 459–462.

Mahler, J., Yi, D., Sacks, M., Dermatis, H., Stebinger, A., Card, C., & Perry, S. (1994). Undetected HIV infection among patients admitted to an alcohol rehabilitation unit. *American Journal of Psychiatry, 151,* 439–440.

Maj, M. (1990). Psychiatric aspects of HIV-1 infection and AIDS. *Psychological Medicine, 20,* 547–563.

Mann, J., Quinn, T. C., Francis, H., Nzilambi, N., Bosenge, N., Bila, K., McCormick, J. B., Ruti, K., Asila, P. K., & Curran, J. W. (1986). Prevalence of HTLV-III/LAV in household contacts of patients with confirmed AIDS and controls in Kinshasa, Zaire. *Journal of the American Medical Association, 256,* 721–724.

Mann, J., Tarantola, D. J. M., & Netter, T. W. (1992). *A global report: AIDS in the world.* New York: Oxford University Press.

Mansfield, S., Barter, G., & Singh, S. (1992). Editorial review: AIDS and palliative care. *International Journal of STD & AIDS, 3,* 248–250.

Mapou, R. L., & Law, W. A. (1994). Neurobehavioral aspects of HIV disease and AIDS: An update. *Professional Psychology: Research and Practice, 25,* 132–140.

Marcus, R., & CDC Cooperative Needlestick Surveillance Group. (1988). Surveillance of health care workers exposed to blood from patients infected with the human immunodeficiency virus. *New England Journal of Medicine, 319,* 1118–1123.

Mariuz, P. R., & Luft, B. J. (1992). Toxoplasmic encephalitis. *AIDS Clinical Review,* 105–130.

Markham, P., Salahuddin, S. Z., Veren, K., Orndorff, S., & Gallo, R. (1986). Hydrocortisone and some other hormones enhance the expression of HTLV-III. *International Journal of Cancer, 37,* 67–72.

Markowitz, J. C., Klerman, G. L., & Perry, S. W. (1992). Interpersonal psychotherapy of depressed HIV-positive outpatients. *Hospital and Community Psychiatry, 43,* 885–890.

Markowitz, J. C., Klerman, G. L., & Perry, S. W. (1993). An interpersonal psychotherapeutic approach to depressed HIV-seropositive patients. In W. H. Sledge & A. Tasman (Eds.), *Clinical challenges in psychiatry* (pp. 37–59). Washington, DC: American Psychiatric Press.

Markowitz, J. C., Klerman, G. L., Perry, S. W., Clougherty, K. F., & Josephs, L. S. (1993). Interpersonal psychotherapy for depressed HIV-seropositive patients. In G. L. Klerman & M. M. Weissman (Eds.), *New applications of interpersonal psychotherapy* (pp. 199–224). Washington, DC: American Psychiatric Press.

Markowitz, J. C., & Perry, S. W. (1992). Effects of human immunodeficiency virus on the central nervous system. In S. C. Yudofsky, & R. E. Hales (Eds.), *The American Psychiatric Press textbook of neuropsychiatry* (pp. 499–518). Washington, DC: American Psychiatric Press.

Markowitz, J. C., Rabkin, J., & Perry, S. (1994). Treating depression in HIV-positive patients. *AIDS, 8,* 403–412.

Marks, G., Bundek, N., Richardson, J., Ruiz, M., Malonado, N., & Mason, H. (1992). Self-disclosure of HIV infection: Preliminary results from a sample of Hispanic men. *Health Psychology, 11,* 300–306.

Marks, G., Richardson, J. L., & Maldonado, N. (1991). Self-disclosure of HIV infection to sexual partners. *American Journal of Public Health, 81,* 1321–1323.

Marks, G., Richardson, J., Ruiz, M., & Maldonado, N. (1992). HIV-infected men's practices in notifying past sexual partners of infection risk. *Public Health Reports, 107,* 100–105.

Marks, G., Ruiz, M. S., Richardson, J. L., Reed, D., Mason, H. R., Sotelo, M., & Turner, P. A. (1994). Anal intercourse and disclosure of HIV infection among seropositive gay and bisexual men. *Journal of Acquired Immune Deficiency Syndromes, 7,* 866–869.

Marmor, M., Weiss, L. R., Lynden, M., Weiss, S. H., Saxinger, W. C., Spira, T. J., & Feorino, P. M. (1986). Possible female-to-female transmission of human immunodeficiency virus. *Annals of Internal Medicine, 105,* 969.

Martin, D. J. (1992). Inappropriate lubricant use with condoms by homosexual men. *Public Health Reports, 107,* 468–473.

Martin, D. (1993). Coping with AIDS and AIDS-risk reduction efforts among gay men. *AIDS Education and Prevention, 5,* 104–120.

Martin, E. M., Robertson, L. C., Edelstein, H. E., Jagust, W. J., Sorensen, D.J ., Giovanni, D. S., & Chirurgi, V. A. (1992). Performance of patients with early HIV-1 infection on the stroop task. *Journal of Clinical and Experimental Neuropsychology, 14,* 857–868.

Martin, E. M., Robertson, L. C., Sorensen, D. J., Jagust, W. J., Mallon, K.F., & Chirurgi, V. A. (1993). Speed of memory scanning is not affected in early HIV-1 infection. *Journal of Clinical and Experimental Neuropsychology, 15,* 311–320.

Martin, E. M., Sorensen, D. J., Edelstein, H. E., & Robertson, L. C.(1992). Decision-making speed in HIV-1 infection: A preliminary report. *AIDS, 6,* 109–113.

Martin, E. M., Sorensen, D. J., Robertson, L. C., Edelstein, H. E., & Chirurgi, V. A. (1992). Spatial attention in HIV-1 infection: A preliminary report. *Journal of Neuropsychiatry and Clinical Neurosciences, 4,* 288–293.

Martin, J. L. (1988). Psychological consequences of AIDS-related bereavement among gay men. *Journal of Consulting and Clinical Psychology, 56,* 856–862.

Martin, J. L., & Dean, L. (1993a). Bereavement following death from AIDS: Unique problems, reactions, and special needs. In M. Stroebe, W. Stroebe, & R. Hannson (Eds.), *Handbook of Bereavement* (pp. 317–330). Cambridge, England: Cambridge Press.

Martin, J. L., & Dean, L. (1993b). Effects of AIDS-related bereavement and HIV-related illness on psychological distress among gay men: A 7-year longitudinal study, 1985–1991. *Journal of Consulting and Clinical Psychology, 61*, 94–103.

Martin, R. L., Cloninger, R., Guze, S., & Clayton, P. J. (1985a). Mortality in a follow-up of 500 psychiatric outpatients. *Archives of General Psychiatry, 42*, 47–54.

Martin, R. L., Cloninger, R., Guze, S., & Clayton, P. J. (1985b).Mortality in a follow-up of 500 psychiatric outpatients. *Archives of General Psychiatry, 42*, 58–66.

Martinez, A., Suffredini, A., & Masur, H. (1992). Pneumocystis carinii disease in HIV infected persons. In G. P. Wormser (Ed.), *AIDS and other manifestations of HIV infection* (2nd ed., pp. 225–248). New York: Raven Press.

Marzuk, P. M., Tierney, H., Gross, E. M., Morgan, E., Hsu, M., & Mann, J. (1988). Increased risk of suicide in persons with AIDS. *Journal of the American Medical Association, 259*, 1333–1337.

Masci, J. R., Poon, M., Wormser, G. P., & Bottone, E. J. (1992). Cryptococcus neoformans infections in the era of AIDS. In G. P.Wormser (Ed.), *AIDS and other manifestations of HIV infection* (2nd ed.). New York: Raven Press.

Mascolini, M. (1994). Glasgow carioca. *Journal of the Physicians Association for AIDS Care, 12*(1), 6–11.

Mastromauro, C., Myers, R., & Berkman, B. (1987). Attitudes toward presymptomatic testing in Huntington disease. *American Journal of Medical Genetics, 26*, 271–282.

Masur, H., Ognibene, F., Yarchoan, R., Shelhamer, J. H., Baird, B. F., Travis, W., Suffredini, A. F., Deyton, L., Kovacs, J. A., & Fallon, J. (1989). CD4 counts as predictors of opportunistic pneumonias in human immunodeficiency virus (HIV) infection. *Annals of Internal Medicine, 111*, 223–231.

Mathews, B., & Bowes, J. (1989). A training model of group therapy with an HIV-seropositive population. *AIDS & Public Policy Journal, 4*, 51–55.

Maxwell, J., Egan, V., Chiswick, A., Burns, S., Gordon, A., Kean, D., Brettle, R. P., & Pullen, I. (1991). HIV-1 associated cognitive/motor complex in an injecting drug user. *AIDS Care, 3*, 373–381.

May, R. M. (1988). HIV infection in heterosexuals. *Nature, 331*, 655–666

Mayou, R., & Hawton, K. (1986). Psychiatric disorder in the general hospital. *British Journal of Psychiatry, 149*, 172–190.

Mays, V. M., & Cochran, S. D. (1987). Acquired immunodeficiency syndrome and

Black Americans: Special psychosocial issues. *Public Health Reports, 102,* 224–231.

Mays, V., & Cochran, S. (1988). Issues in the perception of AIDS risk and risk reduction activities by Black and Hispanic/Latina women. *American Psychologist, 43,* 949–957.

McArthur, J. C. (1987). Neurologic manifestations of AIDS. *Medicine, 66,* 407–437.

McArthur, J. C., Cohen, B. A., Farzedegan, H., Cornblath, D. R., Selnes, O. A., Ostrow, D., Johnson, R. T., Phair, J., & Polk, B. F. (1988). Cerebrospinal fluid abnormalities in homosexual men with and without neuropsychiatric findings. *Annals of Neurology, 23*(Suppl.), S34–S37.

McCann, K., & Wadsworth, E. (1991). The experience of having a positive HIV antibody test. *AIDS Care, 3,* 43–53.

McCorkle, R., & Quint-Benoliel, J. (1983). Symptom distress, current concerns and mood disturbance after diagnosis of life-threatening disease. *Social Science and Medicine, 17,* 431–438.

McCrae, R. R., & Costa, P. T. (1986). Personality, coping, and coping effectiveness in an adult sample. *Journal of Personality, 54,* 385–405.

McCusker, J., Stoddard, A., Mayer, K., Zapka, J., Morrison, C., & Saltzman, S. (1988). Effects of HIV antibody test knowledge on subsequent sexual behaviors in a cohort of homosexually active men. *American Journal of Public Health, 78,* 462–467.

McCutchan, J. A. (1990). Virology, immunology, and clinical course of HIV infection. *Journal of Consulting and Clinical Psychology, 58,* 5–12.

McDonell, J. R. (1993). Judgments of personal responsibility for HIV infection: An attributional analysis. *Social Work, 38,* 403–410.

McGuff, J., & Popovsky, M. A. (1989). Needlestick injuries in blood collection staff. *Transfusion, 29,* 693–695.

McIntosh, J., Santos, J., Hubbard, R., & Overholser, J. (1994). *Elder suicide: Research, theory, and treatment.* Washington, DC: American Psychological Association.

McKeganey, N. P. (1994). Prostitution and HIV: What do we know and where might research be targeted in the future? *AIDS, 8,* 1215–1226.

McKegney, F. P., & O'Dowd, M. A. (1992). Suicidality and HIV status. *American Journal of Psychiatry, 149,* 396–398.

McKegney, F. P., O'Dowd, M. A., Feiner, C., Selwyn, P., Drucker, E., & Friedland, G. H. (1990). A prospective comparison of neuropsychologic function in HIV-seropositive and seronegative methadone-maintained patients. *AIDS, 4,* 565–569.

McKusick, L. (1988). The impact of AIDS on practitioner and client: Notes for the therapeutic relationship. *American Psychologist, 43,* 935–940.

McKusick, L., Horstman, W., & Coates, T. J. (1985). AIDS and sexual behavior reported by gay men in San Francisco. *American Journal of Public Health*, *75*, 493–496.

McShane, R. E., Bumbalo, J. A., & Patsdaughter, C. A. (1994). Psychological distress in family members living with human immunodeficiency virus/acquired immune deficiency syndrome. *Archives of Psychiatric Nursing*, *8*, 53–61.

Medalie, J. H., & Goldhourt, U. (1976). Angina pectoria among 10,000 men: II. Psychosocial and other risk factors as evidenced by a multivariate analysis of a five year incidence study. *The American Journal of Medicine*, *60*, 910–921.

Meichenbaum, D. (1977). *Cognitive behavior modification*. New York: Plenum Press.

Melnick, S. L., Sherer, R., Louis, T. A., Hillman, D., Rodriguez, E. M., Lackman, C., Capps, L., Brown, L. S., Carlyn, M., Korvick, J. A., & Deyton, L. (1994). Survival and disease progression according to gender of patients with HIV infection. *Journal of the American Medical Association*, *272*, 1915–1921.

Melton, G. B. (1988). Ethical and legal issues and AIDS-related practice. *American Psychologist*, *43*, 941–947.

Meyerowitz, B. E. (1980). Psychosocial correlates of breast cancer and its treatments. *Psychological Bulletin*, *87*, 108–131.

Michaels, D., & Levine, C. (1992). Estimates of the number of motherless youth orphaned by AIDS in the United States. *Journal of the American Medical Association*, *268*, 3456–3461.

Miller, D. (1990). Diagnosis and treatment of acute psychological problems related to HIV infection and disease. In D. Ostrow (Ed.), *Behavioral aspects of AIDS* (pp. 187–206). New York: Plenum Press.

Miller, D., & Pinching, A. (1989). HIV tests and counselling: Current issues. *AIDS*, *3*(Suppl.), S187–S193.

Miller, D. & Riccio, M. (1990). Editorial review: Non-organic psychiatric and psychosocial syndromes associated with HIV-1 infection and disease. *AIDS*, *4*, 381–388.

Miller, E. N., Selnes, O. A., McArthur, J. C., Satz, P., Becker, J. T., Cohen, B. A., Sheridan, K., Machado, A. M., Van Gorp, W. G., & Visscher, B. (1990). Neuropsychological performance in HIV-1-infected homosexual men: The multicenter AIDS cohort study (MACS). *Neurology*, *40*, 197–203.

Miller, J. F. (1983). Coping with chronic illness. In J. F. Miller (Ed.), *Coping with chronic illness: Overcoming powerlessness* (pp. 15–36). Philadelphia: Davis.

Miller, R. L., Holmes, J. M., & Auerbach, M. I. (1992, August). *Volunteer experiences of providing AIDS-related educational services*. Paper presented at the 100th Annual Convention of the American Psychological Association, Washington, DC.

Minkoff, H. L., & DeHovitz, J. A. (1991). Care of women infected with the human immunodeficiency virus. *Journal of the American Medical Association, 266,* 2253–2258.

Minkoff, H., Nanda, D., Menez, R., & Fikrig, S. (1987). Pregnancies resulting in infants with acquired immunodeficiency syndrome or AIDS-related complex: Follow-up of mothers, children, and subsequently born siblings. *Obstetrics & Gynecology, 69,* 288–291.

Mondragon, D., Kirkman-Liff, B., & Schneller, E. S. (1991). Hostility to people with AIDS: Risk perception and demographic factors. *Society of Science and Medicine, 32,* 1137–1142.

Monzon, O. T., & Capellan, J. M. B. (1987). Female-to-female transmission of HIV. *Lancet, 2,* 40–41.

Moore, L. H., van Gorp, W. G., Hinkin, C. H., Holston, S. G., Weisman, J. D., & Satz, P. (1994). Frequencies of MMPI-168 code types among asymptomatic and symptomatic HIV-1 seropositive gay men. *Journal of Personality Assessment, 63,* 574–578.

Moore, R., Hidalgo, J., Sugland, B., & Chaisson, R. (1991). Zidovudine and the natural history of the acquired immunodeficiency syndrome. *New England Journal of Medicine, 324,* 1412–1416.

Moos, R. H., & Tsu, V. D. (1977). The crisis of physical illness: An overview. In R. H. Moos (Ed.), *Coping with physical illness* (pp. 3–21). New York: Plenum Press.

Morgan, W. M., & Curran, J. W. (1986). Acquired immunodeficiency syndrome: Current and future trends. *Public Health Reports, 101,* 459–465.

Morin S. F., & Batchelor, W. F. (1984). Responding to the psychological crisis of AIDS. *Public Health Reports, 99,* 4–9.

Morokoff, P. J., Holmes, E., & Weisse, C. S. (1987). The educational model of health care: A psychoeducational program for HIV seropositive persons. *Patient and Education Counseling, 10,* 287–300.

Morrey, J., Bourn, S., Bunch, T., Jackson, K., Sidwell, R., Barrows, L., Daynes, R., & Rosen, C. (1991). In vivo activation of human immunodeficiency virus type 1 long terminal repeat by UV type A (UV-A) light plus psoralen and UV-B light in the skin of transgenic mice. *Journal of Virology, 65,* 5045–5051.

Morrow, R. H., Colebunders, R. L., & Chin, J. (1989). Interactions of HIV infection with endemic tropical diseases. *AIDS, 3,* S79–S87.

Mortimer, P. (1988). Tests for infection with HIV: Slandered goods. *British Medical Journal, 296,* 1615–1616.

Moss. A. R., & Bacchetti, P. (1989). Natural history of HIV infection. *AIDS, 3,* S55–S61.

Moss, V. (1990). Palliative care in advanced HIV disease: Presentation, problems and palliation. *AIDS, 4*(Suppl. 1), S235–S242.

Moss, V. (1991). Terminal care for people with AIDS. *Practitioner, 235*, 446–449.

Moulton, J. M., Sweet, D. M., Temoshok, L., & Mandel, J. S. (1987). Attributions of blame and responsibility in relation to distress and health behavior change in people with AIDS and AIDS-related complex. *Journal of Applied Social Psychology, 17*, 493–506.

Mulder, C., & Antoni, M. (1992). Psychosocial correlates of immune status and disease progression in HIV-1 infected homosexual men: Review of preliminary findings, and commentary. *Psychology and Health, 6*, 175–192.

Mulder, C. L., Emmelkamp, P. M. G., Mulder, J. W., Antoni, M. H., Sandfort, T., & Vries, M. J . (1992, July). *The immunological and psychosocial effects of group intervention for asymptomatic HIV infected homosexual men: The effects of cognitive–behavioral vs. experiential therapy.* Paper presented at the VIII International AIDS Conference, Amsterdam.

Munoz, A., Carey, V., Saah, A., Phair, J., Kingsley, L., Fahey, J., Ginzburg, H., & Polk, B. (1988). Predictors of decline in CD4 lymphocytes in a cohort of homosexual men infected with human immunodeficiency virus. *Journal of Acquired Immune Deficiency Syndromes, 1*, 396–404.

Murphy, D., Bahr, G. R., Kelly, J., Bernstein, B., & Morgan, M. (1992). A needs assessment survey of HIV-infected patients. *Wisconsin Medical Journal, 91*, 291–295.

Murrain, M. (1993). Differences in opportunistic infection rates in women with AIDS. *Journal of Women's Health, 2*, 243–248.

Myers, S. A., Prose, N. S., & Bartlett, J. A. (1993). Progress in the understanding of HIV infection: An overview. *Journal of the American Academy of Dermatology, 29*, 1–21.

Myers, T., Orr, K. W., Locker, D., & Jackson, E. A. (1993). Factors affecting gay and bisexual men's decisions and intentions to seek HIV testing. *American Journal of Public Health, 83*, 701–704.

Naficy, A. B., & Soave, R. (1992). Cryptosporidiosis, isosporiasis, and microsporidiosis in AIDS. In G. P. Wormser (Ed.), *AIDS and other manifestations of HIV infection* (2nd ed.). New York: Raven Press.

Namir, S., Alumbaugh, M. J., Fawzy, F. I., & Wolcott, D. L. (1989). The relationship of social support to physical and psychological aspects of AIDS. *Psychology and Health, 3*, 77–86.

Namir, S., Wolcott, D., Fawzy, F. I., & Alumbaugh, M. J. (1987). Coping with AIDS:

Psychological and health implications. *Journal of Applied Social Psychology, 17,* 309–328.

Namir, S., Wolcott, D., Fawzy, F., & Alumbaugh, M. (1990). Implications of different strategies for coping with AIDS. In L. Temoshok & A. Baum (Eds.), *Psychological perspectives on AIDS: Etiology, prevention, and treatment* (pp. 173–190). Hillsdale, NJ: Erlbaum.

National Task Force on AIDS Prevention. (1990). *A descriptive analysis of AIDS knowledge, attitudes, and risk behaviors for HIV infection among Black males who have sex with other men.* San Francisco: Author.

Navia, B. A., Cho, E. S., Petito, C. K., & Price, R. W. (1986). The AIDS dementia complex: II. Neuropathology. *Annals of Neurology, 19,* 525–535.

Navia, B. A., Jordan, B. D., & Price, R. W. (1986). The AIDS dementia complex: I. Clinical features. *Annals of Neurology, 19,* 517–524.

Neugebauer, R., Rabkin, J., Williams, J., Remien, R., Goetz, R., & Gorman, J. (1992). Bereavement reactions among homosexual men experiencing multiple losses in the AIDS epidemic. *American Journal of Psychiatry, 149,* 1374–1379.

Newmark, D. A. (1984, July). Review of a support group for patients with AIDS. *Topics in Clinical Nursing,* pp. 38–44.

Nichols, S. E. (1985). Psychosocial reactions of persons with the acquired immunodeficiency syndrome. *Annals of Internal Medicine, 103,* 765–767.

Nicholson, W. D., & Long, B. (1990). Self-esteem, social support, internalized homophobia, and coping strategies of HIV+ gay men. *Journal of Consulting and Clinical Psychology, 58,* 873–876.

Nicolosi, A., Leite, M. L., Musicco, M., Arici, C., Gavazzeni, G., & Lazzarin, A. (1994). The efficiency of male-to-female and female-to-male sexual transmission of the human immunodeficiency virus: A study of 730 stable couples. *Epidemiology, 5,* 570–575.

Niederland, W. (1968). Clinical observations of the "survivor syndrome." *International Journal of Psychoanalysis, 49,* 313–315.

Noh, S., Chandarana, P., Field, V., & Posthuma, B. (1990). AIDS epidemic, emotional strain, coping and psychological distress in homosexual men. *AIDS Education and Prevention, 2,* 272–283.

Nolan, K. (1989). Ethical issues in caring for pregnant women and newborns at risk for human immunodeficiency virus infection. *Seminars in Perinatology, 13,* 55–65.

Novick, L. F., Glebatis, D. M., Stricof, R. L., MacCubbin, P. A., Lessner, L., & Berns, D. S. (1991). Newborn seroprevalence study: Methods and results. *American Journal of Public Health, 81,* 15–21.

Nwanyanwu, O. C., Conti, L. A., Ciesielski, C. A., Stehr-Green, J. K., Berkelman, R. L., Lieb, S., & Witte, J. J. (1993). Increasing frequency of heterosexually transmitted AIDS in Southern Florida: Artifact or reality? *Amercian Journal of Public Health, 83,* 571–573.

O'Brien, T. R., Shaffer, N., & Jaffe, H. W. (1992). Acquisition and transmission of HIV. In M. A. Sande & P. A. Volberding (Eds.), *The medical management of AIDS* (3rd ed., pp. 3–17). Philadelphia: Saunders.

O'Donnell, L., O'Donnell, C. R., Pleck, J. H., Snarey, J., & Rose, R. M. (1987). Psychosocial responses of hospital workers to acquired immune deficiency syndrome (AIDS). *Journal of Applied Social Psychology, 17,* 269–285.

O'Dowd, M. A. (1988). Psychosocial issues in HIV infection. *AIDS, 2*(Suppl. 1), S201–S205.

O'Dowd, M. A., Biderman, D. J., & McKegney, F. P. (1993). Incidence of suicidality in AIDS and HIV-positive patients attending a psychiatry outpatient program. *Psychosomatics, 34,* 33–40.

O'Dowd, M. A. & McKegney, F. P. (1990). AIDS patients compared with others seen in psychiatric consultation. *General Hospital Psychiatry, 12,* 50–55.

O'Dowd, M. A., Natali, C., Orr, D., & McKegney, F. P. (1991). Characteristics of patients attending an HIV-related psychiatric clinic. *Hospital and Community Psychiatry, 42,* 615–619.

O'Leary, A. (1990). Stress, emotion, and human immune function. *Psychological Bulletin, 108,* 363–382.

Ong, E. L. C. (1993). The role of aerosol pentamidine prophylaxis. *International Journal of STD & AIDS, 4,* 67–69.

Onorato, I. A., McCray, E., Pappaioanou, M., Johnson, R., Aral, S., Hardy, A. M., & Dondero, T. J. (1990). HIV seroprevalence surveys in sexually transmitted disease clinics. *Public Health Reports, 105,* 119–124.

Osmond, D., Charlebois, E., Lang, W., Shiboski, S., & Moss, A. (1994). Changes in AIDS survival time in two San Francisco cohorts of homosexual men, 1983–1993. *Journal of the American Medical Association, 271,* 1083–1087.

Osmond, D. H., Page, K., Wiley, J., Garrett, K., Sheppard, H. W., Moss, A. R., Schrager, L., & Winkelstein, W. (1994). HIV infection in homosexual and bisexual men 18 to 29 years of age: The San Francisco young men's health study. *American Journal of Public Health, 84,* 1933–1937.

Ostrow, D. (1988). Models for understanding the psychiatric consequences of AIDS. In T. P. Bridge (Ed.), *Psychological, neuropsychiatric, and substance abuse aspects of AIDS* (pp. 85–94). New York: Raven Press.

Ostrow, D. G. (1989). Psychiatry and AIDS: An American view. *Journal of the Royal Society of Medicine, 82,* 192–197.

Ostrow, D. G. (1990). *Psychiatric aspects of human immunodeficiency virus infection.* Kalamazoo, MI: Upjohn.

Ostrow, D. G. (1994). Substance abuse and HIV infection. *Psychiatric Manifestations of HIV disease, 17,* 69–89.

Ostrow, D., Grant, I., & Atkinson, H. (1988). Assessment and management of the AIDS patient with neuropsychiatric disturbances. *Journal of Clinical Psychiatry, 49,* 14–22.

Ostrow, D., Joseph, J., Kessler, R., Soucy, J., Tal, M., Eller, M., Chmiel, J., & Phair, J. (1989). Disclosure of HIV antibody status: Behavioral and mental health correlates. *AIDS Education and Prevention, 1,* 1–11.

Ostrow, D. G., Joseph, J., Monjan, A., Kessler, R., Emmons, C.,Phair, J., Fox, R., Kingsley, L., Dudley, J., Chmiel, J., & Van Raden, M. (1986). Psychosocial aspects of AIDS risk. *Psychopharmacology Bulletin, 22,* 678–683.

Ostrow, D. G., Monjan, A., Joseph, J., VanRaden, M., Fox, R., Kingsley, L., Dudley, J., & Phair, J. (1989). HIV-related symptoms and psychological functioning in a cohort of homosexual men. *American Journal of Psychiatry, 146,* 737– 742.

Ostrow, D. G., Whitaker, R. E. D., Frasier, K., Cohen, C., Wan, J., Frank, C., & Fisher, E. (1991). Racial differences in social support and mental health in men with HIV infection: A pilot study. *AIDS Care, 3,* 55–62.

Ostrow, D. G., & Wren, P. (1992). Module four: Prevention of HIV-1 infection. In P. A. Barr (Ed.), *Mental health aspects of HIV/AIDS: Vol. 1. Curriculum Modules* (pp. 64–114). (Available from D. Ostrow, Medical College of Wisconsin, Milwaukee, WI, 53226)

Ozawa, M., Auslander, W., & Slonim-Nevo, V. (1993). Problems in financing the care of AIDS patients. *Social Work, 38,* 369–377.

Pace, J., Brown, G. R., Rundell, J. R., Paolucci, S., Drexler, K., & McManis, S. (1990). Prevalence of psychiatric disorders in a mandatory screening program for infection with human immunodeficiency virus: A pilot study. *Military Medicine, 155,* 76–80.

Padian, N. S. (1988). Preventing the heterosexual spread of AIDS. *Journal of the American Medical Association, 260,* 1879.

Padian, N. S. (1990). Sexual histories of heterosexual couples with one HIV-infected partner. *Amercian Journal of Public Health, 80,* 990–991.

Padian, N., Marquis, L., Francis, D. P., Anderson, R. E., Rutherford, G., O'Malley, P. M.,

& Winkelstein, W. (1987). Male-to-female transmission of human immuno-deficiency virus. *Journal of the American Medical Association, 258,* 788–790.

Padian, N. S., Shiboski, S. C., & Jewell, N. P. (1991). Female-to-male transmission of human immunodeficiency virus. *Journal of the American Medical Association, 266,* 1664–1667.

Pakenham, K. I., Dadds, M. R., & Terry, D. J. (1994). Relationships between adjust-ment to HIV and both social support and coping. *Journal of Consulting and Clinical Psychology, 62,* 1194–1203.

Pantaleo, G., Graziosi, C., & Fauci, A. S. (1993). The role of lymphoid organs in the immunopathogenesis of HIV infection. *AIDS, 7*(Suppl.), S19–S23.

Pantaleo, G., Menzo, S., Vaccarezza, M., Graziosi, C., Cohen, O. J., Demarest, J. F., Montefiori, D., Orenstein, J. M., Fox, C., Schrager, L. K., Margolick, J. B., Buch-binder, S., Giorgi, J. V., & Fauci, A. S. (1995). Studies in subjects with long-term nonprogressive human immunodeficiency virus infection. *New England Jour-nal of Medicine, 332,* 209–216.

Pearlin, L. I., Mullan, J. T., Aneshensel, C. S., Wardlaw, L., & Harrington, C. (1994). The structure and functions of AIDS caregiving relationships. *Psychosocial Re-habilitation Journal, 17,* 51–67.

Pearlin, L. I., & Schooler, C. (1978). The structure of coping. *Journal of Health and Social Psychology, 19,* 2–21.

Perdices, M., & Cooper, D. A. (1990). Neuropsychological investigation of patients with AIDS and ARC. *Journal of Acquired Immune Deficiency Syndromes, 3,* 555–564.

Pergami, A., Gala, C., Burgess, A., Durbano, F., Zanello, D., Riccio, M., Invernizzi, G., & Catalan, J. (1993). The psychosocial impact of HIV infection in women. *Journal of Psychosomatic Research, 37,* 687–696.

Perkins, D., Davidson, E., Leserman, J., Liao, D., & Evans, D. (1993). Personality dis-order in patients infected with HIV: A controlled study with implications for clinical care. *American Journal of Psychiatry, 150,* 309–315.

Perkins, D. O., Stern, R. A., Golden, R. N., Murphy, C., Naftolowitz, D., & Evans, D. L. (1994). Mood disorders in HIV infection: Prevalence and risk factors in a nonepicenter of the AIDS epidemic. *American Journal of Psychiatry, 151,* 233–236.

Perry, S. (1989). Warning third parties at risk of AIDS: APA's policy is a barrier to treatment. *Hospital and Community Psychiatry, 40,* 158–161.

Perry, S. W., Card, C. A., Moffatt, M., Ashman, T., Fishman, B., & Jacobsberg, L. B. (1994). Self-disclosure of HIV infection to sexual partners after repeated coun-seling. *AIDS Education and Prevention, 6,* 403–411.

Perry, S., & Fishman, B. (1993). Depression and HIV: How does one affect the other? *Journal of the American Medical Association, 270,* 2509–2510.

Perry, S., Fishman, B., Jacobsberg, L., & Frances, A. (1992). Relationships over 1 year between lymphocyte subsets and psychosocial variables among adults with infection by human immunodeficiency virus. *Archives of General Psychiatry, 49,* 396–401.

Perry, S., Jacobsberg, L., Card, C. A., Ashman, T., Frances, A., & Fishman, B. (1993). Severity of psychiatric symptoms after HIV testing. *American Journal of Psychiatry, 150,* 775–779.

Perry, S., Jacobsberg, L., & Fishman, B. (1990). Suicidal ideation and HIV testing. *Journal of the American Medical Association, 263,* 679–682.

Perry, S., Jacobsberg, L., Fishman, B., Frances, A., Bobo, J., & Jacobsberg, B. K. (1990). Psychiatric diagnosis before serological testing for the human immunodeficiency virus. *American Journal of Psychiatry, 147,* 89–93.

Perry, S., Jacobsberg, L., Fishman, B., Weiler, P., Gold, J. W. M., & Frances, A. (1990). Psychological responses to serological testing for HIV. *AIDS, 4,* 145–152.

Perry, S. W., & Markowitz, J. (1986). Psychiatric interventions for AIDS-spectrum disorders. *Hospital and Community Psychiatry, 37,* 1001–1006.

Perry, S., & Markowitz, J. (1988). Counseling for HIV testing. *Hospital and Community Psychiatry, 39,* 731–739.

Perry, S., & Marotta, R. F. (1987). AIDS dementia: A review of the literature. *Alzheimer Disease and Associated Disorders, 1,* 221–235.

Perry, S., Ryan, J., Ashman, T., & Jacobsberg, L. (1992). Refusal of zidovudine by HIV-positive patients. *AIDS, 6,* 514–515.

Perry, S. W. & Tross, S. (1984). Psychiatric problems of AIDS inpatients at the New York hospital: Preliminary report. *Public Health Reports, 99,* 200–205.

Peterson, C., Seligman, M. E. P., & Vaillant, G. E. (1988). Pessimistic explanatory style is a risk factor for physical illness: A thirty-five-year longitudinal study. *Journal of Personality and Social Psychology, 55,* 23–27.

Peterson, J., & Marin, G. (1988). Issues in the prevention of AIDS among Black and Hispanic men. *American Psychologist, 43,* 871–877.

Peterson, L. R., Doll, L., White, C., Chu, S., and the HIV Blood Donor Study Group. (1992). No evidence for female-to-female HIV transmission among 960,000 female blood donors. *Journal of Acquired Immune Deficiency Syndromes, 5,* 853–855.

Pfeiffer, N. (1992, October). Long-term survival and HIV disease: The role of exercise and CD4 response in HIV disease. *AIDS Patient Care,* 237–239.

Phair, J., Munoz, A., Detels, R., Kaslow, R., Rinaldo, C., Saah, A., & Multicenter AIDS Cohort Study Group. (1990). The risk of Pheumocystis Carinii pneumonia among men infected with human immunodeficiency virus type 1. *New England Journal of Medicine, 322,* 161–165.

Piette, J., Mor, V., Mayer, K., Zierler, S., & Wachtel, T. (1993). The effects of immune status and race on health service use among people with HIV disease. *American Journal of Public Health, 83,* 510–514.

Pillard, R. (1988). Sexual orientation and mental disorders. *Psychiatric Annals, 18,* 52–56.

Pinch, W. J., Brown, K., Dougherty, C. J., Allegretti, J. G., & McCarthy, V. (1993). Caregivers' perspectives on confidentiality for mothers and newborns with HIV/AIDS. *Pediatric AIDS and HIV Infection: Fetus to Adolescent, 4,* 123–129.

Pinching, A. J. (1989). Models of clinical care. *AIDS, 3*(Suppl. 1), S209–S213.

Pitchenik, A., & Fertel, D. (1992). Mycobacterial disease in patients with HIV infection. In G. P. Wormser (Ed.), *AIDS and other manifestations of HIV infection* (2nd ed., pp. 277–314). New York: Raven Press.

Pliskin, M., Farrell, K., Crandles, S., & DeHovitz, J. (1993). *Factors influencing HIV positive mothers' disclosure to their non-infected children.* (Available from the authors, State University of New York—Health Science Center, Brooklyn, NY 10465)

Polk, B. F., Fox, R., Brookmeyer, R., Kanchanaraksa, S., Kaslow, R., Visscher, B., Rinaldo, C., & Phair, J. (1987). Predictors of the acquired immunodeficiency syndrome in a cohort of seropositive homosexual men. *New England Journal of Medicine, 316,* 61–66

Polsky, B., Gold, J. W., Whimbey, E., Dryjanski, J., Brown, A. E. Schiffman, G., & Armstrong, D. (1986). Bacterial pneumonia in patients with the acquired immunodeficiency syndrome. *Annals of Internal Medicine, 104,* 38–41.

Poppen, P. J., & Reisen, C. A. (1994). Heterosexual behaviors and risk of exposure to HIV: Current status and prospects for change. *Applied & Preventive Psychology, 3,* 75–90.

Potts, M., Anderson, R., & Baily, M. C. (1991). Slowing the spread of human immunodeficiency virus in developing countries. *Lancet, 338,* 608–613.

Price, R. W., & Brew, B., (1991, May–June). Management of the neurologic complications of HIV-1 infection and AIDS: I. Dementia and diffuse brain disease. *AIDS Reader,* pp. 97–102.

Price, R. W., Brew, B., Sidtis, J., Rosenblum, M., Scheck, A. C., & Cleary, P. (1988). The brain and AIDS: Central nervous system HIV-1 infection and AIDS dementia complex. *Science, 239,* 586–592.

Price, R. W., & Sidtis, J. J. (1992). The AIDS dementia complex. In G. P. Wormser (Ed.), *AIDS and other manifestations of HIV infection* (2nd ed., pp. 373–382). New York: Raven Press.

Price, V., & Hsu, M. L. (1992). Public opinion about AIDS policies: The role of misinformation and attitudes toward homosexuals. *Public Opinion Quarterly, 56,* 29–52.

Pryor, J. B., Reeder, G. D., Vinacco, R., & Kott, T. (1989). The instrumental and symbolic functions of attitudes toward persons with AIDS. *Journal of Applied Social Psychology, 19,* 377–404.

Quadrel, M. J., Fischoff, B., & Davis, W. (1993). Adolescent (in)vulnerability. *American Psychologist, 48,* 102–116.

Quinn, T. C., Glaser, D., Cannon, R. O., Matuszak, D. L., Dunning, R. W., & Kline, M. S. (1988). Human immunodeficiency virus infection among patients attending clinics for sexually transmitted diseases. *New England Journal of Medicine, 318,* 197–203.

Quinn, T. C., Groseclose, S. L., Spence, M., Provost, N., & Hook, E. W. (1992). Evolution of the human immunodeficiency virus epidemic among patients attending sexually transmitted disease clinics: A decade of experience. *Sexually-Transmitted Diseases, 165,* 541–544.

Rabeneck, L., & Wray, N. P. (1993). Predicting the outcomes of human immunodeficiency virus infection: How well are we doing? *Archives of International Medicine, 153,* 2749–2755.

Rabkin, J. G. (1994, January). *Mood and immune effects of pharmacotherapy in HIV illness.* Paper presented at the NIMH Neuroscience Findings in AIDS Research, Rockville, MD.

Rabkin, J. G., & Harrison, W. M. (1990). Effect of imipramine on depression and immune status in a sample of men with HIV infection. *American Journal of Psychiatry, 147,* 495–497.

Rabkin, J. G., Rabkin, R., Harrison, W., & Wagner, G. (1994). Effect of imipramine on mood and enumerative measures of immune status in depressed patients with HIV illness. *American Journal of Psychiatry, 151,* 516–523.

Rabkin, J. G., Rabkin, R., & Wagner, G. (1994). Effects of fluoxetine on mood and immune status in depressed patients with HIV illness. *Journal of Clinical Psychiatry, 55,* 92–97.

Rabkin, J. G., Remien, R., Katoff, L., & Williams, J. (1993). Resiliency in adversity among long-term survivors if AIDS. *Hospital and Community Psychology, 44,* 162–167.

Rabkin, J. G., Williams, J. B., Neugebauer, R., Remien, R., & Goetz, R. (1990). Maintenance of hope in HIV-spectrum homosexual men. *American Journal of Psychiatry, 147,* 1322–1326.

Rabkin, J. G., Williams, J. B., Remien, R. H., Goetz, R., Kertzner, R., & Gorman, J. M. (1991). Depression, distress, lymphocyte subsets, and human immunodeficiency virus symptoms on two occasions in HIV-positive homosexual men. *Archives of General Psychiatry, 48,* 111–119.

Rabkin, J. G., Wilson, C., & Kimpton, D. J. (1993, January). The end of the line . . . when is enough enough? *PAACNOTES,* 25–47.

Ranki, A., Vale, S. L. Krohn, M., Antonen, J., Allain, J. P., Leuther, M., Franchini, G., & Krohn, K. (1987). Long latency precedes overt seroconversion in sexually transmitted human immunodeficiency virus infection. *Lancet, 2*(8559), 589–593.

Raviglione, M. C., Snider, D. E., & Kochi, A. (1995). Global epidemiology of tuberculosis: Morbidity and mortality of a worldwide epidemic. *Journal of the American Medical Association, 273,* 220–226.

Reamer, F. G. (1991). AIDS, social work, and the "duty to protect." *Social Work, 36,* 56–60.

Reed, G. M., Kemeny, M. E., Taylor, S. E., Wang, H-Y. J., & Visscher, B. R. (1994). "Realistic acceptance" as a predictor of survival time in gay men with AIDS. *Health Psychology, 13,* 299–307.

Reed, G. M., Taylor, S. E., & Kemeny, M. E. (1993). Perceived control and psychological adjustment in gay men with AIDS. *Journal of Applied Social Psychology, 23,* 791–824.

Reed, P., Wise, T. N., & Mann, L. S. (1984). Nurses' attitudes regarding acquired immunodeficiency syndrome (AIDS). *Nursing Forum, 11,* 153–156.

Reich, P. & Kelly, M. J. (1976). Suicide attempts by hospitalized medical and surgical patients. *New England Journal of Medicine, 294,* 298–301.

Reidy, M., Taggart, M. E., & Asselin, L. (1991). Psychosocial needs expressed by the natural caregivers of HIV infected children. *AIDS Care, 3,* 331–343.

Remien, R. H., Rabkin, J., Williams, J., & Katoff, L. (1992). Coping strategies and health beliefs of AIDS longterm survivors. *Psychology and Health, 6,* 335–345.

Resnick, L., diMarzo-Veronese, F., Schupbach, J., Tourtellotte, W. W., Ho, D. D., Muller, F., Shapshak, P., Vogt, M., Groopman, J. E., & Markham, P. D. (1985). Intra-blood–brain-barrier synthesis of HTLV-III specific IgG in patients with neurologic symptoms associated with AIDS or AIDS-related complex. *New England Journal of Medicine, 313,* 1498–1504.

Rhoads, J. L., Wright, D. C., Redfield, R. R., & Burke, D. S. (1987). Chronic vaginal candidiasis in women with human immunodeficiency virus infection. *Journal of the American Medical Association, 257,* 3105–3107.

Rich, J. D., Buck, A., Tuomala, R. E., & Kazanjian, P. H. (1993). Transmission of human immunodeficiency virus infection presumed to have occurred via female homosexual contact. *Clinical Infectious Diseases, 17,* 1003–1005.

Richters, J., Donovan, B., & Gerofi, J. (1993). How often do condoms break or slip off in use? *International Journal of STD & AIDS, 4,* 90–94.

Riley, J. L. & Greene, R. R. (1993). Influence of education on self-perceived attitudes about HIV/AIDS among human services providers. *Social Work, 38,* 396–401.

Ritchie, E. C., & Radke, A. Q. (1992). Depression and support systems in male Army HIV+ patients. *Military Medicine, 157,* 345–349.

Robiner, W. N., Melroe, N. H., Campbell, S., Phame, F. S., Colon, E., Chung, J., & Reaney, S. (1993). Psychological effects of participation and nonparticipation in a placebo-controlled zidovudine clinical trial with asymptomatic human immunodeficiency virus-infected individuals. *Journal of Acquired Immune Deficiency Syndromes, 6,* 795–808.

Rodin, G., & Voshart, K. (1986). Depression in the medically ill: An overview. *American Journal of Psychiatry, 143,* 696–705.

Rogers, M. F., & Jaffe, H. W. (1994). Reducing the risk of maternal–infant transmission of HIV: A door is opened. *The New England Journal of Medicine, 331,* 1232–1233.

Rogers, M. F., & Kilbourne, B. W. (1992). Epidemiology of pediatric HIV infection. In G. P. Wormser (Ed.), *AIDS and other manifestations of HIV infection* (2nd ed.). New York: Raven Press.

Root-Bernstein, R. S. (1990). Non-HIV immunosuppressive factors in AIDS: A multifactorial, synergistic theory of AIDS aetiology. *Research in Immunology, 141,* 815–838.

Root-Bernstein, R. S. (1992). AIDS is more than HIV. *Genetic Engineering News, 12*(13), 4–6.

Root-Bernstein, R. S. (1993). *Rethinking AIDS.* New York: Free Press.

Rosenberg, M. J., Holmes, K. K., & the World Health Organization Working Group on Virucides. (1993). Virucides in prevention of HIV infection: Research priorities. *Sexually Transmitted Diseases, 20,* 41–44.

Rosenberg, Z. F., & Fauci, A. S. (1991). Immunopathology and pathogenesis of human immunodeficiency virus infection. *Pediatric Infectious Disease Journal, 10,* 230–238.

Rosse, R. B. (1985). Reactions of psychiatric staff to an AIDS patient. *American Journal of Psychiatry, 142*, 523.

Rothenberg, R., Woelfel, M., Stoneburner, R., Milberg, J., Parker, R., & Truman, B. (1987). Survival with the acquired immunodeficiency syndrome: Experience with 5833 cases in New York City. *New England Journal of Medicine, 317*, 1297–1302.

Royce, R. A., & Winkelstein, W. (1990). HIV infection, cigarette smoking and CD4+ T-lymphocyte counts: Preliminary results from the San Francisco men's health study. *AIDS, 4*, 327–333.

Rozenbaum, W., Gharakhanian, S., Cardon, B., Duval, E., & Coulaud, J. P. (1988). HIV transmission by oral sex. *Lancet, 1*(8599), 1395.

Rundell, J. R., Paolucci, S. L., Beatty, D. C., & Boswell, R. N. (1988). Psychiatric illness at all stages of human immunodeficiency virus infection. *American Journal of Psychiatry, 145*, 652–653.

Ryder, R. W., & Hassig, S. E. (1988). The epidemiology of perinatal transmission of HIV. *AIDS, 2*(Suppl. 1), S83–S89.

Saag, M. S. (1992). AIDS testing: Now and in the future. In M. A. Sande & P. A. Volberding (Eds.), *The medical management of AIDS* (3rd ed., pp. 33–53). Philadelphia: Saunders.

Saag, M. S. (1995). AIDS testing now and in the future. In M. A. Sande & P. A. Volberding (Eds.), *The medical management of AIDS* (4th ed., pp. 65–88). Philadelphia: Saunders.

Saah, A. J., Munoz, A., Kuo, V., Fox, R., Kaslow, R. A., Phair, J. P., Rinaldo, C. R., Detels, R., Polk, B. F., & the Multicenter AIDS Cohort Study (MACS). (1992). Predictors of the risk of development of acquired immunodeficiency syndrome within 24 months among gay men seropositive for human immunodeficiency virus type 1: A report from the multicenter AIDS cohort study. *American Journal of Epidemiology, 135*, 1147–1155.

Sacks, M. H., Dermatis, H., Looser-Ott, S., Burton, W., & Perry, S. (1992). Undetected HIV infection among acutely ill psychiatric inpatients. *American Journal of Psychiatry, 149*, 544–545.

Sadovsky, R. (1991). Psychosocial issues in symptomatic HIV infection. *American Family Physician, 44*, 2065–2072.

Sahs, J. A., Goetz, R., Reddy, M., Rabkin, J. G., Williams, J. B. W., Kertzner, R., & Gorman, J. M. (1994). Psychological distress and natural killer cells in gay men with and without HIV infection. *American Journal of Psychiatry, 151*, 1479–1484.

Sales, E. (1991). Psychosocial impact of the phase of cancer on the family: An updated review. *Journal of Psychosocial Oncology, 9*, 1–18.

Sales, E., Schulz, R., & Biegel, D. (1992). Predictors of strain in families of cancer patients: A review of the literature. *Journal of Psychosocial Oncology, 10*, 1–26.

Sande, M. A., Carpenter, C. C., Cobbs, C. G., Holmes, K. K., & Sanford, J. P. (1993). Antiretroviral therapy for adult HIV infected patients: Recommendations from a state-of-the-art conference. *Journal of the American Medical Association, 270*, 2583–2589.

Sande, M. A. & Volberding, P. A. (1992). *The medical management of AIDS* (3rd ed.). Philadelphia: Saunders.

Sande, M. A., & Volberding, P. A. (1995). *The medical management of AIDS* (4th ed.). Philadelphia: Saunders.

Sarason, I., Sarason, B., Potter, E., & Antoni, M. (1985). Life events, social support, and illness. *Psychosomatic Medicine, 47*, 156–163.

Sarosi, G. A. (1992). Endemic mycoses in HIV infection. In M. A. Sande & P. A. Volberding (Eds.), *The medical management of AIDS* (3rd ed., pp. 311–318). Philadelphia: Saunders.

Saunders, L. D., Rutherford, G. W., Lemp, G. F., & Barnhart, J. L. (1990). Impact of AIDS on mortality in San Francisco, 1979–1986. *Journal of Aquired Immune Deficiency Syndromes, 3*, 921–924.

Saykin, A. J., Janssen, R., Sprehn, G., Spira, T., Cannon, L., Kaplan, J., O'Connor, B., Watson, S., & Allen, R. (1989). Neuropsychological and psychosocial function in two cohorts of gay men: Relation to stage of HIV-1 infection. *International Conference on AIDS, 5*, 389. (Abstract No. W.B.P. 224)

Schaefer, S., & Coleman, E. (1992). Shifts in meaning, purpose, and values following a diagnosis of human immunodeficiency virus (HIV) infection among gay men. *Journal of Psychology and Human Sexuality, 5*, 13–29.

Schaeffer, M. A., & Baum, A. (1984). Adrenal cortical response to stress at Three Mile Island. *Psychosomatic Medicine, 46*, 227–237.

Schechter, M. T., Craib, K. J. P., Le, T. N., Montaner, J. S. G., Douglas, B., Sestak, P., Willoughby, B., & O'Shaughnessy, M. V. (1990). Susceptibility to AIDS progression appears early in HIV infection. *AIDS, 4*, 185–190.

Scheier, M. F., & Carver, C. S. (1987). Dispositional optimism and physical well-being: The influence of generalized outcome expectancies on health. *Journal of Personality, 55*, 169–210.

Scheier, M. F., Matthews, K. A., Owens, J. F., Magovern, G. J., Lefebvre, R. C., Abbott, R. A., & Carver, C. S. (1989). Dispositional optimism and recovery from coronary artery bypass surgery: The beneficial effects on physical and psychological well-being. *Journal of Personality and Social Psychology, 57*, 1024–1040.

Schielke, E., Tatsch, K., Pfister, H. W., Trenkwalder, C., Leinsinger, G., Kirsch, C. M., Matuschke, A., & Einhaupl, K. M. (1990). Reduced cerebral blood flow in early stages of human immunodeficiency virus infection. *Archives of Neurology, 47,* 1342–1345.

Schilling, R., El-Bassel, N., Ivanoff, A., Gilbert, L., Su, K. H., & Safyer, S. M. (1994). Sexual risk behavior of incarcerated, drug-using women, 1992. *Public Health Reports, 109,* 539–547.

Schleifer, S. J., Keller, S. E., Bond, R. N., Cohen, J., & Stein, M.(1989). Major depressive disorder and immunity: Role of age, sex, severity, and hospitalization. *Archives of General Psychiatry, 46,* 81–87.

Schleifer, S., Keller, S., Camerino, M., Thornton, J., & Stein, M. (1983). Suppression of lymphocyte stimulation following bereavement. *Journal of the American Medical Association, 250,* 374–377.

Schleifer, S. J., Keller, S. E., Siris, S. G., Davis, K. L., & Stein, M. (1985). Depression and immunity. *Archives of General Psychiatry, 42,* 129–133.

Schmaling, K. B., & DiClementi, J. D. (1991, October). Cognitive therapy with the HIV seropositive patient. *The Behavior Therapist,* pp. 221–224.

Schmitt, F. A., Bigley, J. W., McKinnis, R., Logue, P. E., Evans, R. W., Drucker, J. L., & the AZT Collaborative Working Group. (1988). Neuropsychological outcome of zidovudine (AZT) treatment of patients with AIDS and AIDS-related complex. *New England Journal of Medicine, 319,* 1573–1578.

Schneider, S. G., Taylor, S. E., Hammen, C., Kemeny, M., & Dudley, J. (1991). Factors influencing suicide intent in gay and bisexual suicide ideators: Differing models for men with and without human immunodeficiency virus. *Journal of Personality and Social Psychology, 61,* 776–788.

Schneiderman, L. J. & Kaplan, R. M. (1992). Fear of dying and HIV infection vs Hepatitis B infection. *American Journal of Public Health, 82,* 584–586.

Schnell, D., Higgins, D., Wilson, R., Goldbaum, G., Cohn, D., & Wolitski, R. (1992). Men's disclosure of HIV test results to male primary sex partners. *American Journal of Public Health, 82,* 1675–1676.

Schoenbaum, E. E., Weber, M. P., Vermund, S., & Gayle, H. (1990). HIV antibody in persons screened for syphilis: Prevalence in a New York City emergency room and primary care clinics. *Sexually Transmitted Diseases, 17,* 190–193.

Schooley, R. (1992). Antiretroviral chemotherapy. In G. P. Wormser (Ed.), *AIDS and other manifestations of HIV infection* (2nd ed., pp. 609–624). New York: Raven Press.

Schoub, B. D. (1994). *AIDS & HIV in Perspective.* New York: Cambridge Press.

Schulz, R., Tompkins, C. A., & Rau, M. T. (1988). A longitudinal study of the psychosocial impact of stroke on primary support persons. *Psychology and Aging, 3*, 131–141.

Schwartzberg, S. S. (1993). Struggling for meaning: HIV-positive gay men make sense of AIDS. *Professional Psychology: Research and Practice, 24*, 483–490.

Schrager, L. K. (1988). Bacterial infections in AIDS patients. *AIDS, 2*,(Suppl. 1), S183–S189.

Selik, R. M., Chu, S. Y., & Buehler, J. W. (1993). HIV infection as leading cause of death among young adults in US cities and states. *Journal of the American Medical Association, 269*, 2991–2994.

Selnes, O. A., & Miller, E. N. (1992). Cognitive impairment of HIV infection. *AIDS, 6*, 602–603.

Selnes, O. A., Miller, E., McArthur, J., Gordon, B., Munoz, A., Sheridan, K., Fox, R., Saah, A. J., & the Multicenter AIDS Cohort Study. (1990). HIV-1 infection: No evidence of cognitive decline during the asymptomatic stages. *Neurology, 40*, 204–208.

Seltzer, E., Schulman, K. A., Brennan, P. J., & Lynn, L. A. (1993). Patient attitudes toward rooming with persons with HIV infection. *Journal of Family Practice, 37*, 564–568.

Selwyn, P. A., Feingold, A. R., Hartel, D., Schoenbaum, E. E., Alderman, M. H., Klein, R. S., & Friedland, G. H. (1988). Increased risk of bacterial pneumonia in HIV-infected intravenous drug users without AIDS. *AIDS, 2*, 267–272.

Sewell, D. D., Jeste, D. V. Atkinson, J. H., Heaton, R. K., Hesselink, J. R., Wiley, C., Thal, L., Chandler, J. L., Grant, I., & the San Diego HIV Neurobehavioral Research Center Group (1994). HIV-associated psychosis: A study of 20 cases. *American Journal of Psychiatry, 151*, 237–242.

Shah, P. N., & Barton, S. E. (1993). Vaginal cytomegalovirus infection in a woman with AIDS. *International Journal of STD & AIDS, 4*, 346–347.

Sharer, L. R. (1992). Pathology of HIV-1 infection of the central nervous system. *Journal of Neuropathology and Experimental Neurology, 51*, 3–11.

Shaw, G. M., Harper, M. E., Hahn, B. H., Epstein, L. G., Gajdusek, D. C., Price, R. W., Navia, B. A., Petito, C. K., O'Hara, C. J., Groopman, J. E., Cho, E.S., Oleske, J. M., Staal, F. W., & Gallo, R. C. (1985). HTLV-III infection in brains of children and adults with AIDS encephalopathy. *Science, 227*, 177–182.

Shearn, M. A., & Fireman, B. H. (1985). Stress management and mutual support groups in rheumatoid arthritis. *American Journal of Medicine, 78*, 771–775.

Sherer, R. (1988). Physician use of the HIV antibody test: The need for consent, counseling, confidentiality, and caution. *Journal of the American Medical Association, 259*, 264–265.

Sherr, L., Davey, T., & Strong, C. (1991). Counselling implications of anxiety and depression in AIDS and HIV infection: A pilot study. *Counselling Psychology Quarterly, 4,* 27–35.

Shinn, M., Lehmann, S., & Wong, N. W. (1984). Social interaction and social support. *Journal of Social Issues, 40,* 55–76.

Siegel, K. (1986). AIDS: The social dimension. *Psychiatric Annals, 16,* 168–172.

Siegel, K., & Krauss, B. (1991). Living with HIV infection: Adaptive tasks of seropositive gay men. *Journal of Health and Social Behavior, 32.* 17–32.

Siegel, K., Levine, M., Brooks, C., & Kern, R. (1989). The motives of gay men for taking or not taking the HIV antibody test. *Social Problems, 36*(4), 368–383.

Siegel, K., Raveis, V. H., & Karus, D. (1994). Psychological well-being of gay men with AIDS: Contribution of positive and negative illness-related network interactions to depressive mood. *Social Science and Medicine, 39,* 1555–1563.

Siegl, D., & Morse, J. M. (1994). Tolerating reality: The experience of parents of HIV positive sons. *Society of Science and Medicine, 38,* 959–971.

Sikkema, K. J., Kalichman, S. C., Kelly, J. A., & Koob, J. J. (in press). Group intervention to improve coping with AIDS-related bereavement: Model development and an illustrative clinical example. *AIDS Care.*

Silva, J. A., Leong, G. B., & Weinstock, R. (1989). An HIV-infected psychiatric patient: Some clinicolegal dilemmas. *Bulletin of the American Academy of Psychiatry & Law, 17,* 33–43.

Silverman, D. C. (1993). Psychosocial impact of HIV-related caregiving on health providers: A review and recommendations for the role of psychiatry. *American Journal of Psychiatry, 150,* 705–712.

Simberkoff, M. S., & Leaf, H. (1992). Bacterial infections in patients with HIV infection. In G. P. Wormser (Ed.), *AIDS and other manifestations of HIV infection* (2nd ed., pp. 269–276). New York: Raven Press.

Sinforiani, E., Mauri, M., Bono, G., Muratori, S., Alessi, E., & Minoli, L. (1991). Cognitive abnormalities and disease progression in a selected population of asymptomatic HIV-positive subjects. *AIDS, 5,* 1117–1120.

Slovic, P., Fischhoff, B., & Lichtenstein, S. (1982). Facts versus fears: Understanding perceived risk. In D. Kahneman, P. Slovic, & A. Tversky (Eds.) *Judgment under uncertainty: Heuristics and biases* (pp. 463–489). New York: Cambridge Press.

Slowinski, J. W. (1989, September). Psychological needs of HIV-positive and AIDS patients. *Medical Aspects of Human Sexuality,* pp. 52–54.

Smith, D. A. & Smith, L. (1989). The isolation of HIV-positive patients. *Journal of the American Medical Association, 262,* 208.

Smith, J. E., Landau, J., & Bahr, G. R. (1990). AIDS in rural and small town America: Making the heartland respond. *AIDS Patient Care, 4,* 17–21.

Smith, M. L., & Martin, K. P. (1993). Confidentiality in the age of AIDS: A case study in clinical ethics. *Journal of Clinical Ethics, 4,* 236–241.

Smith, P. F., Mikl, J., Hyde, S., & Morse, D. L. (1991). The AIDS epidemic in New York State. *American Journal of Public Health, 81,* 54–60.

Snider, W. D., Simpson, D. M., Nielsen, S., Gold, J. W., Metroka, C. E., & Posner, J. B. (1983). Neurological complications of acquired immune deficiency syndrome: Analysis of 50 patients. *Annals of Neurology, 14,* 403–418.

Snyder, S., Reyner, A., Schmeidler, J., Bogursky, E., Gomez, H., & Strain, J. (1992). Prevalence of mental disorders in newly admitted medical inpatients with AIDS. *Psychosomatics, 33,* 166–170.

Solano, L., Costa, M., Salvati, S., Coda, R., Aiuti, F., Mezzaroma, I., & Bertini, M. (1993). Psychosocial factors and clinical evolution in HIV-1 infection: A longitudinal study. *Journal of Psychosomatic Research, 37,* 39–51.

Solomon, G. F., Kemeny, M., & Temoshok, L. (1991). Psychoneuroimmunologic aspects of human immunodeficiency virus infection. In R. Ader, D. Felten, & L. Cohen (Eds.), *Psychoneuroimmunology II* (pp. 1082–1113). Orlando, FL: Academic Press.

Solomon, G. F., & Temoshok, L. (1987). A psychoneuroimmunologic perspective on AIDS research: Questions, preliminary findings, and suggestions. *Journal of Applied Social Psychology, 17,* 286–308.

Somerfield, M., & Curbow, B. (1992). Methodological issues and research strategies in the study of coping with cancer. *Social Science and Medicine, 34,* 1203–1216.

Somlai, A., & Kalichman, S. (1994, August). *The spiritual practices and needs of people living with HIV–AIDS.* Paper presented at the 102nd Annual Convention of the American Psychological Association, Los Angeles.

Soni, S. D., & Windgassen, E. (1991). AIDS panic: Effects of mass media publicity. *Acta Psychiatrica Scandinavica, 84,* 121–124.

Spector, I. C., & Conklin, R. (1987). Brief reports: AIDS group psychotherapy. *International Journal of Group Psychotherapy, 37,* 433–439.

Spielberger, C. D., Gorsuch, R. L., & Lushene, R. (1970). *The state–trait anxiety inventory manual.* Palo Alto, CA: Consulting Psychologists Press.

Srinivasan, A., York, D., & Bohan, C. (1987). Lack of HIV replication in arthropod cells. *Lancet, 1*(8541), 1094–1095.

Stahly, G. B. (1988). Psychosocial aspects of the stigma of cancer: An overview. *Journal of Psychosocial Oncology, 6,* 3–27.

Stall, R., Heurtin-Roberts, S., McKusick, L., Hoff, C., & Lang, S. W. (1990). Sexual risk for HIV transmission among singles-bar patrons in San Francisco. *Medical Anthropology Quarterly, 4*, 115–128.

Stansell, J. D., & Sande, M. A. (1992). Cryptococcal infection in AIDS. In M. A. Sande & P. A. Volberding (Eds.), *The medical management of AIDS* (3rd ed., pp. 297–310). Philadelphia: Saunders.

Stein, M., Miller, A. H., & Trestman, R. L. (1991). Depression, the immune system, and health and illness. *Archives of General Psychiatry, 48*, 171–177.

St. Lawrence, J. S., Kelly, J. A., Owen, A. D., Hogan, I. G., & Wilson, R. A. (1990). Psychologists' attitudes toward AIDS. *Psychology and Health, 4*, 357–365.

Stoneburner, R. L., Chiasson, M. A., Weisfuse, I. B., & Thomas, P. A. (1990). The epidemic of AIDS and HIV-1 infection among heterosexuals in New York City. *AIDS, 4*, 99–106.

Storosum, J. G., Sno, H. N., Schalken, H. F. A., Krol, L. J., Swinkels, J. A., Nahuijs, M., Meijer, E. P., & Danner, S. A. (1991). Attitudes of health-care workers towards AIDS at three Dutch hospitals. *AIDS, 5*, 55–60.

Storosom, J., Van den Boom, F., Van Beauzekom, M., & Sno, H. (1990, June). Stress and coping in people with HIV infection. Paper presented at the VI International Conference on AIDS, San Francisco.

Stowe, A., Ross, M. W., Wodak, A., Thomas, G. V., & Larson, S. A. (1993). Significant relationships and social supports of injecting drug users and their implications for HIV/AIDS services. *AIDS Care, 5*, 23–33.

Stricof, R. L., Kennedy, J. T., Nattell, T. C., Weisfuse, I. B., & Novick, L. F. (1991). HIV seroprevalence in a facility for runaway and homeless adolescents. *American Journal of Public Health, 81*, 50–53.

Strunin, L., Culbert, A., & Crane, S. (1989). First year medical students' attitudes and knowledge about AIDS. *AIDS Care, 1*, 105–110.

Stuntzner-Gibson, D. (1991). Women and HIV disease: An emerging social crisis. *Social Work, 36*, 22–28.

Susser, E., Valencia, E., & Conover, S. (1993). Prevalence of HIV infection among psychiatric patients in New York City men's shelter. *American Journal of Public Health, 83*, 568–570.

Sweeney, J., Peters, B. S., & Main, J. (1991). Clinical care and management. *AIDS Care, 3*, 457–460.

Taerk, G., Gallop, R. M., Lancee, W. J., Coates, R. A., & Fanning, M. (1993). Recurrent themes of concern in groups for health care professionals. *AIDS Care, 5*, 215–222.

Takigiku, S. K., Brubaker, T. H., & Hennon, C. B. (1993). A contextual model of stress among parent caregivers of gay sons with AIDS. *AIDS Education and Prevention, 5,* 25–42.

Tanfer, K., Grady, W. R., Klepinger, D. H., & Billy, J. O. (1993). Condom use among U.S. men, 1991. *Family Planning Perspectives, 25,* 61–66.

Tarasoff v. Regents of the University of California, 131 Cal. Rptr. 14, 551 P.2d 334 (1976).

Taylor, J. M., Schwartz, K., & Detels, R. (1986). The time from infection with human immunodeficiency virus (HIV) to the onset of AIDS. *Journal of Infectious Diseases, 154,* 694–697.

Taylor, M. G., Huo, J. M., & Detels, R. (1991). Is the incubation period of AIDS lengthening? *Journal of Acquired Immunedeficiency Syndromes, 4,* 69–75.

Taylor, S. E. (1983). Adjustment to threatening events: A theory of cognitive adaptation. *American Psychologist, 38,* 1161–1173.

Taylor, S. E., & Aspinwall, L. (1990). Psychosocial aspects of chronic illness. In G. M. Herek, S. M. Levy, S. Maddi, S. Taylor, & D. Wertlieb (Eds.), *Psychological aspects of chronic illness: Chronic conditions, fatal diseases, and clinical care* (pp. 7–60). Washington, DC: American Psychological Association.

Taylor, S. E., & Brown, J. D. (1988). Illusion and well-being: A social psychological perspective on mental health. *Psychological Bulletin, 103,* 193–210.

Taylor, S. E., Helgeson, V .S., Reed, G. M., & Skokan, L.A. (1991). Self–generated feelings of control and adjustment to physical illness. *Journal of Social Issues, 47,* 91–109.

Taylor, S. E., Kemeny, M. E., Aspinwall, L. G., Schneider, S. G., Rodriguez, R., & Herbert, M. (1992). Optimism, coping, psychological distress, and high-risk sexual behavior among men at risk for acquired immunodeficiency syndrome (AIDS). *Journal of Personality and Social Psychology, 63,* 460–473.

Taylor, S. E., Lichtman, R.R., & Wood, J. V. (1984). Attributions, beliefs about control, and adjustment to breast cancer. *Journal of Personality and Social Psychology, 46,* 489–502.

Teguis, A., & Ahmed, P. I. (1992). Living with AIDS: An overview. In P. I. Ahmed & N. Ahmed (Eds.), *Living and dying with AIDS* (pp. 3–18). New York: Plenum Press.

Temin, H. M., & Bolognesi, D. P. (1993). Where has HIV been hiding? *Nature, 362,* 292–293.

Temoshok, L. (1988). Psychoimmunology and AIDS. In T. P. Bridge (Ed.), *Psychological, neuropsychiatric, and substance abuse aspects of AIDS* (pp. 187–197). New York: Raven Press.

Terl, A. H. (1992). *AIDS and the law: A basic guide for the nonlawyer.* New York: Taylor & Francis.

Terragna, A., Mazzarello, G., Anselmo, M., Canessa, A., & Rossi, E. (1990). Suicidal attempts with zidovudine. *AIDS, 4,* 88.

Thomas, C. L. (1977). *Taber's cyclopedic medical dictionary.* Philadelphia: Davis.

Thomas, S., & Quinn, S. C. (1991). Public health then and now: The Tuskegee Syphilis Study, 1932 to 1972: Implications for HIV education and AIDS risk education programs in the Black community. *American Journal of Public Health, 81,* 1498–1505.

Tindall, B., Carr, A., & Cooper, D. A. (1995). Primary HIV infection: Clinical, immunologic, and serologic aspects. In M. A. Sande & P. A. Volberding (Eds.), *The medical management of AIDS* (4th ed., pp. 105-129). Philadelphia: Saunders.

Tindall, B., Imrie, A., Donovan, B., Penny, R., & Cooper, D. A. (1992). Primary HIV infection. In M. A. Sande & P. A. Volberding (Eds.), *The medical management of AIDS* (3rd ed., pp. 67–86). Philadelphia: Saunders.

Tolstoy, L. (1981). *The death of Ivan Ilyich.* New York: Bantam Books. (Original work published 1886)

Treiber, F. A., Shawn, D., & Malcolm, R. (1987). Acquired immune deficiency syndrome: Psychological impact on health personnel. *Journal of Nervous and Mental Disease, 175,* 496–499.

Treisman, G. J., Lyketsos, C. G., Fishman, M., & McHugh, P. R. (1993). *A brief guide to the psychiatric care and evaluation of patients infected with HIV.* (Available from Johns Hopkins AIDS Psychiatry Service, Meyer 4-119, 600 North Wolfe Street, Baltimore, MD 21205)

Triplet, R. G. (1992). Discriminatory biases in the perception of illness: The application of availability and representativeness heuristics to the AIDS crisis. *Basic and Applied Social Psychology, 13,* 303–322.

Triplet, R. G., & Sugarman, D. B. (1987). Reactions to AIDS victims: Ambiguity breeds contempt. *Personality and Social Psychology Bulletin, 13,* 265–274.

Tross, S., & Hirsch, D. (1988). Psychological distress and neuropsychological complications of HIV infection and AIDS. *American Psychologist, 43,* 929–934.

Turner, H. A., Hays, R. B., & Coates, T. J. (1993). Determinants of social support among gay men: The context of AIDS. *Journal of Health and Social Behavior, 34,* 37–53.

Uldall, K. K., Koutsky, L. A., Bradshaw, D. H., Hopkins, S. G., Katon, W., & Lafferty, W. E. (1994). Psychiatric comorbidity and length of stay in hospitalized AIDS patients. *American Journal of Psychiatry, 151,* 1475–1478.

Upchurch, D. M., Ray, P., Reichart, C., Celentano, D. D., Quinn, T., & Hook, E. W. (1992). Prevalence and patterns of condom use among patients attending a sexually transmitted disease clinic. *Sexually Transmitted Diseases, 19,* 175–180.

Valdiserri, E. V. (1986). Fear of AIDS: Implications for mental health practice with reference to ego-dystonic homosexuality. *American Journal of Orthopsychiatry, 56,* 634–637.

Valdiserri, R. O., Tama, G. M., & Ho, M. (1988). A survey of AIDS patients regarding their experiences with physicians. *Journal of Medical Education, 63,* 726–728.

Van Gorp, W. G., Lamb, D. G., & Schmitt, F. A. (1993). Methodologic issues in neuropsychological research with HIV-spectrum disease. *Archives of Clinical Neuropsychology, 8,* 17–33.

Van Gorp, W. G., Satz, P., Hinkin, C., Evans, G., & Miller, E. N. (1989). The neuropsychological aspects of HIV-1 spectrum disease. *Psychiatric Medicine, 7,* 59–78.

Van Servellan, G. M., Lewis, C. E., & Leake, B. (1988). Nurses' responses to the AIDS crisis: Implications for continuing education programs. *Journal of Continuing Education in Nursing, 19,* 4–8.

Velentgas, P., Bynum, C., & Zierler, S. (1990). The buddy volunteer commitment in AIDS care. *American Journal of Public Health, 80,* 1378–1380.

Vermund, S. H., Hein, K., Gayle, H. D., Carey, J. M., Thomas, P. A., & Drucker, E. (1989). Acquired immunodeficiency syndrome among adolescents. *American Journal of Diseases in Children, 143,* 1220–1225.

Viney, L. L., Crooks, L., Walker, B. M., & Henry, R. (1991). Psychological frailness and strength in an AIDS-affected community: A study of seropositive gay men and voluntary caregivers. *American Journal of Community Psychology, 19,* 279–287.

Vitkovic, L., & Koslow, S. H. (1994). *Neuroimmunology & mental health: A report on neuroimmunology research.* Rockville, MD: National Institute of Mental Health.

Vlahov, D., Brewer, F., Munoz, A., Hall, D., Taylor, E., & Polk, B. F. (1989). Temporal trends of human immunodeficiency virus type 1 (HIV-1) infection among inmates entering a statewide prison system, 1985–1987. *Journal of Acquired Immune Deficiency Syndromes, 2,* 283–290.

Voeller, B., Coulson, A. H., Bernstein, G .S., & Nakamura, R. M. (1989). Mineral oil lubricants cause rapid deterioration of latex condoms. *Contraception, 39,* 95–102.

Vogel, J., Cepeda, M., Tschachler, E., Napolitano, L., & Jay, G. (1992). UV activation of human immunodeficiency virus gene expression in transgenic mice. *Journal of Virology, 66*(1), 1–5.

Volberding, P. A., Lagakos, S. W., Grimes, J. M., Stein, D. S., Balfour, H. H., Reichman, R. C., Bartlett, J. A., Hirsch, M. S., Phair, J. P., Mitsuyasu, R. T., Fischl, M. A., & Soeriro, R. (1994). The duration of zidovudine benefit in persons with asymptomatic HIV infection. *Journal of the American Medical Association, 272*, 437–442.

von Overbeck, J., Egger, M., Smith, G. D., Schoep, M., Ledergerber, B., Furrer, H., & Malinverni, R. (1994). Survival of HIV infection: Do sex and category of transmission matter? *AIDS, 8*, 1307-1313.

Wachtel, T., Piette, J., Mor, V., Stein, M., Fleishman, J., & Carpenter, C. (1992). Quality of life in persons with human immunodeficiency virus infection: Measurement by the medical outcomes study instrument. *Annals of Internal Medicine, 116*, 129–137.

Waldorf, D., & Lauderback, D. (1993). Condom failure among male sex workers in San Francisco. *AIDS & Public Policy Journal, 8*, 79–90.

Wallace, B., & Lasker, J. (1992). Awakenings . . . UV light and HIV gene activation. *Science, 257*, 1211–1212.

Wallack, J. J. (1989). AIDS anxiety among health care professionals. *Hospital and Community Psychiatry, 40*, 507–510.

Warner-Robbins, C. G., & Christiana, N. (1989). The spiritual needs of persons with AIDS. *Family & Community Health, 12*, 43–51.

Warwick, H. (1989). AIDS hypochondriasis. *British Journal of Psychiatry, 155*, 125–126.

Watson, M. (1983). Psychosocial intervention with cancer patients: A review. *Psychological Medicine, 13*, 839–846.

Weber, J., & Weiss, R. (1988). HIV infection: The cellular picture. *Scientific American, 101–109.

Weinberger, M., Conover, C. J., Samsa, G. P., & Greenberg, S. M. (1992). Physicians' attitudes and practices regarding treatment of HIV-infected patients. *Southern Medical Journal, 85*, 683–686.

Weiss, R., & Hardy, L. M. (1990). HIV infection and health policy. *Journal of Consulting and Clinical Psychology, 58*, 70–76.

Weisse, C. S. (1992). Depression and immunocompetence: A review of the literature. *Psychological Bulletin, 111*, 475–489.

Weitz, R. (1989). Uncertainty and the lives of persons with AIDS. *Journal of Health and Social Behavior, 30*, 270–281.

Werth, J. L., & Carney, J. (1994). Incorporating HIV-related issues into graduate student training. *Professional Psychology: Research and Practice, 25*, 458–465.

Wicklund, B. M., & Jackson, M. A. (1992). Coping with AIDS in hemophilia. In P. I. Ahmed (Ed.), *Living and dying with AIDS* (pp. 255–268). New York: Plenum Press.

Wilkie, F. L., Eisdorfer, C., Morgan, R., Loewenstein, D. A., & Szapocznik, J. (1990). Cognition in early human immunodeficiency virus infection. *Archives of Neurology, 47,* 433–440.

Williams, J. B. W., Rabkin, J. G., Remien, R. H., Gorman, J. M., & Ehrhardt, A. A. (1991). Multidisciplinary baseline assessment of homosexual men with and without human immunodeficiency virus infection. *Archives of General Psychiatry, 48,* 124–130.

Williams, M. L. (1990). HIV seroprevalence among male IVDUs in Houston, Texas. *American Journal of Public Health, 80,* 1507–1508.

Willoughby, A. (1989). AIDS in women: Epidemiology. *Clinical Obsterics and Gynecology, 32,* 429–436.

Winiarski, M. G. (1991). *AIDS-related psychotherapy.* New York: Pergamon Press.

Wofsy, C. B. (1988). AIDS Care: Providing care for the HIV infected. *Journal of Acquired Immune Deficiency Syndromes, 1,* 274–283.

Wofsy, C. (1992). Therapeutic issues in women with HIV disease. In M. A. Sande & P. A. Volberding (Eds.), *The medical management of AIDS* (3rd ed., pp. 465–476). Philadelphia: Saunders.

Wolcott, D. L., Namir, S., Fawzy, F., Gottlieb, M., & Mitsuyasu, R. (1986). Illness concerns, attitudes towards homosexuality, and social support in gay men with AIDS. *General Hospital Psychiatry, 8,* 395–403.

Wolf, T. M., Balson, P. M., Dralle, P. W., Gaumer, R. H., Morse, E. V., Williams, M. H., & Simon, P. M. (1991). A biopsychosocial examination of symptomatic and asymptomatic HIV-infected patients. *International Journal of Psychiatry in Medicine, 21,* 263–279.

Wolf, T., Balson, P., Morse, E., Simon, P., Gaumer, R., Dralle, P., & Williams, M. (1991). Relationship of coping style to affective state and perceived social support in asymptomatic HIV-infected persons: Implications for clinical management. *Journal of Clinical Psychiatry, 52,* 171–173.

Wong, S. Y., Israelski, D. M., & Remington, J. S. (1995). AIDS-associated toxoplasmosis. In M. A. Sande & P. A. Volberding (Eds.), *The medical management of AIDS* (4th ed., pp. 460–493). Philadelphia: Saunders.

Woo, S. (1992). *Ending the isolation: HIV and mental health in the second decade* (Report of the Federal Centre for AIDS, Working Group on HIV Infection and Mental Health). Ottawa, Ontario, Canada: Minister of National Health and Welfare.

Woodhouse, D. E., Muth, J. B., Potterat, J. J., & Riffe, L. D. (1993). Restricting personal behaviour: Case studies on legal measures to prevent the spread of HIV. *International Journal of STD & AIDS, 4,* 114–117.

World Health Organization. (1979). *International classification of diseases: Clinical modifications* (9th ed.). Geneva: Author.

Worley, J. M., & Price, R. W. (1992) Management of neurologic complications of HIV-1 infection and AIDS. In M. A. Sande & P. A. Volberding (Eds.), *The medical management of AIDS* (3rd ed., pp. 193–217). Philadelphia: Saunders.

Wormser, G. P. (1992). *AIDS and other manifestations of HIV infection* (2nd ed.). New York: Raven Press.

Wu, A. W., Rubin, H. R., Mathews, W. C., Ware, J. E., Brysk, L. T., Hardy, W. D., Bozzette, S. A., Spector, S. A., & Richman, D. D. (1991). A health status questionnaire using 30 items from the medical outcomes study: Preliminary validation in persons with early HIV infection. *Medical Care, 29,* 786–798.

Yalom, I. D., & Greaves, C. (1977). Group therapy with the terminally ill. *American Journal of Psychiatry, 134,* 396–400.

Yarrish, R. L. (1992). Cytomegalovirus infections in AIDS. In G. P. Wormser (Ed.), *AIDS and other manifestations of HIV infection* (2nd ed.). New York: Raven Press.

Yates, J. (1991). AIDS: A Christian view. *International Journal of SID & AIDS, 2,* 38–40.

Zakowski, S., McAllister, C., Deal, M., & Baum, A. (1992). Stress, reactivity, and immune function in healthy men. *Health Psychology, 11*(4), 223–232.

Zamperetti, M., Goldwurm, G. F., Abbate, E., Gris, T., Muratori, S., & Vigo, B. (1990, June). Attempted suicide and HIV infection: Epidemiological aspects in a psychiatric ward. Paper presented at the sixth International Conference on AIDS (Abstract No. S.B. 387).

Zich, J., & Temoshok, L. (1987). Perceptions of social support in men with AIDS and ARC: Relationships with distress and hardiness. *Journal of Applied Social Psychology, 17,* 193–215.

Zich, J., & Temoshok, L. (1990). Perceptions of social support, distress, and hopelessness in men with AIDS and ARC: Clinical implications. In L. Temoshok & A. Baum (Eds.), *Psychosocial perspectives on AIDS* (pp. 201–227), Hillsdale, NJ: Erlbaum.

Ziegler, P. (1969). *The black death.* New York: John Day.

Zigmond, A. S., & Snaith, R. P. (1983). The Hospital Anxiety and Depression Scale. *Acta Psychiatrica Scandinavica, 67,* 361–370.

Zolopa, A. R., Hahn, J. A., Gorter, R., Miranda, J., Wlodarczyk, D., Peterson, J., Pilote, L., & Moss, A. R. (1994). HIV and tuberculosis infection in San Francisco's homeless adults. *Journal of the American Medical Association, 272,* 455–461.

Zonderman, A. B., Costa, P. T., & McCrae, R. R. (1989). Depression as a risk for cancer morbidity and mortality in a nationally representative sample. *Journal of the American Medical Association, 262,* 1191–1195.

Glossary

acquired immune deficiency syndrome (AIDS): The final stage of HIV infection, characterized by clinical symptoms of severe immune deficiency. Although there are several diagnostic systems, the most widely used is the one provided by the CDC that lists opportunistic infections and malignancies that, in the presence of HIV infection, constitute an AIDS diagnosis. In addition, a T-helper cell count below $200/\text{mm}^3$ for people with HIV infection constitutes an AIDS diagnosis.

active immunity: Biological defense to stimulation by a disease-causing organism or other antigen.

acute infection: Any infection that begins suddenly, with intense or severe symptoms.

adverse reaction (side effect): An unwanted negative reaction to an experimental drug or vaccine.

AIDS clinical trials group (ACTG): A nationwide consortium of medical centers carrying out clinical trials to study therapies for HIV–AIDS, sponsored by the National Institute of Allergy and Infectious Disease (NIAID).

AIDS-related complex (ARC): A variously defined term with little clinical value used to identify certain HIV-infected individuals prior to an AIDS diagnosis. Compared with earlier in the epidemic, the term *ARC* is used less often today. Instead, physicians chart HIV disease as starting with no apparent symptoms (asymptomatic) and progressing to symptoms (symptomatic). Fatigue, night sweats, fever, swollen glands, diarrhea, or unintentional weight loss were previously grouped under the term *ARC*.

anemia: A decrease in number of red blood cells or amount of hemoglobin. Commonly called "low blood count."

antibiotic: A chemical substance that kills or inhibits the growth of bacteria.

antibodies: Molecules in the blood or secretory fluids that tag, destroy, or neutralize bacteria, viruses, or other harmful toxins. They belong to a class of proteins known as *immunoglobulins,* which are produced by B-lymphocytes in response to antigens.

antigen: Material that can elicit an immune response.

antiretroviral: Drugs that treat retroviral infection. AZT, ddI, and ddC are examples of antiretrovirals used to treat HIV infection.

antiviral: Drugs that destroy a virus or suppress its replication.

asymptomatic: Having no symptoms; free of sensations of poor health.

attenuated virus: A weakened virus with reduced ability to infect or produce disease. Some vaccines are made of attenuated viruses.

autoimmunization: A self-destructive process characterized by an immune response to one's own cells.

B-cells (also *B-lymphocytes*): Bone-marrow derived precursors of plasma cells that produce antibody.

B-lymphocytes or *B-cells:* One of two major classes of lymphocytes. During infections, these cells are transformed into plasma cells that produce large quantities of antibody directed at specific pathogens. Although HIV specifically infects cells displaying the CD4 receptor, especially T-helper lymphocytes, the disruption of immune function by HIV also affects B-lymphocytes; also, B-cell lymphomas are common among HIV-positive individuals.

bacterium: A microscopic organism composed of a single cell that often causes human disease.

blinded study: A clinical trial in which participants are unaware whether they are in the experimental or the control group.

body fluids: Term usually referring to semen, vaginal fluids, blood, urine, and saliva.

breakthrough infection: An infection that occurs during the course of a vaccine trial.

candida: A yeast-like fungi that is commonly found in the mouth, skin, intestinal tract, and vagina but that can become clinically infectious with immune suppression.

CBOs: Community-based organizations that provide multiple services to people affected by AIDS.

CD4: A membrane protein or receptor of T-helper lymphocytes, mono-cytes, macrophages, and some other cells; is the attachment site for HIV.

CD8 (T8): A membrane protein found on the surface of suppressor T-lymphocytes.

cellular immunity: Biological defense principally mediated by lymphocytes acting directly on invading antigens.

chancre: A sore or ulcer. Presence of a chancre on the genitals apparently increases the probability of being infected with HIV.

chronic infection: Persisting for longer than two weeks or recurring over time.

clinical trial: A medical study usually involving experimental drugs.

clotting factors: Substances in the blood that cause the blood to change from a liquid to a coagulate or a solid to stop bleeding.

cofactors: Substances, microorganisms, or characteristics of individuals that influence disease progression.

cohort: A group of individuals who share one or more characteristics for purposes of a clinical research study.

combination therapy (convergent combination therapies): Combined ad-ministration of drugs that are effective at different stages of the HIV vi-ral cycle or that have an impact on different elements of the virus. Com-bined approaches reduce potential drug resistance.

complimentary treatments: Unapproved substances or procedures used for therapeutic purposes.

contagious: Any infectious disease capable of being transmitted from per-son to person.

controlled clinical Trial: A trial in which one group of subjects is administered an experimental drug or vaccine and another group is administered either a placebo or a standard treatment or vaccine. Participants are usually unaware of which group they are in.

Cryopreservation: A controversial treatment involving freezing cells, such as specific immune cells, for use by the same patient at a later time.

Cytokine: A hormone-like substance produced and released by cells to control other cells.

Cytomegalovirus (CMV): A herpes virus that causes opportunistic diseases in immune-compromised patients. Although CMV can infect most organs of the body, people with AIDS have been most susceptible to CMV retinitis and colitis.

cytotoxic T-lymphocyte (CTL): White blood cell that destroys infected cells directly; nicknamed "killer T-cell."

disseminated: Disease scattered throughout several organ systems.

dormant: Inactive, as in a dormant infection.

encephalitis: Inflammation of the brain, acute or chronic, caused by viruses, bacteria, toxins, etc.

encephalopathy: A broad term used to describe metabolic, toxic, malignant, or degenerative diseases of the brain.

endemic: Continuous presence of a disease in a community or among a group of people.

envelope: In virology, a protein covering of virus genetic material. The HIV envelope is composed of two glycoproteins, *gp*41 and *gp*120, that bind to the CD4 surface molecule.

enzyme linked immunosorbent assay (ELISA): The blood test most often used to screen for HIV infection. ELISA detects HIV antibodies—not HIV itself. Because ELISA is sensitive, it has a high false-positive rate and is therefore confirmed by a more specific test.

epidemic: A disease or condition that affects many people within a population at the same time when they are not ordinarily subject to this condition.

Epstein–Barr virus (EBV): A herpes-like virus that causes mononucleosis; infects the nose and throat, and is contagious; lies dormant in the lymph glands and is associated with Burkitt's lymphoma and hairy leukoplakia.

gastroenteritis: Inflammation of the lining of the stomach or intestines; caused by bacterial or viral infection.

gene therapy: Incorporating genetic material in cells to alter their genetic make-up, such as alteration of T-helper cell genetic information to prohibit HIV infection.

giant cells: Large multinucleated cells sometimes seen in granulomatous reactions and thought to result from the fusion of macrophages.

gingivitis: Swelling, bleeding, or soreness of the gums that can be especially severe in people with HIV infection; treated early, gingivitis can usually be controlled by regular brushing, flossing, and dental care.

gp120: An HIV glycoprotein found on the HIV envelope surface; binds with CD4.

granulocytes: A type of white blood cell that helps kill bacteria and other microorganisms.

hairy leukoplakia: A whitish, slightly raised lesion that appears on the side of the tongue; related to Epstein–Barr virus infection during immune suppression.

helper–suppressor ratio: The number of helper (CD4+) T-cells to suppressor (CD8+) T-cells; suppressor cells outnumber helper cells in advanced HIV infection.

hemophilia: An inherited disease that keeps blood from clotting.

herbal treatments: Small amounts of plants, including roots, bark, leaves, or juices, used for therapeutic purposes.

herpes simplex virus I (HSV I): Causes cold sores or fever blisters on the mouth or around the eyes and can be transmitted to the genital region;

latent HSV I is reactivated by stress, trauma, other infections, or other causes of immune suppression.

herpes simplex virus II (HSV II): Causes painful sores on the anus or genitals; may lie dormant in nervous tissue and can be reactivated to produce symptoms; transmittable to infants during labor and delivery.

herpes varicella zoster virus (HVZ): Causes chicken pox in children; consists of very painful blisters on the skin that follow nerve pathways; may reappear in adulthood as herpes zoster causing shingles.

HIV disease: The spectrum of immunodeficiency and disease associated with HIV infection.

host: An organism harboring an infection.

HTLV-I: Human T-cell leukemia virus, a human retrovirus that causes a rare form of leukemia after a long period of asymptomatic infection. The virus spreads through sexual contact or the sharing of unclean needles by injection drug users.

human immunodeficiency virus (HIV): The AIDS virus; a retrovirus of the lentivirus class; formerly called LAV or HTLV-III. HIV type 1 (HIV-1) is the common cause of HIV disease in the North America; HIV type 2 (HIV-2) is prevalent in some parts of Africa and occasionally occurs in North America and Europe.

humoral immunity: Responses against disease rendered by lymphocytes, where antibodies are produced and circulate in the bloodstream to act against antigens.

immune deficiency: A breakdown or inability of certain parts of the immune system to function; increases susceptibility to certain diseases.

immune suppression: A state in which the immune system is damaged and does not perform its normal functions; can be induced by drugs or result from diseases.

immune system: The complex body function that recognizes foreign agents or substances, neutralizes them, and recalls the response later when confronted with the same antigen.

immunity: Natural or acquired resistance to infection by virtue of previous exposure to a disease-causing organism. Immunity may be partial or complete, long-lasting or temporary.

immunomodulator: A substance capable of modifying one or more functions of the immune system.

immunosuppressed: A weakened state of the immune system.

immunosuppression: Suppression of immune response.

incidence: The number of new cases of disease in a defined population during a specified period of time.

incubation period: The time between infection exposure and the first physical response, such as the production of antibodies.

interferons: Proteins originally defined by their activity against viral infections; Alpha, beta, and gamma interferons have been investigated as therapy for some opportunistic diseases.

invasive: Disease in which organisms or cancer cells are spreading throughout the body; or a medical procedure in which a device is inserted into the body.

in vitro (in glass): An artificial environment created outside a living organism (for example, a test tube or culture plate), used in experimental research to study a disease or process.

in vivo (in life): Studies conducted within a living organism.

Kaposi's sarcoma (KS): A tumor of blood vessel walls or of the lymphatic system; usually appears as pink or purple painless spots on the skin but may also occur on internal organs.

Karnofsky score: A subjective measurement of an individual's functional ability to perform common activities.

latency: The period when a disease-causing agent is in the body and not producing damaging effects.

lentivirus, slow virus: A virus that produces disease with a greatly delayed onset and protracted course, such as HIV.

leukocytes: White blood cells.

lymph nodes (glands): Small bean-sized organs of the immune system, distributed widely throughout the body; lymph fluid is filtered through lymph nodes, in which all types of lymphocytes take up temporary residence; antigens that enter the body find their way into lymph or blood and are filtered out by lymph nodes or the spleen.

lymphadenopathy: Swollen, firm and possibly tender lymph nodes; the cause may be an infection or lymphoma.

lymphocytes: Several types of white blood cells, including helpers, suppressors, and B- and T-lymphocytes.

lymphoma: A cancer that starts in the lymph node; the two major types of lymphoma are Hodgkin's disease and non-Hodgkin's lymphoma (NHL); Lymphoma of the brain is considered an AIDS-defining illness unless HIV infection is ruled out.

MAC (mycobacterium avium complex): A disease caused by two bacteria found in water, soil, and food. In people with AIDS, it can spread through the bloodstream to infect the lymph nodes, bone marrow, liver, spleen, spinal fluid, lungs, and intestinal tract.

macrophage: A type of white blood cell that destroys degenerated cells; function to break down antigens.

malabsorption: Failure of the intestines to properly absorb food or nutrients.

meningitis: An infection of the meninges, the coverings of the brain and spinal cord; cryptococcus is the most frequent cause of meningitis in HIV infection.

monoclonal antibodies: Produced by a single cell, specific to a given antigen; useful as a tool for identifying specific protein molecules.

monocyte: A large white blood cell that acts as a scavenger, capable of destroying bacteria or other foreign material; precursor to the macrophage.

mucocutaneous: Pertaining to the mucous membranes and the skin, e.g., mouth, vagina, anal area.

mycosis: Any disease caused by a fungus.

myelopathy: Any pathological condition of the spinal cord.

myopathy: Any disease or abnormality of voluntary muscle groups.

natural killer cells (NK cells): Large granular lymphocytes that attack and destroy tumors and infected cells; attack without first recognizing specific antigens.

neuropathy: The general term for any disease of peripheral nerves; symptoms include burning pain, loss of sensation, numbness, tingling, and muscle weakness or even paralysis.

neutrophil (polymorphonuclear neutrophils, PMNs): A white blood cell that plays a central role in defense against infection by engulfing microorganisms.

opportunistic infection: An infection in an immune-compromised individual that does not normally occur in healthy people; pathogens that cause dise? ie only with immune opportunity.

p24: An HIV-related protein; indirect measurement of p24 provides an indication of HIV activity; a positive p24 antigen test suggests active HIV replication; p24 antibody levels are usually highest early and late in HIV infection.

palliative: Treatment that provides symptom relief, but not a cure.

pandemic: Denoting a disease affecting the population of an extensive region; i.e., HIV disease is a pandemic disease, affecting an extensive area of the world.

papillovirus (PMV): A virus that may cause oral, skin, anal, and genital warts or nipple-like growths on the skin.

parasite: An organism that feeds on or lives in a different organism; some parasites cause disease.

parenteral: Involving introduction into the bloodstream.

passive immunotherapy: A treatment in which high HIV antibodies from donors are infused into HIV-positive patients.

pathogen: Any virus, microorganism, or other substance causing disease.

peripheral neuropathy: A disorder of the nerves, usually involving the extremities. Symptoms include numbness, a tingling or burning sensation, sharp pain, weakness, and abnormal reflexes. In severe cases, paralysis may result.

phagocyte: A cell that destroys and ingests foreign matter, including bacteria.

phagocytosis: The process by which cells engulf material and enclose it within a vacuole (phagosome) in the cytoplasm.

Pneumocystis carinii pneumonia (PCP): An infection of the lungs caused by a protozoan or fungus that has been the most common life-threatening opportunistic infection in AIDS patients.

polymerase: An enzyme that promotes synthesis of segments of DNA and RNA.

polymerase chain reaction (PCR): A technique for amplifying small amounts of DNA; PCR techniques are useful in identifying HIV infection before an antibody response, such as in young infants.

prevalence: The number of people in a given population with a specified disease at a specified point in time; expressed as a percentage.

prophylactic vaccines: Only work as a preventive and must be given before infection.

prophylaxis: Prevention; a treatment intended to preserve health.

protocol: A detailed plan for a clinical trial that states the trial's rationale, its purpose, drug or vaccine dosages, length of study, route of administration, and who may participate.

provirus: The form of a virus in which its genetic material is incorporated into the host cell's genetic material.

receptor: A cells surface molecule that binds specifically to other particular extracellular molecules.

regulatory genes: HIV genes (e.g., *nef, rev, tat*) that regulate viral replication in infected cells.

resistance (to a drug): The ability of an organism, a microorganism, or a virus to lose its sensitivity to a drug. For example, after long-term use of AZT, HIV can develop strains of virus in the body that are no longer suppressed by this particular drug and are therefore said to be resistant to AZT.

retinitis: Inflammation of the retina; can diminish vision, constrict visual fields, and increase light sensitivity; cytomegalovirus (CMV) infection is a cause in immune-suppressed individuals.

retrovirus: A class of RNA viruses with a complex life cycle that includes an obligatory DNA intermediate and reverse transcription from RNA to DNA and that is almost impossible for the body to eliminate. A retrovirus takes over cells in the body and makes them into factories that produce other infected cells, each with a slightly different retrovirus.

reverse transcriptase: A complex enzyme characteristic of retroviruses; not found in non-HIV-infected human cells.

ribonucleic acid (RNA): A complex nucleic acid responsible for translating genetic information from DNA and transferring it to the cells' protein-making machinery.

seroconversion: When people exposed to an infectious disease develop antibodies to that disease-causing agent; people seroconvert from antibody-negative to antibody-positive.

serologic test: Test performed on the clear, liquid portion of blood (serum); often refers to tests that determine the presence of antibodies to antigens; ELISA and Western Blot are two types of antibody tests.

seropositive or *seronegative*: Implying the presence or absence of antibodies, determined by serological tests.

sign: Observable physical change indicating that a disease may be present. Examples include fever, bleeding, lesions, rash, and swelling.

SIV: Simian immunodeficiency virus.

stem cell: A cell in bone marrow that can grow into many types of immune system cells.

subclinical infection: An infection, or phase of infection, without readily apparent symptoms or signs of disease.

suppressor T-cells (T8, CD8): Subset of T-cells that halt antibody production and other immune responses.

symptom: Feelings or sensations that may indicate disease that are not observable but are reported; examples include, headache, nausea, and pain.

symptomatic: A person who does not feel well and has medical problems that can be observed or measured.

syncytium ("giant cell"): A dysfunctional multicellular clump formed by cell-to-cell fusion.

systemic: Affecting the whole body.

T-helper cell count: The most commonly used laboratory marker for estimating level of immune dysfunction; also known as *lymphocyte count* or *CD4 count*; a measurement of number of T-helper cells per unit of blood.

T-lymphocytes or *T-cells*: The class of lymphocytes derived from the thymus and involved in cell-mediated immune responses. The T-helper/inducer lymphocyte displays the CD4 membrane protein on its surface and is susceptible to HIV infection.

T-suppressor lymphocytes (T-8 cells): A group of T-lymphocytes that regulates the antibody production of B-lymphocytes.

therapeutic vaccines: Used to treat disease after infection occurs.

thrush: Caused by candidiasis, a yeast infection occurring in the mouth.

thymus: The central lymphoid organ that is present in the thorax and controls the ontogeny of T-lymphocytes.

toxoplasmosis: An opportunistic infection caused by the protozoan *Toxoplasma gondii*; frequently causes focal encephalitis (inflammation of the brain); may also involve the heart, lung, adrenal gland, pancreas, and testis.

transcription: The synthesis of RNA molecules from a DNA template.

vaccination: Immunization with antigens, administered for the prevention of infectious diseases.

viremia: The presence of virus in the bloodstream.

virion: A virus particle existing freely outside a host cell.

virus: A group of infectious agents characterized by their inability to reproduce outside of a living host cell; may subvert the host cell's normal functions, causing the cell to behave in a manner determined by the virus.

wasting syndrome: Progressive, involuntary weight loss associated with advanced HIV infection.

Western Blot: A test for detecting specific antibodies to a particular pathogen; in testing for antibodies to HIV, a Western Blot test confirms a positive ELISA screening blood test.

SELECTED LIST OF MEDICATIONS COMMONLY USED IN HIV INFECTION

The following list contains only the most commonly used medications. It is not meant to be comprehensive and does not include many drugs currently used to treat people with HIV infection and AIDS. For more complete information about treatments for HIV infection, please refer to the volumes of *AIDS Treatment News*, published by John S. James, P.O. Box 411256, San Francisco, CA 94141.

Antivirals and Antiretrovirals

Acyclovir (Zovirax): Antiviral medication used to control herpes simplex and other viruses.

AZT (Retrovir, Zidovudine): The first drug approved for control of HIV infection; disrupts HIV genetic processes.

BI-RG-587: An experimental anti-HIV drug that blocks the reverse transcriptase enzyme.

d4T (Stavudine): An anti-HIV drug currently in human testing; d4T belongs to the same family of drugs as AZT, ddI, and ddC. Adverse side effects may include peripheral neuropathy, headaches, and nausea.

ddC (Hivid): An antiretroviral approved for use in combination with AZT.

ddI (Videx): An antiretroviral drug approved for control of HIV infection.

Foscarnet (Foscavir): Treatment for CMV.

Ganciclovir: The first drug approved for treating CMV.

Hypericin: An experimental treatment for hepatitis B and CMV infections.

protease inhibitors: Compounds that block the ability of HIV to produce the enzyme protease, an essential enzyme for the HIV replication process.

tat inhibitors: Experimental agents that block HIV's *tat* gene; for possible use in combination therapies.

Medications for Opportunistic Diseases

Amikacin: One of the drugs used to control MAC infection.

Amoxicillin: A form of penicillin commonly used for sinus and respiratory infections.

Amphotericin B: An antibiotic for severe fungal infections.

Ampicillin: A common form of penicillin.

Azithromycin (Zithromax): An antibiotic for sinus and lung infections.

Bactrim: Used as a prophylactic and treatment of PCP.

Ciprofloxacin (Cipro): An antibiotic commonly used for lung and urinary infections and possibly MAC infections.

Clarithromycin: A drug used for treating MAC infection.

Clindamycin: An antibiotic commonly used for PCP and toxoplasmosis.

Clotrimazole (Lotrimin, Mycelex): Used to treat skin and vaginal fungal infections.

Dapsone: A prophylaxis for PCP.

Diclazuril: An antiprotozoal agent available by compassionate use for treatment of patients with cryptosporidiosis.

Erythromycin: An antibiotic commonly used for respiratory infections.

Erythropoietin: A substance that stimulates bone marrow to produce red blood cells.

Ethambutol: An approved anti-TB drug being used experimentally against MAC.

Etoposide (VP-16): An approved anticancer drug that is being used experimentally for Kaposi's sarcoma.

Fluconazole (Diflucan): Used for control of or to prevent thrush and other fungal infections.

Heptavax: A vaccine for hepatitis B.

Isoniazid (INH): A common anti-TB drug.

Itraconazole: An experimental antifungal drug that is being studied for treatment of histoplasmosis and cryptococcal meningitis.

Megestrol (Megace): A drug used to stimulate appetite and weight gain.

Nystatin (Mycostatin): A drug used to control fungal infections.

Pentamidine: Used for prevention or treatment of PCP.

Pneumovax: A vaccine to prevent pneumococcal pneumonia.

Prednisone: An approved steroid used to reduce inflammation.

Pyrazinamide: An anti-TB agent.

Pyrimethamine (Fansidar): Used for treatment of toxoplasmosis.

Rifampin: An approved antibiotic being used experimentally as a treatment for MAC.

TMP/SMX (Bactrim, Septra): Used for prevention or treatment of PCP.

Trifluridine: Approved for the treatment of a viral eye infection; it is also being studied for the treatment of herpes infections that are resistant to acyclovir.

Trimethoprim: An approved antibiotic that is used in combination with other drugs for the treatment and prevention of PCP.

HIV-Related Resources

AIDS Action Bulletin: Directory of clinical research in AIDS for Baltimore and Washington, DC. Published by AIDS Action Baltimore, Inc., 2105 North Charles St., Baltimore, MD 21218. Phone (410) 837-2437.

AIDS Drug Assistance Program (ADAP): Administered by the New York State Department of Health. ADAP provides access to specific drugs for the treatment of HIV infection and various opportunistic infections. Phone (518) 459-1641.

AIDS Education General Information System (AEGIS): A 24-hour AIDS information bulletin board system and on-line database. International conferences and full text articles from a number of newsletters and papers are available. P.O. Box 184, San Juan Capistrano, CA 92693.

AIDS/HIV Treatment Directory: Published by the American Foundation for AIDS Research (AmFAR) and updated quarterly. The directory is also available on a searchable database. Phone (800) 39-AmFAR, ext. 106.

AIDS Link: Published by East Central AIDS Education & Training Center (covering Ohio, Michigan, Tennessee, and Kentucky), for health care professionals. AIDS Link University of Cincinnati, Medical Center Information and Communications (MCIC), 231 Bethesda Ave., Cincinnati, OH 45267.

AIDS Medicines In Development: An annual chart of medications as well as information on diagnostics and vaccines. Pharmaceutical Manufacturers Association, Communications Division, 1100 15th St. NW, Washington, DC 20005. Phone (202) 835-3400.

AIDS Treatment Data Network Inc.: The Network provides HIV treatment and research information, educational resources, and training to professionals, service providers, and the individuals and communities that they serve. It also assists individuals with lower English and Spanish literacy levels, in addition to those with little or no scientific background or expertise. 259 W. 30th St., 9th Floor, New York, NY 10001. Phone (212) 260-8868.

AIDS Treatment News: Developments in AIDS research, experimental therapies, and treatment options. John S. James, P.O. Box 411256, San Francisco, CA 94141. Phone (415) 255-0588.

AIDS Update: Newsletter includes general information on AIDS issues and treatments. Dallas Gay Alliance, P.O. Box 190712, Dallas, TX 75219. Phone (214) 528-4233.

AIDS Weekly: A weekly newsletter with short abstracts of AIDS-related news items, journal articles, and conference reports. P.O. Box 830409, Birmingham, AL 35283-0409. Phone (800) 633-4931.

Association for Drug Abuse, Prevention and Treatment (ADAPT): AIDS-oriented outreach, support groups, and education resources for users of injectable drugs. 552 Southern Boulevard, Bronx, NY 10455. Phone (718) 665-5421.

Being Alive: Medical updates plus information on AIDS advocacy, a calendar of local events, listing of AIDS support groups, peer support, and counseling. Published by the LA Action Coalition, 3626 Sunset Boulevard, Los Angeles, CA 90026. Phone (213) 667-3262.

Body Positive: This newsletter provides a European perspective on treatment information not seen in similar U.S. publications. Published by Body Positive Group, 51B Philbeach Gardens, London, SW5 9EB, Great Britain. Information can be requested by mail or by fax at 011-71-373-5237. (212) 721-1346.

Bulletin of Experimental Treatments for AIDS (BETA): Mainly covers current AIDS research and developments in mainstream medicine. The newsletter devotes whole issues to specific topics. San Francisco AIDS Foundation, BETA Subscription Department, P.O. Box 2189, Berkeley, CA, 94702. Phone (510) 596-9300, (800) 327-9893.

Canadian AIDS News: A newsletter focusing on AIDS education in Canada, published by the Canadian Public Health Association, AIDS Education and Awareness Program, 400-1565 Carling Avenue, Ottawa, ON, Canada K1Z 8R1. Phone (613) 725-3769.

Canadian HIV Trials Network: Includes brief description of trials and locations of trial centers. 200-1033 Davie St., Vancouver, BC V6E 1M7. Registry of Canadian HIV Clinical Trials. Phone (604) 631-5327 or fax (604) 631-5210.

Center for Natural and Traditional Medicines (CNTM): Promotes and disseminates information on indigenous and natural medicines. Resources include *Ancient Roots: A Modern Medicine, Vol. 1: A Cross Cultural Discussion on AIDS*. CNTM, P.O. Box 21735, Washington, DC 20009. Phone 202-234-9632.

Clinical Trials: Talking It Over: Published by the National Institute of Allergy and Infectious Diseases. An educational pamphlet designed for those considering participation in an AIDS/HIV clinical trial. NIAID, Office of Communications, National Institutes of Health, Building 31, Room 7A32, Bethesda, MD 20892.

The Common Factor: A newsletter of the Committee of Ten Thousand, an organization by, for, and of people infected with HIV through blood and blood products. Includes treatment articles, early intervention, and resource list. The Committee of Ten Thousand, c/o The Packard House, 583 Plain St., Stoughton, MA 02072. Phone (617) 344-9634.

Critical Paths AIDS Project: Publishes in-depth information about treatments, research, and related political issues. Also contains an extensive listing of community events and support services in the Philadelphia area. 2062 Lombard St., Philadelphia, PA 19146. Phone (215) 545-2212.

Directory of HIV Clinical Research in the Bay Area: The San Francisco Community Consortium, 3180 18th St., Suite 201, San Francisco, CA 94110. Phone (415) 476-9554.

Facts on Alternate AIDS Compounds and Treatments (FAACTS): Provides summaries and reprints from the scientific and popular press concerning emerging treatments for HIV disease. 111 Gates St., San Francisco, CA 94110. Phone (415) 648-1357.

Gay Men's Health Crisis: 129 W. 20th St., New York, NY 10011. Phone (212) 807-7517.

Healing Alternatives Foundation: A nonprofit buyers club organized to assist people with AIDS in obtaining medications. Alternative and not-yet-approved treatments are available, mail orders accepted. 1748 Market St., Suite 204, San Francisco, CA 94102. Phone (415) 626-2316.

HIV Frontline: Published by the University of California San Francisco Center for AIDS Prevention Studies, this newsletter specifically targets mental health and health care professionals who serve HIV-infected people. Discussions and commentary are directed at human service and clinical issues pertinent to individuals with HIV. Articles emphasize practical approaches to complex clinical problems. Contact UCSF-CAPS, 74 New Montgomery, Suite 600, San Francisco, CA 94105. Phone (415) 597-9100.

I Heard It Through the Grapevine: Newsletter gives a strictly subjective yet insightful perspective on alternative treatments and is adept at finding research about little-known or -studied treatments. Recent topics have included garlic, bitter melon, shark cartilage, PCM-4, and others. AIDS Project Los Angeles, 6721 Romaine St., Los Angeles, CA 90038. Phone (213) 993-1600.

Institute for Traditional Medicine and Preventive Health Care (ITM): Provides literature, catalogs, and video programs describing Chinese herbs and other aspects of traditional medicine. ITM, 2017 S.E. Hawthorne, Portland, OR 97214. Phone (800) 544-7504.

Life Link: Newsletter from the People With AIDS Coalition, includes AIDS information and local resources. PWAC also provides support groups, education, and a hotline for current AIDS/HIV information and service referrals. PWA Coalition of Long Island, 1170 Route 109, Lindenhurst, NY 11757. Phone (516) 225-5700.

National AIDS Manual: A comprehensive and extensively cross-referenced guide to information about AIDS treatments, prevention, and services in

Great Britain. NAM Publications, Unit 407, Brixton Enterprise Centre, 444 Brixton Road, London, England SW9 8EJ. Phone 011-71-737-1693.

The News: A newsletter reporting on treatment issues and community outreach programs. Atlanta Gay Center, 63 12th St., Atlanta, Georgia 30309. Phone (404) 876-5372.

Notes From the Underground: This newsletter reports on issues pertaining to AIDS treatments, including background information about particular alternative therapies and their use. Also covered are experimental pharmaceutical treatments, including those already approved but not indicated for HIV-associated diseases. The PWA Health Group (the New York City buyers' club), 150 W. 26th St., Suite 201, New York, NY 10001. Phone (212) 255-0520.

The Orphan Project: Dedicated to caring for children and families affected by AIDS. 121 Avenue of the Americas, 6th Floor, New York, New York 10013. Phone (212) 925-5290.

PAACNOTES: A news journal of the Physicians Association for AIDS Care. Features articles on clinical management, scientific research, and a diverse range of legal, ethical, psychosocial, and economic issues directly affecting the care of people with HIV disease. 101 W. Grand Avenue, Suite 200, Chicago, IL 60610. Phone (800) 243-3059.

PI Perspective: Newsletter covers allopathic treatment information including pharmaceutical drug development and clinical trials, vaccine development, and AIDS research policy. It addresses broad-based community needs like standard of care, early intervention strategies, and prophylaxis for opportunistic infections. Project Inform, 1965 Market St., Suite 220, San Francisco, CA 94103. Phone (800) 822-7422.

Positive Directions News: Published by Positive Directions, 140 Clarendon St., Suite 805, Boston, MA 02115. Phone (617) 262-3456.

Positively Aware: Community-based newsletter covers many aspects of the AIDS epidemic. It focuses on research, mainstream and alternative treatment information, funding alerts, public policy issues, social concerns, and community events. Each edition also includes a Spanish-language section.

Test Positive Aware Network, 1340 West Irving Park, Box 259, Chicago, IL 60613. Phone (312) 404-8726.

Prisoners With AIDS Rights Advocacy Group (PWA Rag): Newsletter containing articles, treatment updates, and resources for prisoners. P.O. Box 2161, Jonesboro, GA 30327. Phone (404) 946-9346.

Psychology and AIDS Exchange: Updates the American Psychological Association's education, policy, and practice activities regarding AIDS. American Psychological Association, Office on AIDS, 750 First St., NE, Washington, DC. Phone (202) 336-5500.

PWA Health Group: A nonprofit buyers club organized to assist people with AIDS in obtaining medications. 150 W. 26th St., Suite 201, New York, NY 10001. Phone (212) 255-0520.

PWA Newsline: Committed to including diverse opinions of the many different people affected by the AIDS epidemic. Newsline Coalition, 50 W. 17th St., 8th Floor, New York, NY 10011. Phone (212) 647-1415.

Seasons: A quarterly newsletter of the National Native American AIDS Prevention Center featuring articles and artwork by Native Americans affected by HIV/AIDS. American AIDS Prevention Center, 3515 Grand Avenue, Suite 100, Oakland, CA 94610.

SIDAhora: Original material published in Spanish. Each edition focuses on specific aspects of the AIDS epidemic and its effect within the Latino/Latina community. Comprehensive coverage includes treatment information, women's issues, pediatric concerns, public policy, art, and literature. Newsline Coalition, 50 W. 17th St., 8th Floor, New York, NY 10011. Phone (212) 647-1415.

Southern California Treatment Directory: A listing of clinical trials being conducted in Southern California. Southwest Community-Based AIDS Treatment Group (ComBAT), 1800 North Highland, Suite 610, Los Angeles, CA 90028. Phone (213) 469-5888.

STEP Perspective: Newsletter primarily covers treatment information including both mainstream and alternative approaches. Some articles address insurance and other practical concerns. A general information packet and a variety of fact sheets are available. Magazine-style format allows topics to be examined thoroughly by an extensive scientific review committee. Seattle Treatment Education Project, 127 Broadway East, Suite 200, Seattle, WA 98102.

Treatment and Data Digest: This newsletter is essentially the report of the treatment and data committee of ACT UP/New York. Very current information about public policy, clinical trials, and research issues. Newsletter often covers first reports about issues not yet thoroughly known by the larger AIDS community, which usually leads to further investigations by others. ACT UP/New York, 135 W. 29th St., New York, NY 10001. Phone (212) 564-AIDS.

Treatment Issues: Covers experimental treatment research for HIV disease and related opportunistic infections, including advances in prophylaxis and prevention strategies. Gay Men's Health Crisis, Medical Information, 129 W. 20th St., New York, NY 10011. Phone (212) 807-7517.

Treatment Update: Follows activities in the U.S. and Europe. Newsletter covers a broad range of treatment issues abstracted from peer-review journals. Community AIDS Treatment Information Exchange, Suite 324, 517 College St., Toronto, Ontario, Canada M6G. Phone (416) 944-1916.

Vancouver PWA: By the Vancouver Persons with AIDS Society, the newsletter includes short medical updates, local news, and a listing of upcoming events. 1107 Seymour St., Vancouver, BC V6B 5S8. Phone (604) 681-2122.

WORLD: Written by and for HIV-positive women to address concerns specific to HIV disease and women, including treatment information and psychosocial issues. Newsletters also include forums for personal testimonies, activist alerts, and events calendar. P.O. Box 11535, Oakland, CA 94611. Phone (510) 658-6930.

DIRECTORY OF LOCAL AND NATIONAL RESOURCES FOR HIV/AIDS

ALABAMA

Birmingham	AIDS Outreach	205 322-4197
Huntsville	AIDS Action Coalition	205 533-2437

Mobile	AIDS Support Services	334 433-6277
Montgomery	AIDS Task Force	334 269-1432

ARIZONA

Phoenix	Phoenix Body Positive	602 264-7414
Tucson	La Frontera Center / Positively Native	602 741-2351
	PWA CoalitionTucson	602 770-1710

CALIFORNIA

Fresno	ACT UP	209 843-2748
Long Beach	Being Alive Long Beach	310 495-3422
Los Angeles	Being Alive / PWA Coalition	213 667-3262
	AIDS Project Los Angeles	213 993-1600
Oakland	ACT UP	510 836-4401
Redondo Beach	Being Alive South Bay	310 544-2702
San Diego	Being Alive San Diego	619 291-1400
San Francisco	AIDS Treatment News	415 282-0588
	Multicultural AIDS Resource Center	415 861-2142
	San Francisco AIDS Foundation	415 864-4376
	Women's AIDS Network	415 864-4374
San Mateo	San Mateo County AIDS Program	415 573-2385
West Hollywood	Being Alive	310 854-1327

COLORADO

Boulder	Boulder County AIDS Project	303 444-6121
Denver	Colorado AIDS Project	303 837-0166
	PWA Coalition Colorado	303 837-8214

CONNECTICUT

Bethel	AIDS Project Greater Danbury	203 778-2437
Hartford	AIDS Project—Hartford	203 247-2437
New Haven	AIDS Project New Haven	203 624-0947

DELAWARE

Wilmington	Friends Against AIDS	302 655-8334

DISTRICT OF COLUMBIA

Washington	Lifelink	202 547-7813

| | National Women's Health Network | 202 347-1140 |
| | Whitman-Walker Clinic | 202 797-3560 |

FLORIDA

Clearwater	AIDS Coalition Pinellas	813 449-2437
Ft. Lauderdale	PWA Coalition	305 565-9119
	Center One	305 537-4111
Jacksonville	PWA Coalition	904 398-9292
Miami	Body Positive	305 576-1111
	Cure AIDS Now	305 375-0400
	PWA Coalition	305 573-6010
Orlando	LUCHA	407 932-4482
Palm Beach	PWA Coalition	407 697-8033
Sarasota	AIDS Manasota	813 954-6011
Tampa	DACCO	813 223-4648

GEORGIA

Albany	Give For Life Association	912 883-1290
Atlanta	AIDS Survival Project	404 874-7926
	Grady AIDS Clinic	404 616-2440
	NAPWA Atlanta	404 874-7926

HAWAII

| Honolulu | Hawaii AIDS Task Force | 808 956-7400 |
| | PWA Coalition | 808 948-4792 |

IDAHO

| Boise | Idaho AIDS Foundation | 208 345-2277 |
| Hailey | Idaho AIDS Foundation | 208 788-4372 |

ILLINOIS

Chicago	Chicago Area AIDS Task Force	312 467-6370
	Chicago Women's AIDS Project	312 271-2070
	Howard Brown Clinic	312 871-5777
	Test Positive Aware Network	312 404-8726

INDIANA

| Fort Wayne | AIDS Task Force | 219 424-0844 |
| Indianapolis | Damien Center | 317 632-0123 |

| | Indiana Cares | 317 632-0123 |
| | PWA Coalition | 317 636-2134 |

IOWA

Davenport	Quad Cities AIDS Coalition	319 324-8638
Sioux City	Siouxland AIDS Coalition	712 252-4081
Waterloo	Cedar AIDS Support	319 292-2437

KANSAS

| Topeka | Topeka AIDS Project | 913 232-3100 |

KENTUCKY

Lexington	AIDS Crisis Task Force	502 288-2445
Louisville	Kentucky Minority AIDS Council	502 585-1254
Middlesboro	Tri-State AIDS Response Project	606 248-2378

LOUISIANA

New Orleans	New Orleans AIDS Project	504 523-3755
	PWA Coalition	504 945-4000
	NO/AIDS Task Force	504 522-2458
Shreveport	NW LA AIDS Task Force	318 221-8219

MAINE

| Portland | PWA Coalition | 207 773-8500 |

MARYLAND

| Baltimore | AIDS Response Center | 301 837-2437 |
| | PWA Coalition | 410 625-1677 |

MASSACHUSETTS

Boston	AIDS Action Committee	617 437-6200
	Boston Living Center	617 236-1012
	PWA Coalition Boston	617 266-6422
	Positive Directions	617 262-3456
Hyannis	Cape Cod AIDS Council	508 778-5111
Provincetown	Provincetown Positive	508 487-3049

MICHIGAN

| Detroit | Friends Alliance | 313 836-2800 |

Ferndale	Friends Detroit	313 543-8310
Grand Rapids	Grand Rapids AIDS Resource Center	616 459-9177

MINNESOTA

Minneapolis	The Aliveness Project	612 822-7946
	Coalition for People With Color/AIDS	612 870-1193
Moorehead	West Central AIDS Project	218 299-5220

MISSISSIPPI

Hattiesburg	Hattiesburg Area AIDS Coalition	601 544-6333
Jackson	PWA Project	601 353-7611

MISSOURI

Columbia	Mid-Missouri AIDS Project	314 875-3592
St. Louis	Positive Voices	314 361-6918

MONTANA

Billings	AIDS Task Force	406 256-6821
Glendive	AIDS Task Force	706 365-5213
Helena	AIDS Support Network	706 449-1071

NEBRASKA

Omaha	Nebraska AIDS Project	402 342-4233

NEVADA

Las Vegas	AID for AIDS in Nevada	702 369-2326
Reno	Nevada AIDS Foundation	702 329-2437

NEW HAMPSHIRE

Hanover	AIDS Community Resource Network	603 536-2232

NEW JERSEY

Atlantic City	South Jersey AIDS Alliance	609 347-8789
Collingswood	AIDS Coalition	609 854-7578
Fort Lee	PWA Coalition N.J.	201 944-6670
Jersey City	AIDS Support Project	201 944-0346

NEW MEXICO

Albuquerque	NMAPLA	505 266-0342
Santa Fe	Rosina AIDS Center	505 892-5995

NEW YORK

Albany	Damien Center	518 449-7119
Buffalo	AIDS Alliance of Western New York	716 852-6778
Long Island	PWA Coalition	516 225-5700
New York City	AIDS Resource Center	212 481-1270
	Brooklyn AIDS Task Force	718 638-2437
	Gay Men's Health Crisis	212 337-3656
	Hispanic AIDS Forum	212 966-6336
	HIV Center—Community Core	212 740-7292
	PWA Coalition New York	212 629-3075
	NY AIDS Coalition	212 675-7750
Syracuse	Central New York AIDS Task Force	315 475-2430

NORTH CAROLINA

Asheville	Western NC AIDS Project	704 252-7489
Durham	Durham AIDS Network	919 560-7768
Wilmington	GROW AIDS Resource Center	919 675-9222
Winston-Salem	Community AIDS Coalition	919 723-3601

NORTH DAKOTA

Bismark	ND Department of Health AIDS Project	701 224-8378

OHIO

Athens	Athens AIDS Task Force	614 592-4397
Cincinnati	SHARE	513 861-0755
Cleveland	Cleveland Area AIDS Task Force	216 844-1000
Columbus	AIDS Task Force	614 488-0695

OKLAHOMA

Oklahoma City	Other Options	405 728-3222
Tulsa	SHANTI	918 749-7898

OREGON

Portland	Cascade AIDS Project	503 223-5907
	Oregon Minority AIDS Coalition	503 293-5870
Salem	Mid-Oregan AIDS Support	503 363-4963

PENNSYLVANIA

Philadelphia	Action AIDS	215 981-0088
	AIDS Task Force	215 545-8686
	We The People	215 545-6868
Pittsburgh	AIDS Task Force	412 363-6500

PUERTO RICO

Rio Piedras	Coalition of Positive People	809 753-9443

RHODE ISLAND

Providence	HIV Clinic, Rhode Island Hospital	401 277-4741

SOUTH CAROLINA

Columbia	Palmetto AIDS Life Support	803 779-7257
Greenville	Palmetto AIDS Life Support	803 271-9308
Hilton Head	Low Country AIDS Community Education Task Force	803 686-4567

SOUTH DAKOTA

Pierre	SD Department of Health AIDS Program	605 773-3364

TENNESSEE

Knoxville	AIDS Response	615 523-AIDS
Nashville	Nashville Cares	615 385-AIDS
	Vanderbilt AIDS Project	615 322-AIDS

TEXAS

Austin	AIDS Services of Austin	512 451-2273
	PWA Coalition	512 472-3792
Dallas	AIDS Resource Center	214 521-5124
	AIDS Services of Dallas	214 941-0523
	Dallas Legal Hospice	214 522-8064
	PWA Coalition	214 941-0523

Houston	Houston AIDS Foundation	713 639-6796
	PWA Coalition	713 522-5428
San Antonio	AIDS Foundation	512 821-6218
Tyler	Community Assistance for AIDS Relief	903 566-3539

UTAH

Salt Lake City	PWA Coalition Utah	801 484-2205

VERMONT

Brattleboro	Vermont PWA Coalition	802 257-9277
Burlington	Vermont Cares	802 863-2437

VIRGINIA

Norfolk	AIDS Network	804 622-0837
Richmond	Richmond AIDS Information Network	804 358-AIDS
Woodstock	AID for AIDS	703 459-4021

WASHINGTON

Olympia	AIDS Task Force	206 352-2375
Seattle	Chicken Soup Brigade	206 328-8979
	People of Color Against AIDS Network	206 322-7061

WEST VIRGINIA

Morgantown	Mtn. State AIDS Network	304 292-5789
Wheeling	AIDS Task Force of the Upper Ohio Valley	304 232-6822

WISCONSIN

Madison	Madison AIDS Support Network	608 238-6276
Milwaukee	Milwaukee AIDS Project	414 273-1991
	PLWA Coalition of Wisconsin	414 273-7592

WYOMING

Casper	Wyoming AIDS Project	307 237-7833
Cheyenne	Southeast Wyoming AIDS Project	307 635-6199

STATE HOTLINES

For information about HIV-specific resources and counseling and testing services, call your state AIDS hotline:

Alabama	800-228-0469
Alaska	800-478-2437
Arizona	800-548-4695
Arkansas	501-661-2133
California (No.)	800-367-2437
California (So.)	800-922-2437
Colorado	800-252-2437
Connecticut	800-342-2437
Delaware	800-422-0429
District of Columbia	202-332-2437
Florida	800-352-2437
Georgia	800-551-2728
Hawaii	800-922-1313
Idaho	208-345-2277
Illinois	800-243-2437
Indiana	800-848-2437
Iowa	800-445-2437
Kansas	800-232-0040
Kentucky	800-654-2437
Louisiana	800-922-4379
Maine	800-851-2437
Maryland	800-638-6252
Massachusetts	800-235-2331
Michigan	800-827-2437
Minnesota	800-248-2437
Mississippi	800-537-0851
Missouri	800-533-2437
Montana	800-233-6668
Nebraska	800-782-2437
Nevada	800-842-2437
New Hampshire	800-324-2437
New Jersey	800-624-2377
New Mexico	800-545-2437

New York	800-541-2437
North Carolina	800-733-7301
North Dakota	800-472-2180
Ohio	800-332-2437
Oklahoma	800-535-2437
Oregon	800-777-2437
Pennsylvania	800-662-6080
Puerto Rico	800-765-1010
Rhode Island	800-726-3010
South Carolina	800-322-2437
South Dakota	800-592-1861
Tennessee	800-525-2437
Texas	800-299-2437
Utah	800-366-2437
Vermont	800-882-2437
Virginia	800-533-4148
Virgin Islands	809-773-2437
Washington	800-272-2437
West Virginia	800-642-8244
Wisconsin	800-334-2437
Wyoming	800-327-3577

NATIONAL CENTERS AND HOTLINES

AIDS Clinical Trials, Information Service, P.O. Box 6421, Rockville, MD 20850; (800) TRIALS-A, (800) 874-2572.

American Foundation for AIDS Research (AmFAR), 1515 Broadway, 36th Floor, New York, NY 10036; (212) 719-0033.

Burroughs Welcome Drug Information, 3030 Cornwallis Road, Research Triangle Park, North Carolina 27709; (800) 443-6763.

Center for AIDS Prevention Studies (CAPS), University of California at San Francisco, 74 New Montgomery, Suite 600, San Francisco, CA 94105; (415) 597-9100.

Gay Men's Health Crisis (GMHC), 129 W. 20th St. New York, NY 10011; (212)807-6655.

Hemophilia/HIV Peer Association, P.O. Box 931, Nevada City, CA 95959; (800) 800-5154.

Names Project—The AIDS Quilt, Box 14573, San Francisco, CA 94114; (415) 863-1966.

National AIDS Hotline (24 hours/day), (800) 342-AIDS (800-342-2437), (800) 344-SIDA, (800) 344-7432 (Spanish).

National AIDS Information Clearinghouse, (800) 458-5231.

National Hotline for Experimental Drug and Treatment Center, (800) 874-2572.

Native American Indian AIDS Hotline, (800) 283-2437.

People with AIDS Hotline, (800) 828-3280.

Project Inform Hotline (Treatment), 347 Delores St., Suite 301, San Francisco, CA 94110; (800) 334-7422 (within California), (800) 822-7422 (outside California).

Sexually Transmitted Disease Hotline, (800) 227-8922, Test Positive Aware Network, 1340 W. Irving Park, Box #259, Chicago, IL 60613; (312) 404-8726.

AIDS Risk Knowledge Test

Please answer each question by circling either **TRUE** or **FALSE**. (Correct answers are indicated in boldface.)

1. The AIDS virus cannot be spread through kissing.	**True**	False
2. A person can get the AIDS virus by sharing kitchens and bathrooms with someone who has AIDS.	True	**False**
3. Men can give the AIDS virus to women.	**True**	False
4. The AIDS virus attacks the body's ability to fight off diseases.	**True**	False
5. You can get the AIDS virus by someone sneezing, like a cold or the flu.	True	**False**
6. You can get AIDS by touching a person with AIDS.	True	**False**
7. Women can give the AIDS virus to men.	**True**	False
8. A person who got the AIDS virus from shooting-up drugs cannot give the virus to someone by having sex.	True	**False**
9. A pregnant woman can give the AIDS virus to her unborn baby.	**True**	False
10. Most types of birth control also protect against getting the AIDS virus.	True	**False**
11. The AIDS virus cannot be spread through kissing.	**True**	False
12. A person can get the AIDS virus by sharing kitchens and bathrooms with someone who has AIDS.	True	**False**
13. Condoms make intercourse completely safe.	True	**False**
14. Oral sex is safe if partners "do not swallow."	True	**False**
15. A person must have many different sexual partners to be at risk for AIDS.	True	**False**
16. It is more important to take precautions against AIDS in large cities than in small cities.	True	**False**

17. A positive result on the AIDS virus antibody test often occurs for people who do not even have the virus.   True   **False**

18. Only receptive (passive) anal intercourse transmits the AIDS virus.   True   **False**

19. Donating blood carries no AIDS risk for the donor.   **True**   False

20. Most people who have the AIDS virus look quite ill.   True   **False**

Author Index

Subject Index

413

About the Author

Seth C. Kalichman is an assistant professor in the Department of Psychiatry and Behavioral Medicine at the Medical College of Wisconsin and a senior scientist at the Center for Aids Intervention Research. Dr. Kalichman has published extensively on the psychological aspects of the HIV–AIDS epidemic. His research focuses on identifying factors that determine HIV risk behavior, testing theoretically derived intervention models, and examining the psychological adjustment of people with HIV infection. His AIDS research has been published in the *Journal of Consulting and Clinical Psychology*, the *American Journal of Public Health*, the *American Journal of Psychiatry*, *Health Psychology*, and the *Journal of Personality Assessment*. Dr. Kalichman is also the author of *Mandated Reporting of Suspected Child Abuse: Ethics, Law, and Policy*, published by the American Psychological Association. He serves on the editorial boards of several scientific journals, including *Health Psychology* and the *Journal of Personality Assessment*.

Dr. Kalichman received his PhD in Clinical–Community Psychology from the University of South Carolina and did his undergraduate work at the University of South Florida. His research and clinical interests include the psychosocial aspects of AIDS, human sexuality, sexual violence, child maltreatment, and public policy. Dr. Kalichman currently dedicates all of his effort to developing behavioral strategies to impede the spread of HIV infection in urban settings and to addressing the psychological needs of people affected by HIV and AIDS.